12 THEORIES OF AGING
THAT REALLY MATTER
&
WHAT YOU CAN DO ABOUT THEM

12 THEORIES OF AGING THAT REALLY MATTER

&

WHAT YOU CAN DO ABOUT THEM

An interview with Dr. Tessler
and his historical view on
health and aging.

TERENCE L. REED

ISBN-13: 978-1494761844

For information, please contact:
Terence L. Reed
17310 Farmington Rd.
Livonia, MI 48152

http://www.12theories.com

Although the author and publisher have made every effort to ensure the accuracy and completeness of information contained in this book, we assume no responsibility for errors, inaccuracies, omissions, or any inconsistency herein.

Cover and interior design by Michael Park
Cover photograph by Henrik Jonsson
Editing by Rob Bignell

*To healers and educators Doug Tessler and Simm Gottesman
and their prized pupil Daina Reed. Kudos to David Derenzo for
his pursuit of all things true.*

Educate yourself now and realize there is a different path. Strive instead from being treated for sickness, to being cured, by utilizing a common sense holistic approach. Read on how the author questions what real health can be in today's immense medical system conflicting itself with an over-abundance of advice, drugs, tests and health care protocols, in which he finds too many things that do not really benefit us.

While the format is told in a fictional conversational tone, the information is very real.

Terence L. Reed

Contents

Preface

MOST PEOPLE DO not understand our medical system. We have countless individuals committing their lives to healing people, yet their care and efforts often are stymied. So much has gone astray. The current model is influenced too much by drug companies, medical device makers, and profits. The current status is neither normal nor healthy. We have become a country of "being treated" instead of "being cured."

Common sense and compassion have been left by the wayside. Instead, cold data, profit margins, harmful protocols, invasive procedures, and unproven treatment options need to be addressed. Many of these unproven treatments are promoted as being state of the art medicine and talked about as if they were saving thousands and thousands of lives, when in fact, the truth is the opposite. These misguided treatment protocols are killing Americans by the thousands each day. Yet, there seems to be no outrage. Why is that? People are purposely kept in the dark and fed misinformation. Their expectations for good health have been set so low that almost all people are truly kept ignorant of what real health can offer—a high energy level and a lifetime free of major maladies. Only now are scientists realizing the true possibility of how long humans can live. Hopefully our current medical system will change soon and open the door to accommodate the new era of long and healthy living.

Modern science's newly discovered data, along with insights from the past, are the key to great leaps in health and longevity in the years to come. Taking the best from the past and wedding it to what we now know could deliver a state-of-the-art medical system that could finally meet the needs of humankind. All of this and much more is possible in the near future. Lives will be extended and joy placed into the hearts of millions of people if modern, proven protocols are implemented to treat the whole person.

The outcome, however, is not assured. Three major problems face us. First, there are very powerful special interest groups who have consistently placed their profits and influence above people's welfare. It will take both the public at large to change their own thoughts on what proper medical care should be and decisive government intervention to break the monopoly of medical governance that controls healthcare in this country. Secondly, people need to be weaned off of inactivity where watching television five hours a day is considered normal, where texting 3000 messages a month for average teenagers is considered OK, and where too many people sit surfing the Internet senselessly for thousands of hours a year. Finally, food issues will have to be addressed, as consumers have grown use to dead food, overly processed food, and nutrient-poor food choices.

Longevity and good health are not a mystery. They are simply a matter of cause and effect. Hopefully readers of this book will start taking steps to rule their destiny instead of being cheated out of their most precious asset, their health.

Society needs to evaluate what truly does work best and utilize this knowledge. It does not matter that many of these truths stem from a bygone era. What works is what works. We humans have not evolved as much as we think we have. We are still the same beings that we were thousands of years ago. That is our collective vanity and ego, along with special interest groups placing their profits and interests ahead of others, holding us back. Use the stepping stones of health outlined in this book to pave your way and your family's way to good health and longer lives.

Terence L. Reed

Heal Thyself

A JUMBO JET CRASHING EVERY DAY

ACCORDING TO AN article printed in the Journal of the American Medical Association during the year 2000, Dr. Barbara Starfield noted that studies indicate that 225,000 people pass away yearly from their medical treatment. She breaks down those numbers indicating 12,000 die from unnecessary surgery, 7,000 due to medication errors in hospitals, 20,000 due to other hospital errors, 80,000 from hospital caused infections and 106,000 due to negative effects of drugs given.

In my view, this estimate is very concerning as it does not include all the deaths caused by doctors and smaller clinics practicing the art and science of medicine. Nor does it include all the numerous deaths caused by prescription drugs due to their long-term effects on our kidneys, brains, hearts and livers.

In short, our current medical system is killing hundreds of people per day, if not thousands. How would the American public feel if a fully loaded 747 jumbo jet were crashing each day, killing everybody on board? Would you want to fly an airline under those conditions? Would you let your loved ones board a plane? Well, the current medical system may be killing almost twice that many people each day and yet nothing is being done about it.

So off we go to the doctor's office, the clinics, the hospitals, taking their advice, using their drugs, having medical procedures done, exposing ourselves to medical tests all the time knowing that the treatment may be worse than the ailment we are suffering from, as the treatment may kill us. Does this strike you as a little insane?

Yes, at various times you may need medical treatment. Often, these will be live saving: antibiotics, emergency medicine, hernia repairs, heart attack and stroke treatments, congenital heart correction procedurs, brain surgery for aneurysm repairs, etc. But too often we have too many procedures performed without a proper risk/reward evaluation. One really needs to think before having procedures and treatments.

The question you should be asking yourself each time you interact with our medical system is the same one I would ask if I were about to take a flight. Do the potential rewards outweigh the very real risks involved? When you look at it this way you will never be the same. Why is that? Gone will be the days of just following a doctor's orders. Gone will be the days of just submitting to their tests. Gone will be the days of just taking their drugs and gone will be the days of blindly having invasive procedures and numerous operations.

The upside is that if you start to question the medical community you may find that many of these things should be gone, as too many were never needed in the first place! Your first rule for self preservation of yourself and your loved ones is to never fully abdicate your healthcare over to anybody else, regardless of how tempting it may seem. You must always stay involved and examine all that they tell you, otherwise you may find yourself walking down the tarmac to one of those jumbo jets I mentioned.

How to Use this Book

FIRST, REALIZE THAT there is a lot of information presented here. Much of it may appear unbelievable, as it is information that only recently has been discovered. Other information will appear more familiar, as it is based on observations of what works in folk medicine, which has been with us for hundreds of years. Some people prefer to skim the chapters before reading straight through. Others who are more methodical prefer to start at the beginning and progress one chapter at a time. Within a short while they realize that they should be applying this information to their lives to obtain the maximum health benefits. In that case, they may find themselves proceeding slowly as they want to apply the knowledge they have gained.

My advice: Give yourself permission to move slowly, as you will get the maximum gains and benefits. Live the information and in doing so change your habits, eating patterns, and health behavior.

The information is conveyed using two fictional characters, Dr. Tessler and his soon to be pupil, a science reporter named David. While the format is told in a fictional conversational tone, the information is very real.

Prudence and liability laws in the United States require that we tell you to consult with your medical doctor before starting any supplement program, diet or reduction in current medications. If on medication, inquire and confirm that any supplements mentioned in this book do not interfere with any medications you may be taking. Hopefully you are working with a doctor who specializes in preventive medicine or anti-aging medicine, otherwise you may not find them very supportive.

12 THEORIES OF AGING THAT REALLY MATTER

&

WHAT YOU CAN DO ABOUT THEM

Part I

History & Perspective

1
The Introduction

THE DEADLINE FOR his article was only a short time away. No problem, David thought, as he would have it ready to go. This time he would be more prepared and would work well ahead of any looming deadlines. The bad part of being a writer, David knew, was the ease in delaying a project. After all, wasn't it human nature to put off until tomorrow what you were suppose to do today? Not this time, David thought. He would work well in advance and have the next several articles ready to go and not find himself working under a demanding deadline.

This thought process is what brought David to his next stop. He found himself on the doorstep of a Dr. Tessler. Hopefully this doctor would have a story for David, and he could take his time in reporting it. This was the doctor he had heard good things about from several different people in the sleepy town of Lexington, Virginia. David was always looking for stories on health or science since he made his living providing articles to various health magazines.

This Dr. Tessler was relatively new to that town, but already his reputation was attracting a slew of new clients and patients. Word had it that this elderly doctor had the manner of an old country doctor mixed with a success rate of a television doctor in which almost all medical problems seemed cured or figured out by the end of the show. In short, the doctor was getting real results.

David wanted to see this doctor and determine what techniques he might be using with his patients. He suspected the good country doctor might be employing the placebo effect either knowingly or unknowingly. This can occur when a medical practitioner uses their medical presence complete with their white coat and prescriptions, or in the case of a country doctor, with their charm, knowledge, and folksy manner. David had seen this placebo effect before when a doctor believes in what they are doing and conveys that to a patient along with a treatment or medication.

Often the patient gets better on their own accord just based on faith and confidence in the doctor or treatment. That is why many doctors may prescribe a sugar pill or a harmless substance just to make the patient feel that something proactive was being done. He had seen it before at clinics where such treatments were given to several ill patients. As crazy as it was, many of the patients' health improved, often dramatically. Of course, in some of the more severe cases like terminal cancer, patients were misled, and while the placebo medication extended the patients expectations and hope, it did nothing to extend their actual lives. In short, David wanted to make sure he wasn't dealing with a quack doctor.

David approached a white Victorian home, which sat on a crowded boulevard of similar homes all built about a hundred years ago. The address was easy to find as it was almost directly across from a famous historical Southern cemetery that contained the remains of Stonewall Jackson and other notable sons and daughters of the Confederacy.

David paused outside of the door, standing on the porch of a well-maintained home, which sported the large porches of yester-year, porches big enough for families to gather during special events or to cool off from the hot Virginia summers. The cool breeze would make its way down from the surrounding green mountains toward evening, and families would congregate there to enjoy the cooling off period and to wave at neighbors as they made their way by. It was time well spent with each other. Nowadays with air conditioners and television sets in each room, and computers and electronic games to distract us, those neighborly moments were long gone. What a shame he thought as he glanced up to the door. Imagine your neighbors being more available both physically and emotionally. What a loss, he thought.

He noted the friendliness of an old wooden bench-swing hanging from the porch ceiling. Also, he noted the welcoming effect of many robust, tall, purple flowers he recognized as Echinacea and a bounty of well maintained rose bushes surrounding the porch. They created a cascade of flowering dark red blooms that flowed like a deep living ribbon around the home. David felt better already in his decision to interview the doctor. Seeing so many well maintained plants also hinted to David many things. Perhaps, it showed that someone who appreciated life, love, and beauty lived here.

TOO OFTEN

Too often many medical professionals have big screen televisions in their waiting rooms or old magazines dealing with cars, hunting, or worse, dating advice from Cosmopolitan. They left no room to truly express their tastes or real personalities. Too many doctors hide behind their professional demeanor. No, David did not expect to find any of this stuff here. A simple porch with heartfelt decorations told him that a real person lived here. Hopefully that would lead to a more rewarding interview. A quick interview would be a real bonus, but he didn't want to get his hopes up.

As David's fingers reached for the door knocker, he suddenly felt off balance. At that precise moment someone was opening the door. Standing before him stood a beautiful lady dressed in a white laced blouse and a simple long dark skirt. Her black hair was pulled back in a bun but did not look old fashioned as much as it did elegant. She had a bright smile along with radiant hazel eyes. She was full of life and good energy, beaming with apparent good health. David suddenly realized he must be staring at his host just a little too intensely.

Sensing he was startled by her actions, she quickly responded, "Sorry to have surprised you! You must be David. I heard someone coming up the steps, and I didn't want to keep you waiting. Please come in; my husband's expecting you."

"Thanks," said David, not knowing what else to add.

Sensing his hesitation she added, "Well, my name is Esmeralda. Please have a seat and make yourself comfortable, won't you? Can I grab you a cup of tea or coffee? Water perhaps?"

"Sure, make mine a cup of black tea with a hint of sugar, if you have it."

David was shown to a set of chairs that lined the large entryway to the home's many rooms. As the doctor's wife made her way down a hallway, David took the time to explore the waiting area in more detail. He noticed a lack of diplomas and certificates on the wall. Once again, many doctors had taken to the practice of showing all their certificates including the mini courses they took for continuing education. David used to be impressed by these, but that faded away as soon as he realized that just because you attended the event doesn't mean that you really learned much. Some courses were so much better than others, David had found. Why was it that some courses conveyed real knowledge while other courses were more of the same stuff that really didn't promote good health? Stuffy courses just prolonging procedures and theories that didn't really seem to be curing anyone.

David had covered many medical conventions over the years for various science publications and health magazines looking for stories, yet was only impressed by a few, like the anti-aging workshops, disease prevention workshops, and alternative healing protocols that seem to work. David noted that from the last anti-aging conference he attended that he felt he had gained more from that conference than he had garnered from a whole semester of biology in college. He wondered how much real information is out there and who really knows it all.

Esmeralda entered the room and delivered his tea, presented on a tray complete with sugar, cream, and small spoons, all the small niceties of a bygone era. She excused herself with a genuine smile. David felt very comfortable here.

GETTING TO KNOW YOU

Just then a tall man entered the room. He stood about six-feet-one with black hair laced with streaks of pure gray. He had a wide smile projecting warm sincerity. Obviously this Dr. Tessler was comfortable with himself. David suspected the doctor was quite a bit older than his wife. Well, he guessed, perhaps having money allows for that privilege.

"David, I'm glad you came," the doctor said. "I have to admit I was reluctant to talk with anybody regarding my practice as I find it's too easy to be misrepresented or misunderstood, especially by the press community."

Smiling, David replied, "So what changed your mind, Doctor?"

"Well," said Dr. Tessler, "I've read several of your past articles and sense you are a fair person, someone who will search for the truth and know that truth when you find it. Is that right, David?"

David once again was at a loss for words. Twice in one day, an event that rarely occurred to him at anytime. "Yes, Doctor, I believe you know me better than most of my associates, unless you are trying to butter me up for some reason, but I don't sense that from you at all. So am I right as well, Doctor?"

"Yes, David, we both are correct, which gives us a good basis for moving ahead. Now tell me, what you would like to know about our small, humble practice? What would you like to discuss?"

"Well, Doctor, let's start with what you do here and why your patients seem to like you so much. Are you giving them happy pills or something?"

"Not quite," replied the doctor, "we are here to help people... but really we rarely ever send anyone home with medication. I will explain that later. Tell me first, David, what is the thrust of your article? How can I contribute best, where it might really make a difference to your readers?"

WHAT MAKES YOU DIFFERENT

"Well, Doctor, I need some fresh insight into how smaller communities are doing without the big clinics, special practices, and jumbo hospital networks that seem to be springing up all over the place. I want to write about the view of a country doctor and their take of what's going on nowadays in the world of medicine."

"I see, David. Well, I will try to not disappoint you, but first you need to understand that I am not your typical country doctor and my views of medicine run deep. I've been ready for a long time to tell someone on how a real medical practitioner should be helping others and not hurting them."

"How's that, Doctor?"

"Well, in years past I did perform pretty much as a typical country doctor going home to home, bringing new souls into this world and caring for the sick and needy. Been paid more in apple pies and homemade stews than I care to remember to...but I found out a long time ago that it was not really the best use of my time and energy. Nor was it really in the best interests of my patients."

"Jeez, Doctor, you don't look that old, I mean to be making house calls and all that, but then again, I'm a city boy, doctors there haven't made house calls in years."

"Nor here," replied the doctor, "but let's stick to your story. If I told you my theories of health and well-being, and they really made sense to you, would you put it in print?"

David said, "Of course, Doctor, if I really felt your theories made sense and if it isn't the same old mumbo jumbo we have been hearing about for years. You know, like eat a well-balanced diet, exercise, get your checkups, and see your doctor before doing anything. Well, if it was different from that and made sense, then I would be totally open to writing about it. Of course, Doctor, I would have to make sure your advice and methods, or magic bullets, work first."

"No, no, David, it's not that I have magic bullets to share with you. It's more a series of steps that, if followed, almost assures a long life, free of most disease. Also, if those steps are followed, it offers a full life that's worth living...because you will be full of energy. But having said that, David, I would need you to make a real commitment here."

2
The Commitment

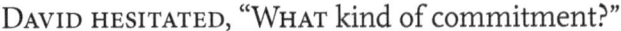

David hesitated, "What kind of commitment?"

Dr. Tessler continued, "A commitment that, as you learn the steps to health, you follow those steps as close as possible yourself. I need someone who will live and breathe the process. Someone who can stick to the steps to health that we share with our patients. But also, David, let me stress that I need someone in your position that can keep an open mind, and just as important, someone who can free their mind of all the misinformation and misconceptions that people have come to believe about the way to real health."

"How's this, Doctor? If what you show me makes sense, then I will follow your steps as you call them, but first let me ask if any of these steps involve using mumbo jumbo or worse, colonics?"

The doctor's smile grew wider, "No colonics or colon irrigation as they call it, David, unless you really want it? I mean, you may not know what you've been missing." They both laughed.

FIRST, DO NO HARM

The hours passed on as David and the doctor conferred. The doctor covered several topics. Of the most interest to David was when the doctor laid out the first step in his health program which was, "First, do no harm."

David replied, "Yeah, Doctor, we all know that doctors should do no harm, I mean it is the Hippocratic Oath and all. All physicians take the oath, right? So what you are saying is what any doctor would say."

"Well, David, yes and no, what you are saying is partially correct, most physicians take the oath then promptly go about circumventing it. It's similar to complaints ministers have about people that follow the Bible. You know what they say, David?"

"No, Doc."

"They say that too many people look upon the Bible like you would a menu. They pick and chose what they like and ignore the rest."

David smiled. "How's that related to the Hippocratic Oath?"

"Well, many of the practices, procedures, and standards of care protocols doctors follow are really not beneficial to the patient's well-being. For instance, many doctors perform invasive tests and procedures that absolutely may lead to a negative outcome."

"What do you mean by negative?"

"How about death at the top of the list for negative outcomes, but if the patient is more fortunate they may just be maimed, overexposed to toxins, or deprived of their true health potential. That just about covers it, except I didn't mention the expenses financially, emotionally, time spent, or the trauma and fear that many patients and their families have to go though."

Cautiously, David responded, "Doctor, are you saying that too many physicians are hurting people out there? Because that's what it sounds like you are saying..."

"Yes, David, that's exactly what I'm saying, but let me add quickly, if it is any comfort, that much of the harm they do is not intentionally done, at least not at first and not in most cases."

"Wow," David replied. "Why don't you outline exactly what is harming people so I can report on that?"

"That's just it, David, so many things done in the name of medicine are not really quote, good medicine, real medicine, or things that should be done."

"Yeah, I get your message, but I need real life examples, in plain English, please," said David.

"David, I could give you a long list of stuff and we will cover a lot more of it as we go along. Let me just say that a quick example is the unnecessary radiation exposure involved in a mammogram, full body scans, cat scans, and radioactive tracers that are used in so many tests. Add to this the damage to the kidneys caused by sodium phosphate enemas used before colonoscopies." He paused. "How about the potential death that can result from invasive heart tests like the angiogram and the angioplasty procedure that many times follows? Not to mention how many patients die of hospital-contracted infections or the side effects of too many physician-prescribed drugs."

David just nodded and continued taking notes.

DON'T GET ME STARTED

The doctor continued, "And don't even get me started on the many cancer treatments that do no good but ruin the patient's body and take away any chance of their health being restored. The facts are that chemo only works on a select few cancers and not on the majority. Some cancers like pancreatic and mesothelioma are probably better off without chemo. Also, many of the cancer treatments are cancer-causing themselves. I have seen patients treated for one cancer and end up dying years later from another cancer caused by that treatment. Blood cancers and testicular cancer may respond well to chemo and lymphomas often respond well to chemo and radiation, but many cancers don't respond at all to

11

these treatments. It's like going to an auto mechanic who insists on changing your engine at great expense when really it's your tires that need fixing. It just doesn't make sense the way many doctors are treating some patients.

"Most types of lung cancers and brain cancers are treated with heavy chemo even when the doctor knows it seldom cures those types of cancer. Having the patient boost their own immune function would prove a better bet. I mean make these doctors show you their success rates. They can't and they won't. They will talk about the cancer responding to treatment, but that is not curing cancer. If you radiate a tumor or inject chemo into it, it will shrink. So great, now you have a smaller but more virulent tumor growing in you. And the sad fact is, most doctors never ask the question of why you have cancer in the first place. An important question needs to be asked: if you don't know how you got it, then how can you get rid of it, or effectively treat it, to eradicate it or keep it from reoccurring? Attention needs to be on how to stop it in its tracks and prevent it from coming back. Stating this, prevention is the key and is only given lip service by the medical community and society at large. Too many people are getting cancer nowadays, and academics and doctors are not really addressing why. I have to tell you that it is out of control. We need to look at what people are doing today that they were not doing a hundred years ago. Also, people really need to question their doctors before submitting to their treatments, as many treatments simply don't add years to your life or life to your years."

David spoke up, "Why would so many people submit to such treatments if they weren't really necessary? I mean really?"

The doctor looked David in the eyes. "Most patients assume someone has established this protocol or treatment and it must be advantageous, so whatever the doctor says, it must be the best possible treatment available. That is simply not true. I mean they also think that their insurance company wouldn't approve such a treatment if it didn't work. The insurance companies do approve a lot of treatments that don't extend life due to that treatment being deemed common for that illness. So it isn't about what really is working out there. Patients simply don't understand how the medical system works."

"No, Doctor, I mean, why would a patient go along with a proposed treatment without checking out all of their options first?"

ASSUMED CONSENT

The doctor said, "First off, people are scared. Second, there is so much information overload out there along with so many opinions, people are confused. To move treatment along, many doctors use a strategy called assumed consent. It's very powerful."

"How's that?" David asked, "I mean I never heard of assumed consent."

"It's simple, David, a doctor just assumes you will go along with their treatment plan and directs you down that path on a program of care that is presented to you as the only option. Most people are too afraid to ask too many questions let alone question the doctor's treatment plan. Sad but true. Doctors learn this in their residency program in hospitals, to assume the patient's permission so they can get on with their workload."

David responded, "OK, Doctor, you're right. I mean I agree to all kinds of things in the doctor's office. With me it doesn't even have to be the doctor telling me what to do, but I even follow the staff's instructions often to the letter. Like I take off my clothes when told to do so or use a certain product like I'm told to before a certain procedure."

"That's common, David, and that is the part of assumed consent that allows important things to get done. I'm sure that we have to take off our shirts to get examined and all of that, but the assumed consent doesn't stop there. The medical community has you in a vulnerable position. You are sick, hurting or scared, and they are in the power position and are supposed to be true professionals. Well, that's when a lot of the mischief can happen. A doctor may do things to you that are not in your best interest. They may do this for money or out of ignorance, but regardless of the motive a negative outcome is a negative outcome. Now, here is what I get upset about. Not only do they assume permission but they also fail to get your intelligent informed consent before doing a procedure, test or treatment. When you hear of a doctor or hospital getting sued, the lawsuit often mentions this lack of informed consent. Many doctors don't feel it's in the patient's best interest to have so many tests done, but feel forced to do so to protect themselves from potential lawsuits. They often can't really offer you the treatment they personally would use because it may be viewed as not enough."

"I hear you, Doctor. So the doctors are victims too."

"Right, David, many doctors blindly follow protocols of treatments as they may be deemed common for that ailment. Many years ago a doctor had much more leeway to practice medicine!"

KEY POINTS

- First, do no harm. Keep this in mind when dealing with medical personnel. Often, they get so wrapped up with processes and procedures that they exceed boundaries of safety, reasonableness and common sense.

- Watch out for assumed consent. Many times medical staff use this technique to proceed with procedures or tests without explaining all the real risks. This also pertains to financial costs involved. Most patients are never told up front what the true costs will be.

- Take a knowledgeable and trusted friend or family member with you when you are being asked to do an invasive test, surgical procedure, or before undergoing radiation treatments or chemotherapy. In all of these cases, seek a second and third medical opinion.

- Ask about all risks and all costs of any procedure or treatment beforehand and keep detailed records. Only by keeping the medical system accountable in both of these areas can we affect meaningful change.

3
Immunizations

THE DOCTOR PAUSED only briefly then continued, "And if you look at too many immunizations for our younger population, it ought to create more concern, especially when most of those vaccines are bundled together with toxic substances and are injected directly into very immature immune systems, often with side effects. For instance, what child really needs a Hepatitis B vaccine at such a young age? That is a vaccine that a health care worker may want to get if they are working around needles or medical waste, or seriously, if they are having unprotected sex with an infected person. These types of people need a hepatitis B shot, but our babies, at birth? Really, where does this recommendation stem from?"

"Yeah," responded David, "but that whole immunization schedule thing and the pros and cons of vaccines has already been reported on, hasn't it? I mean there is no real harm from it, is there?"

"Well, yes and no," responded the doctor. "Too many companies that profit from these vaccines have constantly over reported the need for most vaccines and have intentionally misled us about the adverse effects that are impacting our population. Also, common sense has gone out the window. Why would you inject a newborn with a hepatitis B shot during the first week of life? Unless their mother tested positive for hepatitis. Otherwise, medical people have no business giving this shot. When the baby becomes a young adult they can make their own mind up about getting this vaccine. It reminds me of forced circumsion on most boys in the U.S. They have no say in this procedure, yet spend their lives with the irreversible outcome. Also, who really needs three vaccines combined in one shot like DTaP or MMR, given over and over again? At a minimum, it seems prudent to wait three to four years between shots. If just one shot gives 80% immunity, why have three shots in such a short time span just to increase that immunity a little bit more? David, simply stated, the medical community is advocating too many shots, too early in many cases and too often."

"You know, I've wondered about that myself, but the drug companies must know what they are doing, right?"

"I really don't think so," replied the doctor. "Remember they have a huge profit motive here; let me explain a little. Vaccines can vary from $25 a shot to over $150 a shot. Now, assuming an average of $50 per vaccine and a total of over 20 shots given, you have a cost of about $1,000 per child, not counting the cost of the office visits."

"Really? I don't think they give that many shots, do they?"

"Well, let's walk through it a little. The DTP shot for diphtheria, tetanus, and pertussis is given in a series of four shots. The Hib vaccine is given two or three times. Hepatitis B is given three times. The MMR vaccine for measles, mumps and rubella is given at least twice, and the polio vaccine is given four times. Many communities also require the HPV vaccine for human papilloma virus, especially in young ladies."

"Wow, that is a lot."

"Yes, it is, but that is not all. Usually pediatricians recommend a pneumococcal vaccine, chicken pox vaccine, and a seasonal flu shot. Not to mention an encephalitis shot as they grow older. By the way, some states require booster shots along the way. It begs the question: Should we really be injecting all these vaccines into our children's systems?"

"But don't we need these?"

"Need? Yes and no. If they caused no harm, and we were sure of that, then yes. However, we are not clear on that point. Anyone who says we are is misinformed, unaware or in denial. And do we need all these shots to be given at such a young age? Let's start with the diphtheria, tetanus and pertussis shot, known as DTP, or the newer DTaP vaccine. We know that pertussis, also known as whooping cough, is a rough, 100-day sickness, especially for infants, yet the other two vaccines usually are given at the same time, they don't even give you a choice. Tetanus and diphtheria are not so common here in the United States, so why can't people elect to get those later? They could wait on those two until the child's immune system has matured a little. For prevention purposes, I feel it is far better to have family members such as parents and older siblings vaccinated against potentially deadly diphtheria. You can vaccinate the children after they become much older, say age 5. And tetanus, why vaccinate at such a young age, unless warranted by a puncture, deep wound, or contamination of a wound? At the very least, I would hold off on that vaccine until the children are older."

"So, Doc, you are in no rush to vaccinate babies in the U.S. for tetanus unless the situation calls for it?"

"Pretty much, David, I'm a minimalist when it comes to injecting vaccines into our babies. In most cases, the substances and by-products they place into the vaccine concern me more than the active ingredient that produces the immune response."

"Are there any vaccines you feel children need?"

MAYBE NEEDED?

"Here in the United States, perhaps for babies, the Hib vaccine which protects against the bacterium Haemophilus influenzae type b, which in plain English, is the bug that can lead to a high fever and vomiting in most cases and can even lead, in some cases, to pneumonia or meningitis, an infection of the membranes covering the brain."

"Why this vaccine?"

"Because this affliction Hib is sure to come into a baby's life. But understand, doctors want to give repeated inoculations of this and other vaccines over and over again. I am open to this vaccine, but only one time and not over and over again as they are currently given. Multiple vaccine injections may improve the effectiveness of the body developing an immune response but it is simply too many injections for most babies."

"So this vaccine is acceptable?"

"Perhaps, David, but there have been side effects for many of the babties receiving this vaccine. However, it certainly makes a lot more sense than a hepatitis B vaccine. Also, pediatricians want to place a lot of other vaccines into our babies at such a young age and I feel it overburdens the body's ability to overcome such toxins that are mixed in with those vaccines. Also, the government accepts all of these vaccines into our society without asking for constant improvements in these products or rigorous ongoing studies as to their safety and effectiveness."

"So, Doc, are you saying, 'Slow down with all the vaccine stuff already?'"

"Yes, David. The Hib vaccine can be given to a young baby to protect them from something they are almost always going to contract. Saying this, most but not all children that do contract the bugs that Hib vaccine is protecting them from, do fine. The tetanus vaccine should be given to most children sooner or later. It's the time frame we are talking about. A two month old baby can be given a tetanus shot, but should they? One shot of tetanus is enough to give immunity from tetanus for many years, so why keep giving it over and over again as they do when they combine the tetanus vaccine in with the DTaP shots. They want you inject the DTaP vaccine into your children repeatedly. These are the type of questions we need to address."

"But it sounds like you have a healthy respect for the tetanus vaccine?"

"Yes, David, and for a good reason."

"OK, Doc, fill me in."

NEONATAL TETANUS

"It is a sad fact that tetanus is still robbing our world of at least 60,000 to 80,000 babies a year. A real tragedy."

"Really, Doc? I've not heard of that; fill me in."

"David, many newborns in Third World countries are exposed to the spores of the bacterium which cause tetanus. It's found naturally in the soil, so it finds its way to wounds or umbilical cords, which can easily be contaminated by unsanitary conditions."

"Like found in these countries?"

"Right, David. Transmittal of tetanus this way can be diminished greatly by having clean birthing centers, education, and vaccinating the mothers."

"The mothers, Doc? How does that save the babies?"

"David, when we vaccinate the mothers against tetanus we protect them from contracting maternal tetanus and also provide some passive immunity to the babies, especially during the first few weeks of life when the babies are most likely to be exposed to this tetanus bacterium by a dirty or contaminated umbilical cord."

"Wow, Doc, that's impressive. So this an example on how to intelligently deploy vaccines?"

"I think so, David. You can't argue with its success rate."

"How so?"

"David, the World Health Organization, usually just called WHO, estimated that during the 1980s an average 800,000 babies were dying of tetanus each year. Now, after their vaccination campaign, that number has dropped by over 80% per year."

"So, Doc, this was a huge vaccine success story."

"Yes, David, but along with the vaccines was an educational program that really helped."

"What was that, Doc?"

"The WHO educated people on clean baby delivery."

"Such as?"

"The WHO, and various other organizations, set up numerous sanitary birthing centers. They put the word out on the three C's of birthing."

"Which are?"

"Clean hands, clean surfaces and clean cord cutting. This clean environment for the birth process has dramatically cut infant mortality and also saved a lot of mothers. In short, clean sanitation saves lives!"

"So, Doc, refresh my mind on why the Third World would have so much tetanus exposure in the first place."

"It's simple, David. Dirt, dust and animal droppings. In many situations mothers and infants are exposed to the spores of the bacterium Clostridium tetani, found mostly in dirt or in the digestive tract of animals."

"So when was a vaccine developed?"

"Great question. It's been less than 100 years and a lot has been accomplished in regards to deadly tetanus. A vaccine was developed around 1924, but before that, a tetanus anti-toxin was developed by the famous German bacteriologist Emil von Behring. This anti-toxin allowed many injured soldiers to survive the tetanus infections acquired during dirty trench warfare. Behring's work on anti-toxins for tetanus and, especially, diphtheria won him the first Nobel prize ever given for medicine. Before World War I, too many soldiers died of tetanus. However, during World War I, the medical corps started giving tetanus anti-toxins to the wounded. They would mark an injured soldier with a large T on their forehead to acknowledge that they indeed were given the anti-toxin. This greatly improved survival for soldiers exposed to tetanus. Later, around 1924, a proven vaccine was available to all troops before they even went into battle. So the effects of tetanus during World War II and beyond were negligent."

"I see, Doc. I guess with trench warfare during World War I, many soldiers were exposed to tetanus."

"That's right, David. It could have been one of the leading causes of death behind sepsis and gangrene had it not been for the tetanus anti-toxins. So many soldiers were spared the agony of tetanus due to the anti-toxins being available. Now, at the start of the war, many troops did get tetanus, especially with the battlefronts taking place in dirty cow pastures and such. It wasn't until the medical corps understood where the tetanus was coming from did they implement the necessary preventive measures."

"So what about the Civil War? The same conditions, the same causes of death?"

"Right, David. Any war before the tetanus vaccine would find many of the combatants dying of tetanus. A horrible way to go as your body tightens up so much, causing great pain and exhausting the victim. Countless men, women, and animals have died from tetanus."

"Animals?"

A HORSE STORY

"Of course, David. Perhaps you don't know it, but right here in Lexington, Virginia, Robert E. Lee's horse Traveller is buried. He stepped on a rusty nail, developed tetanus and had to be shot. Nobody could bare to see the horse die from the paralyzing effects of tetanus. He's buried right up at the Washington and Lee University."

"I never thought about that. It's great to know we have such a powerful vaccine against such a common enemy."

"Right you are, David. Unlike some other diseases and afflictions, we will always have to defend ourselves against tetanus, since it is found all over. It's not likely we can eliminate it like we did with smallpox and, perhaps soon, polio."

"So, Doc, you would not immediately give a baby a DTaP shot, but would wait longer and stretch out the needed doses over time, as long as a child gets at least one tetanus shot. Would you say the same about the measles, mumps and rubella vaccine?"

"Likewise, I feel the same way about the MMR vaccine. I know we all want to spare our children from the danger of measles, but instead, inoculate the family and caretakers first. Same for mumps, and rubella or German measles as they call it. I would worry more about measles than mumps. However, stating that, adults do poorly with mumps. With German measles, it is more about protecting unborn children, as German measles in pregnant women lead directly to birth defects. So having everybody getting a rubella shot later in life just makes sense."

David responded, "I am a little confused; you are not saying you are against all vaccines, just the schedule of how the vaccines are being given?"

A MIRACLE TOOL

The doctor took a deep breath and continued, "David, no one should argue that vaccines are not a miracle tool that can be used to prevent sickness and can be a benefit to our society. Up to the late 1930s, diphtheria caused many childhood deaths. But today vaccines are being totally misused and in my view, abused. They are injecting into babies a combination vaccine for DTaP at 2 months of age, again at 4 months, then again at 6 months, again at 18 months, and then also around ages 4-6. Too many shots and too often! What most people don't realize is that many of these vaccines contain preservatives that are harmful and contain too much aluminum, which is often used to illicit a stronger immune response. A lot of these vaccines are also made using animal parts, human parts, and their fluids. And contrary to what drug companies have you believe, seldom are those vaccines produced in the best fashion for our children. I mean it may cost a lot more, but I want vaccines that are free of unnecessary animal products and other agents. Don't you agree our children are worth the additional costs?"

David said, "OK, I hear what you are saying, Doc, but do you feel the same way about all the other vaccines?"

"I feel the same way about almost all the current vaccines. Of course, vaccines can be wonderful tools, but like all tools they must be used carefully and for a specific purpose. When our country faces an epidemic, then vaccines can be a godsend, depending on exactly what specifically we are facing. Not all vaccines for different diseases or afflictions work as well as the drug companies will have you believe. And often, the side effects are not factored in completely or at all. If vaccines worked like the drug companies would have you believe, then you could vaccinate your child and not worry at all about them contracting anything from a social setting, but that is not the way it works. Many times in outbreaks like measles, the vaccinated children get the illness anyways."

OVER & OVER

The doctor reflected only for a moment before continuing, "And, if immunizations worked like they insinuate, you would only need one shot and only a small amount. Yet often you must take a series of shots for one vaccine exposing you over and over again to hidden toxins that most vaccines contain. So clearly, they are not communicating everything fully to us."

David replied, "I think I understand your position, Doctor, but just to be clear, what is your main point about vaccines I should write about for my readers?"

MY POINT

"I will get to that in a moment, David. However, first let me reiterate that vaccines should stand ready to assist us when an epidemic hits or is pending. No doubt about that. However, the current system is to inoculate everybody upfront to keep an epidemic from happening in the first place. Health officials know this so they go the route of least resistance and vaccinate all of our children, especially since they can't say no. This is logical since many adults may have already been exposed to many of the infectious agents such as measles, mumps, chickenpox, and other ailments. This early inoculation or giving of vaccines to children acts as a strong barrier to the spreading of new infections. As I said, this indeed does make sense, but only if we are sure our babies immature immune systems and bodies can handle these vaccines. I contend they cannot. At least not in the form many vaccines are given nor in the manner given."

"So, Doctor, please explain, as you just said it makes sense to vaccinate children and you even gave me several good reasons to do so?"

"Let me explain, David. Like many things in life you can find reasons for or against something. Four important reasons against are: there are too many junk ingredients in most vaccines, too many vaccines are given, they are given too early, and they are given too often. We need vaccine reform. Parents should be the young babies' advocates and not just conform to what health departments tell us. I believe these health departments direct their efforts at babies since they cannot speak up or weigh the pros and cons of each vaccine recommended. They bully parents into getting too many shots in a very short time period without giving full disclosure of what ingredients are contained within those vaccines, the real rate of side effects, the breadth of those side effects, or how those vaccines are really manufactured. This may be causing some real problems within the babies' delicate system. Also, as I said earlier not all countries give so many vaccines to their children, hence, the reactions people are seeing like attention deficit problems, personality changes, withdrawal behavior, fevers, autism, immune problems, etc., which are much higher here in the United States."

"Ok, Doctor, when you say it that way, it makes sense. So you agree vaccines indeed do work?"

WATCHFUL WAITING

"David, yes vaccines are miracle tools and often do work, but at a cost. That cost is what the drug companies, the Centers for Disease Control, and the medical community seldom discuss in an open manner. You only hear the good attributes but the not the bad. Even most anti-vaccine advocates admit vaccines do indeed work. What most of them are against is how vaccines are given in this country, the junk ingredients, and how they are abused. So, I would absolutely practice watchful waiting."

"Which is?"

"Which simply is giving just one shot at a time to your child and waiting a few months before giving another. This would allow time for the parent to observe if there are any changes in their child's personality. They should look for negative reactions such as high fevers or, worse, things like the child becoming noticeably less responsive or withdrawing from normal behaviors. Pay attention if your child becomes less responsive or develops repetitive behaviors of any sort. Especially note if they become less active or if they start withholding their affection. All of these are signs that the vaccine ingredients could be impacting your child's mental, physical, and social development. I feel many children can tolerate numerous shots, but not all. That is why one vaccine schedule does not suit all children. Be especially wary of clinics that want to over-vaccinate your children by giving multiple vaccines on the same day. This would concern me greatly. The Centers for Disease Control states this should not be an issue, yet my response would be, "To who?" Following the guidelines blindly is not the path I would pursue.

"So let me be clear, vaccines have their place; history would have been totally different had vaccinations been around for a longer period of time. For instance, if the Native Americans in North America and the American civilizations of Central and South America had vaccines available over the last six hundred years the world would be very different today."

PARADISE LOST

"How so, Doc?"

"David, when the Spaniards landed in the West Indies, Cuba, and other areas of the New World they unleashed a series of afflictions of biblical proportions, namely, plagues.

"These plagues decimated the native populations. Smallpox alone wiped out entire populations. Cortez, the Spanish conqueror, invaded the Aztec capital, where Mexico City now sits, and found thousands of bodies floating in the canals of the city. It seems that when the Spaniards landed further away they brought with them smallpox which immediately made its way to the heart of the Aztec city. It beat them there by spreading from the coast where they landed to the heart of the Aztec kingdom very quickly, moving faster than Cortez's army, a case of unintentional germ warfare being used to win a war. Otherwise, it is doubtful that Cortez and his small army could have made much progress, but with the entire city's population inflicted with dreaded smallpox, its resistance was muted tremendously.

"Likewise, millions of Native Americans perished from these infectious diseases. It's known that diseases brought by Europeans spread all throughout North America. Pilgrims landing in New England found entire Indian villages piled high with bones and bodies from infections that were sweeping through the Indian nations. It seems that the Spanish and their germs inadvertently had infected tribes far away and the infections spread like a wild fire. This decimation of native tribes and future further population die off made it impossible for Native Americans to offer any real resistance as their numbers were so much less now. The native people had no resistance against smallpox or measles as they were never exposed to these. It is estimated that small pox alone wiped out fifty percent of the New World's population, if not greater. This was followed up by measles which may have been even more deadly. So, now their numbers dwindled by an estimated eighty percent. Now you add to this other new diseases that they were never exposed to such as mumps, yellow fever, chickenpox, diphtheria, etc. and it's a wonder that any native people survived at all."

"So they had not developed any real immunity to these afflictions?"

"No, David, these germs were new to their systems and their societies had not built up any real immunity. These viral and bacterial infections were dramatic and deadly to them. Had they had vaccines available like we do today, most of them would have survived. A lesson that must not be lost on us as a modern society."

"But they had no vaccines back then, right, Doctor?"

"Sadly no, David, that's what I am pointing out, vaccines are really important to mankind and the course of history both in the past, the present, and going forward. No one should doubt that."

"Continue, Doc, this is fascinating."

The doctor continued, "But I should note that early colonists in North America commented that often they noticed that many slaves from northern Africa had small scars from being inoculated for smallpox through a process known as variolation. This is when a small amount of dried up pox skin-scrapings from a recovering smallpox victim are transferred to a healthy person by scrapping their skin and rubbing the skin-scraping into them conferring partial or full immunity to smallpox, often for many years. This is what gave many slaves protection from smallpox. It was a practice done by some African tribes, Arabic people, and other people in places like India and China."

"Why did Native Americans not figure this out?"

"Timing, David, timing, the Indians never had a chance to learn this inoculation technique as they were impacted not only by smallpox but by a host of many different diseases. Imagine smallpox, measles, mumps, yellow fever, typhus, new forms of malaria, the flu, and on and on, it would be tremendously overwhelming to say the least. The other populations of the world had thousands of years to figure out some immunizations techniques like variolation but even then, is was not used by all of those peoples."

"So what about the vaccines being given to our children nowadays?"

"Well, David, many diseases were not as virulent in European descendants, since past Europeans that reacted badly to these viruses had died off during prior epidemics. Also, remember, the Native American populations were never before exposed to these germs. There was no herd immunity from having had a good portion of the population contracting the virus causing diseases before. Over the years, wave after wave of such things as measles, chickenpox, smallpox, and mumps allowed many Europeans to develop some herd immunity, meaning the diseases did not impact the entire population at one time and those that were impacted often did not get as sick as native populations. For instance, younger people do better with smallpox and Europeans were often exposed when they were younger. Add to the equation that these viral diseases adapted to surviving Europeans somewhat, becoming less virulent. Viruses especially, have been known to do this as a survivor mechanism or adaptive measure, since a disease that kills its host often loses its home. At least that is the theory."

"So I ask the same question, Doctor, what about today's vaccines for children? Are you saying you are against most of them or just the timing of when they are given?"

VACCINE COURT

"That's a difficult question to answer, David. As I said, children are given too many vaccines, too often, and exposed to a lot of garbage ingredients. The whole vaccine industry needs to be investigated. We are allowing them to make injections for our children that, in many cases, are full of toxins. They are given blanket immunity from liability as well. As you may know, David, it's difficult to sue drug companies for vaccine related side effects or even death because of laws passed in the 1980s."

"I'm familiar with a little of that, Doctor, but don't the drug companies need that protection? I mean, look at all the frivolous lawsuits nowadays and the really expensive class action lawsuits."

"I hear you, David, but our country did fine without these laws for years up until the mid 1980s. We had, at that time, many children reacting badly to the DTP vaccine. This caused the drug companies to ask congress for relief and protection or else they threatened to stop making many vaccines available. The vaccine court came first followed soon after by the National Childhood Vaccine Injury Act. This act limits the amount a victim, or family of the victim, can get, even if that victim dies, to a relatively low limit. These laws take away the incentive for lawyers to expose the side effects of vaccines."

"Do we really need the lawyers to expose these types of things, Doctor?"

"I know what you mean, David, but yes, in my humble view we do. I saw the lawyers bring to everyone's attention on how asbestos used in the shipyards, auto plants, and building trades was killing thousands of workers. Without the lawyers I don't think much would have happened to stop the common use of dangerous asbestos in our lives. Likewise, look at cigarette smoking, benzene, coal dust, etc. The list goes on and on. We do need someone besides the drug companies investigating these products in more depth. Of course, the problem is that we have a few attorneys who sue anybody for any reason as long as there is money involved. So we need some protection against these types of lawsuits. However, giving blanket protection like the National Childhood Vaccine Injury Act does is not the right answer. If you note, this act applies specifically to children. It affirms the concept that if you give vaccines to children you are protected as a drug company. Hence, the incentive to say all children need so many vaccines. This creates an atmosphere of giving all these vaccines to children when they are young and also while you, as a drug company, are protected against using an inferior product. Vaccine laws that fully protect drug companies are not the answer, safer vaccines are."

THE LINK

"So, Doctor, you are in the medical camp that believes vaccines may be causing us some harm. It sounds as if you see a connection between vaccines and the increase in autism and other problems such as hyperactivity in our children?"

29

The doctor paused and was deep in thought. David knew enough from hundreds of interviews not to interrupt this process. He would just sit and wait for the doctor to resume his answer.

The doctor inhaled. "Well, as a medical writer you know that several studies show no correlation between vaccines and rising autism rates. However, let me just state a known correlation between two items called 'cause and effect.' Many times, if you do something, it will produce an outcome. Like if I hit my thumb with a hammer, it will hurt, I guarantee it. You know, cause and effect. If you inject so many non-natural substances directly into the body, you are going to see many repercussions. I mean, these modern vaccines are not like the simple dried up flakes of cowpox pustules that were given to people to prevent smallpox at the dawn of the vaccination era. No, these current vaccines can be a cesspool of vile animal products, fluids, viruses, and heavy metals, a lot of it being total nonsense."

The doctor rose out of his chair and spoke in a clear but stronger voice, "So back to your question, could current vaccines being given, the amounts they are given in, and at such early ages, be responsible for an increase in autism? Then my answer would be, it seems very possible to me. Why not? Especially if you really understand the history of medicine, as modern medicine is descended from ancient medicine more than people realize. Over the last 500 years a substance has been widely used in allopathic, or what we refer to as modern medicine, which we now know to be unsafe in any amount."

David was quick to probe into this more, "What's that?"

KEY POINTS

- Vaccines are miracle tools, but like most tools, they must be used correctly.

- The medical community is under pressure from the drug companies to vaccinate children while they are young. The reason? Vaccine manufacturers are protected more due to federal law against the effects of a vaccines given to a minor. Children also can't speak up for themselves.

- Consider practicing watchful waiting. Observe your child after receiving a vaccine. Give it some time (two to three months). If no negative reactions are seen, it may be deemed safer to proceed. This is only recommended if there are no deadly outbreaks currently occurring.

4
Quicksilver

"DAVID, DID YOU ever here of something called quicksilver?"

"Of course, Doctor, that's mercury, right?"

"Right, David, and mercury has been used in medicines since the Roman times, maybe even longer. The real shame is that it is still being used in medicine without most people realizing it."

"No way. You have got to be kidding me, I mean they shut down my daughter's school because some kid had broken a thermostat with mercury in it and they were worried about the health hazards."

"Well, that type of mercury is actually safer than the mercury they are using in our medicines."

David stared in disbelief; he could not believe what he was hearing. "Doctor, you will have to back that one up because my doubting, logical mind doesn't process this. How could we still be using mercury in our medicines? I mean, why would we being doing something like that?"

The doctor proceeded to tell David the history of quicksilver, or mercury as we now call it. He explained how mercury generated a powerful reaction from the body when given internally or when placed on the skin. The doctor talked about the history of medicine and how most bacteria-caused diseases were not really treatable before the advent of antibiotics.

A BRIEF HISTORY LESSON

The doctor explained that for hundreds of years mercury was used to treat one of the worst diseases people could imagine, syphilis. The disease was a life-long ailment to people who contracted it. Millions of people have gone to their death due to syphilis. It was the AIDS of their day. It was called the Great Pox to distinguish it from smallpox.

It was spread through sexual contact, so it naturally made its way amongst the human population. The amount of people in our history that contracted syphilis is far more than most people can imagine. Many doctors were specialists in that field even going by the name of syphilologist. Alexander Exquemelin, the author of *The Illustrated Pirate Diaries*, wrote on how prevalent syphilis was in the 1600s – so common that the infamous pirate Blackbeard blocked ship traffic from entering the port of Charleston, South Carolina, as he wanted to obtain a medical chest of mostly mercury compounds to treat syphilis that inflicted his crew. Of course, syphilis was around for many years and was thought to have been brought back to Europe by Columbus's crew. It only came under control in the 1940s when antibiotics came into use. In the United States, most traditional doctors used mercury compounds to treat syphilis up to just 70 years ago. Not only for syphilis but many other disorders as well. Syphilis, along with smallpox and tuberculosis, were major afflictions for countless generations.

Years back, doctors were not aware of the germ theory of disease nor of sanitary conditions. The result was that most doctors used whatever means they could to try to control diseases and disorders. This lead to some very bizarre treatments like bleeding, or releasing humours as it was called, a process mistakenly based on the ancient medical belief that the fluids of the body need to be balanced, along with the thought that taking some very toxic poisons into the body could alter those fluids. Some of the more enlightened ones were using arsenic, considered a serious poison but less life destroying than mercury.

Why was mercury used? Compounds with mercury were used for over a thousand years to treat leprosy. Mercury is so toxic that it kills bacteria when applied to the skin. When syphilis first made its appearance, it was a very deadly strain that killed many people quickly, but not before causing their skin to fester with ugly sores and such. It appeared at first to look like a form of leprosy, and indeed many who had syphilis were treated as lepers. The skin lesions many times would show a response to mercury ointments, hence the treatments continued. It's easy to relate mercury to modern chemotherapy treatments, as both do not usually cure more than just treat the symptoms. In fact, you could argue that mercury was one of the first chemo drugs used. The parent of modern chemotherapy, it involved taking a known toxin to suppress symptoms but seldom curing the real underlying condition.

THE WALKING DEAD

The doctor continued to explain, "Thousands and thousands of patients suffered from insanity, or hysteria as it was called, from mercury poisoning. Mercury compounds under various names were used for treatment either by ingesting the toxic stuff or applying it to the skin for lesions caused by syphilis. The names were many, such as Mercurial, golden elixir, and later by names such as Calomel. Unfortunately, for too many people the treatment of choice was mercury. This toxic substance produced mental problems in many of its users. The mental degeneration and craziness it produced sometimes would not strike until years later, giving the impression it was the syphilis causing the illness. However, in many cases it really was the mercury causing the mental illness.

David interrupted, "Are you saying that medical doctors supported this treatment?"

"More than that, they thought it was really working, and this logic only just slowed down recently. I mean the president of the American Medical Association proclaimed in a speech made during 1903, 'Drugs, with the exception of quinine in malaria and mercury in syphilis, are valueless as cures.' So in effect, doctors thought mercury was one of their most valuable medicines."

David said, "So mercury in medicine has been going on for centuries. Most people are not aware of that, I guarantee you."

The doctor continued, "Not only did the patients suffer from the toxic effects of mercury poisoning, but the doctors, nurses and family members helping to take care of the sick people suffered as well. The treatment they gave was killing them, but slowly in many cases. Daughters taking care of their sick parents would have been exposed to the mercury compounds as they applied ointments. Surgeons in prior years used mercury compounds to sterilize their instruments. They also use mercury paint to cover incision areas both before and after cutting in surgery.

"The sad fact is that we all have been exposed to mercury. The very air we breathe is polluted with mercury from the power plants and factories burning coal, as coal naturally contains mercury. That pollution is spread through the air and makes its way into our food supply, especially the fish population. Worse, is that the mercury from the air pollution goes through a chemical change once it is exposed to bacteria. It becomes a more toxic form of mercury called methylmercury. It accumulates in lake fish and larger ocean fish, especially predator fish that live by consuming other fish. Mercury makes its way up the food chain, in stronger doses as it proceeds."

David said, "So that's why they tell pregnant women not to eat swordfish or too much tuna?"

"Yes, once a human consumes any mercury, the toxic metal becomes cumulative, interfering with normal cellular activity, and this mischief promotes illness. The body can only get rid of so much mercury at one time. The liver and kidneys try, but if impaired at all or undeveloped as in infants, they fight a losing battle. Almost always, people can't even associate the symptoms they are having to any exposure. Many diseases and disorders are linked to this mercury contamination. To add insult to injury, we still have medical people placing more mercury in our bodies."

"More mercury?"

"Yes," responded the doctor. "Many people can remember having mecuricome used on their wounds. Now you may recognize the mercury sounding name, or how about those silver fillings in your mouth? Sorry, but the dentist lied. Those are not silver anymore than lead is gold. You can mix lead and gold together, but that still leaves lead as lead. A major ingredient of a silver amalgam filling is mercury. That's right, they are silver mixed with a large dose of mercury. Referring to my notes, one silver/mercury amalgam critic pointed out that 'The container this material is delivered in clearly states this material is toxic. The container that your dentist will place a loose silver amalgam filling in after they extract it from your mouth states it is a hazardous waste. So the only safe place for these mercury fillings according the dentists that use such fillings, is in your mouth.' Now imagine, a lifetime of chewing and how the mercury from those fillings leak out. Where do those leaks go? In your body and in your brain."

David could not keep quiet any longer, and his voice quivered with anger. "Doc, my children just had fillings, and our dentist said that silver amalgam fillings were safe. Now what you are telling me is that these are not really silver but toxic mercury?"

"That's right, David. Amalgam simply means mixture, and in this case it is mercury mixed with other metals like silver, copper, zinc and more. Now when they first came up with this concept of mixing metals together to repair cavities in someone's mouth, it was actually quite cutting edge technology. I mean over 175 years ago when you got a cavity they usually had to pull the tooth or find some expensive gold metal to place into that cavity to keep the decay at bay or from spreading. It works in this respect, so millions and millions of these fillings have been put into people's mouths. And, David, don't feel stupid; thousands of doctors have had this toxic sludge put into their mouths as well."

"But, Doc, we all know that mercury is bad for us so why are they still using this stuff?"

The doctor inhaled then said, "Yes, many people are waking up to the fact that just because something has always been done that way doesn't make it right.

Too bad, but it takes time for these things to work themselves out. Many in the dentistry business believe that the amount of mercury used is so little that it couldn't possibly have much of a negative effect. They are wrong, of course. They believe somehow that the mercury gets locked up because it is mixed with other metals. This is wishful thinking and not very scientific, I am sad to say. For too many people, most mercury contamination comes from the inside of their mouths due to these toxic fillings rather then outside pollution sources. It reminds me of what the Romans did."

"What's that?"

"They use lead pipes for collecting rain water and lead vessels for cooking, and they slowly poisoned themselves. It may account for their slip in intelligence as lead blunts the IQ of people. Yet now we have the luxury of time and knowledge to look back at how ignorant they were – I mean poisoning themselves and not knowing it! Yet we are doing the same thing in modern times with our misuse of one of nature's most toxic metals, mercury."

REMOVAL

"But Doctor," asked David, "shouldn't I get those fillings out of their mouths?"

"Of course, but let me tell you, David, just taking them out like most conventional dentists would do, may be worse. They typically drill out the fillings, spewing the toxic mercury into the patient's bloodstream or allowing the vapors to enter the patients system via the respiratory tract. Be careful; only use a dentist that specializes in mercury extraction techniques. They will use a small device that extracts the toxic vapors while they are working on the tooth. Also, you should not remove too many mercury fillings at one time as it may be too much for your body to deal with, I mean the detoxification process of your body trying to eliminate all those mercury toxins at one time."

Forcefully, David said, "OK, Doc, you're not making me feel a whole lot better about this process. I mean how the hell did we end up in this position, trying to get out something so toxic that a doctor put in?"

"Remember, David, dentists have one of the highest suicide rates of any profession. Many of them may not really know it, or are rationalizing, but mercury is a horrible product to be working with. It messes with the body, the immune system, the brain. And it is so subtle that most people never connect the dots of why they are sick and what caused it. I mean, if mercury made you sick right away, then people would see the cause and effect. But even lethal exposure to mercury may take months to kill you, so people just don't see the correlation. Now, I am not saying mercury fillings are going to kill your children; they won't. In fact, many cutting edge doctors and dentists feel the best policy is to leave silver/mercury amalgam fillings as is in children, since they grow so quickly and during ages 6 through 12, their second teeth will push out those older teeth anyways. There might be less exposure in letting it sit there until a later time. A small amount of mercury will leach into the body, especially when chewing such things as nuts and such, but it still may be less mercury exposure then removing it all at once. Sorry, David, but I know how you feel."

"How's that, Doctor?"

"Well, early on in my life I had a mouth full of silver/mercury fillings. It took me years to get rid of them. When I did, my health slowly improved. I have seen this over and over again in my patients."

"So, Doc, what did you see improve?" said, David.

"For me, I noticed right away that my anxiety levels dropped. I used to have a sense of impending doom, and I have not felt that in years since I had those mercury fillings removed. I also had more of a bad temper, which I slowly moved away from, and even had an irregular heartbeat. Now, I have to tell you that I had a lot of mercury in my mouth back in the day. I also suffered from a strange upper back pain that could not be remedied. I saw countless specialists and nothing helped. I tried medications, physical therapy, getting my back and neck manipulated, but it just took time. A few years after having the fillings removed I no longer suffer with any major afflictions. And that is my point, mercury toxicity comes in many forms and in many disguises. It is too hard to pin down on what may be causing problems in your body when mercury is involved. It is a very disruptive substance, one that should never knowingly be put into anyone's body."

What disorders have you seen clear up in your patients, Doctor?"

"Irritability, lack of concentration, anxiety, and dizziness in the short term. Long term, I have seen fatigue, headaches, nervousness, allergies and such clear up."

"Unbelievable," said David. "That's quite a list of symptoms clearing up. Any other things you have seen get better?"

"Yes," with a chuckle, the doctor replied, "Ironically, David, quite often mouth disorders like gum disease and such. Which shouldn't be surprising, I guess, since mercury is a strong toxin, and it's sitting there in your mouth. But re-member, while mercury fillings are really bad from my viewpoint, removing them will only remove the problems they may have been causing, not solve problems that were there before they were put in."

David smiled and responded, "Of course, Doctor, that makes perfect sense."

CAUSE AND EFFECT

The doctor and David rose and made their way from the study lined with books to an outer seating area just outside the doors of the room. The doctor contin-ued with his dialogue pausing, as he repeated several times, "Cause and effect, cause and effect..." Then he resumed, "I remember the same garbage being said about cigarette smoking, leaded gas, leaded paint, asbestos, cotton fibers, Teflon, aluminum, fabric protector, DDT, mercury-based fungicides, exces-sive amounts of prenatal vitamins most of which contain synthetic forms of vitamins, and a host of other items. Those producing the products were always able to hire medical spokespeople or advertising agencies to confuse people. They would throw studies out there that seemed to show their products to be harmless. And you know what I think about lots of studies? They can be done for or against almost anything. Causing confusion and uncertainty is relatively easy to do. We all need to use common sense, which is not common anymore."

THE STUDY SAYS

The doctor said, "If a study comes out showing ill effects of something, you better believe that the manufacturer of a product will come out with a study that seems to show the opposite. I mean, if you throw some articles out there stating the opposite view of what may be the truth, it can keep people guessing about who is right and who is wrong for years."

David just continued to nod to show he was listening, as he kept busy writing. He didn't want to miss any item. The doctor looked directly at David, and his voiced lowered in volume just a little, "David, I mean it's just like people looking around at all of our fat children and wondering why they are getting fatter...I mean wake up, it's cause and effect. Too many calories, junk food, high fructose corn syrup, trans fats, along with no exercise, and children will get fat. Now, here's what I mean about cause and effect and the vaccine connection. If you are giving a lot of shots or immunizations at birth and every year thereafter, which our children are getting, then yes, as I said before, I think it's possible that these vaccines are contributing to the huge increase of developmental disorders. However, saying this, who knows what's really behind such an increase in autism rates?"

Before David could answer, the doctor continued, "While many feel overuse of vaccines, especially those containing the mercury-based preservative thimerosal or the immune provoking metal aluminum, are causing developmental problems within our children, others think it is the toxic overload in our food, fluoride in our water, mercury in our fish, arsenic in our eggs, lack of vitamin D, additives in our milk, too many plastic products and packaging, copper pipes, MSG or its cousins in so much of our prepared food, or bromide in our flour products. It's back to cause and effect.

"Someone will figure it out some day, and hopefully be able to bring it to the forefront...But also, quite honestly, I feel there are other items that may be contributing to the developmental problems as well."

David jumped on that last sentence, "What items are those?"

ULTRASOUNDS

"Quite honestly, David, I feel that all the ultrasounds given to babies while they are in the womb may be a problem and, well, a real possible reason for increasing developmental problems. I mean, it is just an additional item being added to the toxic burden that our undeveloped children are dealing with."

David sat back and took in what the doctor was saying; he was uncertain how to deal with what the doctor had just said. All he could respond with was his muted, "Doctor, to be frank with you, I have never heard anyone mention that ultrasounds may be causing problems."

"It's a consideration, David. This country allows too many ultrasounds, and no one I know is speaking out about this diagnostic tool being overused...and in my view, it is really being misused. It reminds me of how X-rays were used on pregnant women in the 1930s and 1940s, especially in England. A large increase in children's cancer was the result and their medical community was in denial about it for decades."

"Yeah, Doc, but the ultrasound isn't an X-ray, so how could it be hurting the baby?"

"Remember, David, we started off saying that a physician's first duty is to do no harm. Let me explain how this test may be hurting babies. Nowadays doctors have lost control over the practice of medicine. The attorneys, government, medical boards, HMOs, insurance companies, drug companies, hospital management, and God knows who else are becoming a wedge between doctors and their patients. As a doctor, you are no longer really free to voice your real opinion on what a patient should do because of all the other considerations. It's the perfect recipe for inferior care and treatment, and sadly, too often, a tragedy. So what I am trying to say, David, is nowadays a doctor has to do what others expect from them and not what they feel is really needed. That is why I broke away from so many of their influences. You have to be ready to take a heck of a pay cut but sometimes a person just has to do what they have to do."

"I understand that entirely, Doctor, I really do. In fact, all the doctors I talk to voice the same concerns that you just mentioned. Medicine is no longer fun or rewarding. They are too busy covering their backsides from potential law suits or dealing with getting paid for their services from insurance companies or Medicare. But please, can we deal with what you were just saying about ultrasounds?"

PROFIT MARGINS

"Of course, David. An obstetrician office makes money from office visits, procedures, and the actual birthing process. With today's rising rates of malpractice insurance, a medical practice needs all the money they can generate. An easy way to do this is to do ultrasounds and do a lot of them. If you are charging let's say $300 a test and if the average patient has three to four of them, then you have added $900 to $1,200 in revenue for each pregnant patient. Take an office of four doctors, and you have just produced enough revenue to take care of their office rent and most of their nursing staff for the year." The doctor paused for a moment. "The mother gets a cute sonogram photo, but God only knows how these ultrasounds may impact the babies' mental and emotional development. I've reviewed work done at several universities like the University of Dublin for one, and a Patrick Brennan and his team of researchers noticed that ultrasound can increase the temperature within various cells and impact their normal function. Other researchers note that ultrasounds can affect the baby's brain development, since the ultrasound itself may create harm or the heating up of the surrounding fluid by the effect of the pulsed Doppler energy that is produced by the ultrasound machine. The bottom line, for me, is not to do an ultrasound unless deemed necessary."

"I see, but what about for detecting birth defects? Isn't that a valid enough reason, Doctor?"

The doctor shifted in his chair a little and looked out the window for a moment. It was still mid-day, and the bright sunshine was flowing into the room, casting windows of bright light throughout the room. "Yes, David, it will detect various abnormalities, but patients should not be exposing their unborn babies to three, four, sometimes five, ultrasounds unless those congenital birth defects run in their family. And even then I wonder about the wisdom of doing that."

"I see," said David, "but won't these tests help detect Down's syndrome and such? Early detection could allow mothers to abort the fetus. Right, Doctor?"

"Wrong," replied Dr. Tessler. "What you refer to as a fetus in reality is a developing baby, and remember what I told you about the Hippocratic Oath, 'First, do no harm.'" The doctor's voice dropped an octave as he said, "What part of that isn't clear or shouldn't be followed by doctors these days?" Before David could respond, the doctor added, "Medical doctors really need to do some real soul searching in these situations."

"I'm sorry," said David, trying not to anger the doctor who clearly had his opinion about this topic, "I didn't mean to stray into a religious area, Doctor, so forgive me."

"I'm sorry, too," replied Dr. Tessler, stern and firm of his view, but seemingly not offended. "I don't think religion is really applicable here, David. I oppose the taking of any life not on religious grounds but on moral principles. My oath does not say, 'Do no harm unless it proves convenient for someone, etc.'

"Now back to ultrasounds and vaccinations, something is clearly causing a huge spike in autism and other development disorders like attention deficit disorders, dyslexia and such, and I think we need to look at everything we are doing today that we did not do 30-40 years ago when we didn't have so many cases. What are we doing different today? Doesn't it make sense to look at things that way, David?"

THE ARGUMENT IS

"Of course, but, Doctor, could it be that we are just more accurately diagnosing these cases now, where in the past we were overlooking them?"

"Sorry, David, that argument has been thrown out there, but if you ask any doctor who has been around for a while, or older parents, none of them are buying that story. I mean all you have to do is say something like that and make others spend their energies disproving it. A huge waste of time and energy for that argument. Look at school records, social service records, medical records, and that argument is just a false road that many people demand that you walk down as you try and explain the huge increase in autism today. The numbers of our children affected these days are off the charts."

David replied, "OK, it seems easy enough to test this theory, right? So what are the results?"

"Good question. I know of no major studies being done here in the U.S. on ultrasounds, but as you know, some vaccine studies have been done. However, there is a major problem. Most vaccine program studies have had drug company ties to begin with, and many people state that they have tested the vaccine theory and its relationship to autism, but in reality there haven't been viable studies for a host of reasons. Often, the researchers looking into this have their own agendas or biased view to begin with. Also, many times vaccinated patients get side effects that go unreported. I have seen children develop seizures after having the older DTP vaccine, and those cases were seldom ever reported to any organization as a side effect. So in practice, many side effects are not even being reported, especially those like high fevers, children being lethargic for days, or pain at the injection site."

JADED RESULTS

The doctor continued, "Now, back to those studies. I would not call such studies done by drug companies who sell such vaccines, or by federal panels who initiated such broad vaccine programs to begin with, unbiased, would you? I've seen doctors' and researchers' reputations harmed for even questioning such studies. If you get in their way, they will discredit you sooner or later. I am not convinced that it is the MMR vaccine causing increases in autism but perhaps it is the total amount of all vaccines given in such a tight time period that may be producing symptoms.

"I want to see a third party study done that examines children whose parents have opted out of all vaccines and compared that to children who are getting all their shots. How hard could that be? But they state that would be unethical, as the unvaccinated children would be doomed to suffer diseases that can be easily prevented. So if the children and their parents have opted out, how can that be a problem, really, and for whom? Do the study that way, and we might find some true answers, if it is in fact, done the right way. I will sum it up this way, who are these people that say we must inject these products into our babies at such a young age. I see vaccines being used in countries in South America, and they give far fewer shots. They also appear to have much lower rates of autism."

CHURCH OF VACCINATIONS

The doctor paused. "Too many medical professionals want everyday people to abdicate their total responsibility for their own health care over to them. Really? At times I feel like I am fighting the church of vaccinations. Don't dare question them or their methods. So enough about that topic, David; the bottom line is don't overdue anything medical unless you really have strong justification."

THE DOSE

"Doctor, have you taken any shots yourself? I mean vaccines."

"Of course, David, I have taken a tetanus shot after stepping on a nail, I've used yellow fever vaccine before traveling to the mountains of Peru, since yellow fever was so prevalent there at the time I traveled, and I don't think anyone should suffer a health crisis from Hepatitis A, which is so common in India and South East Asia. I would, however, be very leery of any vaccine containing mercury. You have to find out what's in your vaccine before letting them inject it into your body. Many contain aluminum and formaldehyde as well."

"But, Doctor, haven't they been taking mercury containing preservatives like thimerosal out of our vaccines?"

"David, like I was saying, the dose makes the poison. They are starting to take thimerosal out of some vaccines, which is great, but it still is being used in almost every flu shot I know of. Also, it is still sitting on the shelves of many doctors' offices, hospitals and health clinics. I have to tell you, if we had a food product that was hurting our children, we would recall it and destroy all of it. Not so with these vaccines that still contain mercury preservatives. We hold on to them. That is truly the definition of being crazy. We allow these dangerous preservatives and current stocks of it to be held on to and used up by the medical community that is still warehousing it, and just tell the medical community not to order any more of that stuff in the future. And if that is not crazy enough for you, our children are getting more and more shots today. If you follow the recommended amount of vaccines, including the annual flu shots, you are looking at over 70 shots. Amazing. This makes no sense in anybody's book except those that are producing the vaccines."

KEY POINTS

- Mercury is still used in the medical field. It is unsafe in any amount.

- Avoid unnecessary medical tests.

- Keep always in mind that you are in charge of your own health. Delegate tasks but never abdicate total authority to medical staff. Yes, you may have to place yourself in their hands for life-saving procedures. However, make sure you are making an informed decision and not reacting to needless pressure. It's not easy to speak out and politely demand that everything be explained to you in simple English, but the reward can be less medical procedures and less risk from those procedures.

5
Polio Scare

"So," said David, "you do use vaccines and are not against all of them. You are just suggesting that they be used in moderation. I am sorry, Doctor, I could not really judge where you were coming from. So then, let me ask you. What is one vaccine you would never take yourself?"

"Well, it's too late, but if I could do things differently, I would never have taken the initial polio vaccine that was peddled to Americans back in the early Sixties."

"Why is that, Doctor?"

"David, let me state that the polio vaccine was rushed to market. You can imagine their excitement when they finally had a vaccine. The best we can figure, the vaccine was contaminated with a herpes-type virus found in monkeys. This is called monkey B virus. We are close relatives, so naturally the virus would impact us. They found another monkey virus strain SV40, and let's just say it could be implemented in a host of current medical conditions such as autoimmune disorders and even cancers that are facing so many Americans today."

David's voice expressed surprise when he responded, "Doctor, are you saying that anyone who took the polio vaccine may be contaminated by monkey viruses?"

The doctor replied, "I expect so. I mean the sterilization methods used then and the process of using monkeys to produce the vaccine all point in that direction. In fact, David, let me give you a few books to take with you. I know I have them over here."

David waited as the doctor got up and made his way to an adjoining room. The doctor walked over to a huge bookcase with hundreds of books all lined up in what appeared to be alphabetic order. Grabbing several books, he made his way back to David.

"Here, David, two books I want you to review. One is an easy-to-read book titled *The Vaccine Book*, by medical doctor Robert Sears. In that book, he does a fine job of discussing what is in most of our current vaccines and the odds of contracting some of the more common ailments. He puts things in perspective, I believe, on what vaccines might be considered needed. The only negative is he doesn't address the real degree of danger that thimerosal represents to our helpless children. If a child gets too many shots, they most likely will have too much exposure to the mercury preservatives used and other toxins like aluminum. There is a wise saying in the drug and medical industry, 'The dose is the poison.' Too much thimerosal is in too many vaccines. It exceeds the Environmental Protection Agency's limit in far too many cases for mercury exposure.

"The other book is more controversial. It is by a Dr. Cass Ingram. Many folks listen to his radio show. He published this book called *The Cause for Cancer Revealed*, and in his book he links several cancers directly to the polio vaccine. His book led me to do my own research, and I was shocked to find out that scientists have known for years that the SV40 virus was showing up in many lung and brain tumors. In fact, during a medical talk, I think in the middle of the 1950s, a Bernice Eddy spoke on such matters. She and Sarah Stewart had done solid research that no one disputed at the time. I recall Eddy giving a talk in New York City on this connection. She went public with her findings and was quickly silenced. So like many doctors of the day, I thought about it a little before losing myself in work."

David said, "That was over 50 years ago. You mean they knew then the vaccine was faulty?"

"Yes, not only were humans contracting this monkey virus by vaccination, but since these types of viruses take on their own lifecycle and are almost impossible to eradicate from the human body, those infected people can possibly end up passing on the virus to their children. I think more people need to look at and really read these two books before forming their opinions on vaccines. It's strange to me, David, how people don't want to believe that viruses can cause cancer when one of the most common cancers dogs get are passed as a virus. In fact, I find it a little humorous, that since they came up with a partial vaccine for a few papilloma virus strains for cervical cancer, they are now letting us know that this type of cancer has been spreading as a virus for years. Leave it to them to educate the public once they have a product for them. Anyways, keep the books, David, as I have several copies."

David grabbed the books and placed them to his side; he had already filled up a small notepad with notes and was working on his second pad, "Thanks, Doctor, but just be aware, I will do my own research on these items as I am a confirmed information junkie by nature and it also happens to be in my job description." He smiled at Dr. Tessler, letting the doctor know that he was not a pushover for anyone's point of view. "Good, OK, Doc, so where were we, I mean on the first step to health?"

"Yes, we seem to have gotten off track a little, but not really, as we first have to practice prevention. So, David, the first step is the same as my medical oath, 'First, do not harm.' Of course, David, that is a tenet of medicine and actually a first step on the path to successful aging. It is the prevention theory of health and starts with, 'First, do no harm.'"

David made his notation, "So, that is your first step to health then, Doctor?"

"Absolutely. I will explain a little bit about preventative medicine in context with recent history."

KEY POINTS

• Many older adults were exposed to polio vaccines containing active monkey viruses as both the dead polio type vaccine and live type vaccine were grown within monkeys' kidneys. These viruses, including SV40, have been found in many cancerous tumors and could also be the cause for several severe medical disorders. These contaminated vaccines occurred during the years 1955 through 1963. Even today, polio vaccine manufacturers still use monkey kidneys to culture polio vaccines, but they do inactivate potential viruses by using powerful agents to kill them. Hopefully, that is enough. Thousands of monkeys have been killed in the manufacturing of the polio virus and millions of humans have been exposed to viruses that previously only were found in monkeys. You have to question the science and the justification of all of this.

• Generally, you are best to avoid new vaccines until you have had the time to analyze the risk and return of such vaccines. Also, wait until researches have had time to see what the real long-term effects of any vaccine are going to be. Don't always assume your doctor knows best, as your doctor may have been misled by misinformation, conflicting studies, drug companies and sales people.

6
Great Mysteries Solved

"David, let me fill you in on some things that occurred in the 1900s. First, a brief historical reference. For thousands of years, corn has successfully been used as a staple grain by many cultures. These ancient cultures learned corn had two unique traits. First, by itself, corn is an incomplete protein. However, these ancient cultures figured out that when you combine beans with corn it gives a perfect protein at meal time. The second major point about corn is that it must be prepared a certain way to unlock its true nutrient power.

"Failure to follow proper corn storage and preparation can lead to a life-threatening disease that tragically and needlessly killed thousands and thousands of Europeans and Americans."

"Really, Doc? Fill me in."

"Native tribes knew two major things about corn. First, don't let it sit in dampness where it can collect mildew, and secondly, the really important thing, corn must be processed correctly."

"How so?"

"Native societies in the Americas, including in South America, Central America and North America, knew that they must prepare corn a certain way. We call that way, or method, nixtamalization."

"Nixta-what?"

"Nixtamalization, a word derived by Native Americans that lived in Mexico. They discovered that corn was much more nutritious and easier to work with if they soaked the corn in an alkaline solution. They used lime, usually from heated limestone or seashells. Native Americans in North America also used potash. They allowed the corn to soak in this alkaline solution. This made it much easier to grind the corn, and gave it a much fuller flavor. It also unlocked the corn's enzyme potential. Now, this processing method also allowed the niacin contained within to become much more available. It also helped deactivate the fungus contamination that periodically occurred."

"OK, Doc, why was this so important?"

"Well, when I tell you of one of medicine's greatest detective stories, you will understand."

"I'm ready."

PELLAGRA

"You've heard of the disease pellagra?"

"Of course. It was a major disease throughout the southern part of the U.S. for many years. Thousands died from it."

"Right you are, David. Now that pellagra is behind us, people have forgotten how bad it really was. It not only caused thousands of deaths in the U.S. but caused thousands of deaths in Europe as well. All because modern people dismissed the ways of Native Americans."

"How so?"

"They assumed they knew better. Native Americans used their preparation methods of soaking their corn grain in an alkaline solution. It freed up the niacin, or as many call it, vitamin B-3. When Europeans and Americans sent their corn to modern grain mills, the corn was simply ground up into corn meal, missing a vital step. That step being nixtamalization."

"It made that big of a difference?"

"David, recall that I mentioned that Indians soaked grains to unleash their enzyme potential?"

"Right."

"Well, it also can activate the vitamin potential and increase the availability of minerals and amino acids. Ironically, with so many people relying on corn for a major part of their diet, a normally life-promoting and nutritious grain was turned into a horrible, health-destroying grain because it was not processed correctly. Soaking also increased the availability of its small amount of tryptophan, an essential amino acid."

"Go on."

"Pellagra is a disorder that has everything to do with an overreliance on an improperly processed corn product."

"So what did pellagra do to people?"

"David, it produces a host of symptoms. Many of those symptoms would mimic other diseases as well. But once pellagra took hold of a person, it was a horrible thing to see unfold."

"Like?"

"The skin would become very sensitized to the sun. Common parts of the skin that got a lot of sun exposure like necks, faces, and hands, would develop a horrible red rash. The scaly skin often forms a band around the neck. This intensifies with sun exposure. This would have increased the redness many Southerners already had from working outdoors, leading possibly to them first being called rednecks! Their overreliance on improperly refined corn in their diet gave them pellagra. Not only did they develop horrible rashes, but many developed diarrhea, dementia, and far too often, death."

"Really? That is horrible. How long was this disease around?"

"At least two hundred years, if not longer, David. But I do recall reading that pellagra epidemics were reported in Spain, Italy, Russia and South Africa. Some of those occurred in the 1700s."

"But, Doctor, you think they would have figured it out sooner."

"Not really, I mean, look at some of the things we do today."

"Such as?"

"We hydrogenate our oils causing them to be health destroying, we strip nutrients out of many processed foods before consuming them, and we add junk forms ot minerals to our cereals. We even poison our water with chlorine and drink it without a second thought."

"But, Doc, it seems so obvious what their problem was, doesn't it?"

"No, David, it doesn't. For years, doctors could not pin down what was causing pellagra. Most assumed it was a communicable disease like smallpox. After all, it seemed to come and go with some people while intensifying in others, leading to death. Medical people saw whole families affected as well as entire communities. Deemed a communicable disease, people suffering from it were often ostracized. Their homes were quarantined. Well meaning neighbors would often drop off food. You guessed it, cornbread, grits, and corn cakes."

"So what was the fatality rate?"

"The fatality rate for pellagra sufferers could reach 40%, David. And this disease did not care if you were a woman, man, or child. It especially impacted poor black families in the deep south who were on restricted diets, not by choice, but because of their work and life situation. Mill towns and cotton workers were more prone to pellagra because of a lack of diversified diet."

"How sad, Doctor. How did this madness end?"

AN INDEPENDENT THINKER

"An independent thinker named Dr. Joseph Goldberger correctly figured out that pellagra was caused by diet, in this case the overconsumption of corn meal. This hundreds-of-years affliction that had troubled so many for so long had finally been figured out. Too late, of course, for thousands of people who suffered needlessly and died. Dr. Goldberger found yeast extract supplements to be largely preventative for pellagra. Obviously, something in yeast was having a huge impact. That something was niacin. In 1937, a chemist by the name of Conrad A. Elvehjem used nicotinic acid to cure pellagra in dogs, confirming the value of niacin."

"So, Doctor, I guess no one should rely on one grain too much."

"Right, especially when processed incorrectly."

"So improper processing of grains. Doc, it seems obvious looking backwards."

"Sure does, David, but corn wasn't the only problem."

"Really?"

"How about rice, David?"

"Really? How's that?"

"Another disease, David, which also caused misery and death."

"Its name?"

BERIBERI

"David, let me give you a little perspective, actually from recent history, 1896 was not that long ago. During that time tens of thousands of people were dying in China, India, Japan, and Indonesia, many of them just infants. They were dying from a slow debilitating and painful disease named beriberi. At times, one third of the Japanese navy suffered from this debilitating and deadly disease. Imagine having a large segment of your population immobilized with this affliction. They were incapable of moving without severe pain and left with numbness and exhaustion. They most often lost the use of their legs, suffered pain in their limbs, swelling of their legs, stomach pains, confusion, destruction of their heart muscle, and for too many, death.

"Observing this disease and its horrendous impact on so many people, Christiaan Eijkman, after much research and observation, made a profound statement, 'White rice can be poisonous.'"

"How's that, Doctor?" said David, "I heard white rice in excess can cause higher blood sugar but never that it could be poisonous?"

"Let me explain more, David, and what led Eijkman to this startling conclusion. Stationed at a Dutch research institute on the large island of Java, located in what then was called the Dutch East Indies, he observed a huge wave of beriberi cases impacting the local population. Death from this affliction and other diseases were all around him.

"Eijkman knew this disorder plagued Asia for hundreds of years. What he did not know initially was the incidence of beriberi was increasing dramatically due to a modern convenience intended to simplify and improve our lives, which was modern milling techniques. That's right modern methods of de-husking normal rice and creating a whiter, polished product was the root cause of thousands and thousands of painful deaths. Interestingly, beriberi not only affected humans but animals as well."

David responded, "So, Doc, it wasn't a germ or virus spreading malady but another nutrient disaster?"

"I am afraid so, David. Let's follow the research on this a little. Eijkman, at first, was convinced the culprit was a bacterium since that was the current thinking going around. The concept of germ theory, illustrated by scientists Louis Pasteur and Robert Koch around the 1850s, was just recently discovered to be the culprits behind countless diseases. Eijkman was sure he was on the right track. Remarkably, an experiment he was doing with chickens at the institute led him to the real culprit.

"In an experiment to test his germ theory, Eijkman had kept chickens near the institute and had exposed them to what he thought were germs causing beriberi. He obtained these samples from diseased tissue of deceased animals that had died recently from beriberi. Interestingly, all his test chicken subjects developed beriberi. However, unlike most victims, his test chickens suddenly got better. This astounded Eijkman because he had not provided any medical treatment to them."

"What was it then, Doctor?"

"Luckily for humanity, David, Eijkman had held a conversation with the worker whose job it was to feed the chickens daily. The worker informed him that he had started feeding unpolished, uncooked rice to the chickens instead saving the more sought after polished, white rice for another purpose, as it was deemed much more valuable. This information gave Eijkman insight and, through a series of experiments, he was able to introduce beriberi in his test subjects at will. Give them a predominate diet of polished, white rice and the animals developed beriberi. Change their diet to the more wholesome unpolished rice and the disease reversed itself. At first, Eijkman assumed there must be some poison or toxin created by processing the normal rice into polished rice."

"Incredible, Doctor, all that death due to food?"

"Yes, David, and think about it, that was just one food causing so much death. With years of research and with so many doctors studying beriberi, you would have thought that they would have figured it out much earlier, but the disease was so common and seemed to affect areas just as a virus or bacteria would.

Many scientists had conducted elaborate experiments and thought they had ruled out any possibility of a deficiency causing such destruction. They saw so many people eating rice with their food that they were convinced it could not simply be the rice, but what they failed to see was many people relied on too much white rice to make up their protein needs and they relied on the rice processed in the wrong way. Using brown rice or parboiled rice did not induce beriberi, only the polished white rice did, and not in everybody as each person may have been consuming a slightly different diet. In areas where processed rice was not available there was no beriberi disease."

"But, Doctor," said David, "It seems so obvious."

"Perhaps with our perspective, but try and place yourself in the past. There were simply too many diseases to deal with; you had cholera, malaria, and typhoid, to name a few. Each disease caused by something different. However, Eijkman also may have heard that the Japanese navy had reduced incidence of beriberi dramatically by forcing their sailors to consume more meat and vegetables with their primary rations of white rice. It was reported that the Japanese military consumed massive amounts of white polished rice with low incidence of beriberi but only after forcing their soldiers to focus more on increasing their intake of other food groups. They had figured out that white rice must be combined with other food groups such as meat or vegetables in the right portion. What they did not articulate was why it worked. They had observed that as long as this was done one could continue to consume white rice with a low incidence of ill effects. What the Japanese had figured out is variety of foods really does matter. Eijkman now labeled the problem. Something was lacking in white polished rice that wasn't missing in unprocessed rice, some vital nutrient that our bodies require. That something was vitamin B-1, also known as thiamine."

"Yes, I am familiar with that vitamin. It is added to our white rice now, isn't it?"

"Yes, David, Thankfully"

The doctor added, "While Eijkman did not identify the exact vitamin missing within polished white rice, he was the first Westerner to indentify the lack of some vital nutrient, thereby earning him a Nobel Prize. A major observation here: just because millions of people consume a food product, thereby giving it the appearance of something healthy and nutritious, does not make it so. Having a varied diet is crucial in providing the body with the tools it needs to maintain, repair, and nurture itself. The lack of just one nutrient can have a devastating result."

"You know, it makes you wonder what we might be missing in our diets."

"Great point, David. I feel you are on the right track. Perhaps it is iodine, boron, lithium or some other trace mineral."

"So, Doc, you gave me a few examples of vitamin B deficiencies that afflicted people in the good old days. Do you have any more?"

"Well, David, I do. I know you have heard the term 'miracle cure.' I am going to explain an instance where that really was true."

A MIRACLE CURE

"But, David, as bad as pellagra was, a lack of another B vitamin had killed even more people throughout history. Worse than a lack of vitamin B-3 or niacin is a lack of vitamin B-12 or your body's inability to utilize it correctly, causing much sickness and death over the past centuries. The disorder is called pernicious anemia. In fact, the very word pernicious means lethal. Years ago, being diagnosed with pernicious anemia was equivalent to a death sentence. It was more prevalent in people as they entered their 50s and 60s. Saying that, however, any person, at any age, could develop this pernicious anemia. I recall one American celebrity passing away from this many years ago; she was Annie Oakley, who died in 1926 at age 66, ironically the same year the first successful 'liver treatment' for her condition was made public."

"Was pernicious anemia common?"

"It was fairly common. I remember people dying from this condition. If you look at death certificates from the 1800s and 1900s, you will see it listed too often."

"What causes it?"

"The body's lack of vitamin B-12 or an inability of the body to process B-12. It was found that many people could not absorb the vitamin B-12 from their diet as they aged due to their intestinal tract having an autoimmune reaction, or from them having weak stomach acid, ulcers, or other factors. The body can store vitamin B-12 for a long time, however, you still need to find food sources or supplement. I advise older people to use a weekly B-12 supplement that you place in your mouth, where it dissolves, getting absorbed directly into your system and avoiding your digestive tract, or better yet, get vitamin B-12 shots periodically if your B-12 levels are too low."

"How long did it take to kill people, Doctor?"

"David, usually death occurred within about three years."

"Ouch, I am glad you don't hear of people dying from this today."

"Really, David, you are so correct, at least in our country. In poor countries, I am sure people are still dying from this condition. Before I forget, let me tell you about the liver treatment. Years ago, several researchers shared a Nobel Prize for their insight of how a diet high in liver could prevent death in most cases, if caught early enough."

"So, I get it, just eat liver every day to keep the anemia at bay. I could handle that, I love liver and onions."

"Sorry, David." He smiled. "The diet required raw liver."

"OK, Doc, that is a different story."

"In 1934, Dr. Murphy showed a movie on the effects of a liver diet on patients. They literally got better in front of your eyes within a few weeks of treatments. In fact, Murphy, Minot and Whipple were all awarded the Nobel Prize in medicine. The first time I ever heard of this prize being shared. Solving B-12 deficiency was a great detective story. William Castle, doing work at Harvard, found that people who had their stomachs removed would eventually die of vitamin B-12 deficiency. He figured out correctly that something in the stomach provided an intrinsic factor, allowing the vitamin B-12 to be absorbed properly. In 1928, Edwin Cohn, a chemist, created a condensed liver extract that was much easier to consume. It wasn't until 1971 that a chemist by the name of Robert Woodward finally announced the synthesis of vitamin B-12."

"So lack of the intrinsic factor within our stomachs led to pernicious anemia?"

"Right, David, of course many people suffer a more subtle form or lack of vitamin B-12 that can be a different form of anemia. But still, a major concern, as it may cause confusion, depression, fatigue and nerve damage. This can be caused by a lack of stomach acid, intestinal problems, etc. Keep in mind that liver is high in B-12 and iron. So it proved effective in treating two major types of anemia: pernicious anemia and iron-poor blood anemia. People that had to use the liver diet back in the late 1920s, which all things considered, was a real godsend, especially considering the alternative."

"Any more on that story?"

"Yes, David, many vitamins were synthesized in the 1900s, like vitamins D, C, E, and K. In addition to this we had a revolution in vaccines and antibiotics. Diphtheria, a major killer of children, was dealt with first by an antitoxin, then later prevented by vaccine, and later yet treated with antibiotics if contracted."

HOW DOES THIS RELATE?

"So how does all this relate to theories of aging, Doctor?"

"David, I am showing you that we are moving quickly to the future with these miracle cures. Some were discoveries that we were not consuming a proper diet or the proper nutrients, causing such disorders as pellagra and beriberi – discoveries that various forms of anemia were caused by a lack of various B vitamins or finding out that pernicious anemia was being caused by something our body failed to do properly. A goldmine of discoveries were made and are still being made. Understanding nutrient issues, utilization issues, and how our bodies really function will unlock many new mysteries and add countless years to our lives. Solving nutritional deficits, no matter how small, may be the key to longevity. These discoveries and research are going on as we speak. Also, diseases that seem incurable now may have cures waiting for them just around the corner."

"So Doc, you are saying that perhaps several maladies or illnesses nowadays may really be nutrient disorders or shortages that we just haven't realized yet? And that we are on the fast track to increasing longevity as soon as we figure more of this stuff out? I mean, based on the relatively recent discoveries you just told me about, this could really be the situation. I have heard some scientists believe that excess dairy consumption could be the reason we have so much breast cancer and prostate cancer in our country today. If that turns out to be true, then that would be a huge advance in our knowledge and an even deeper acknowledgement of our current ignorance."

THE GOLDEN AGE

"Right, David, so many advances have been made. Looking back with a historical perspective, it is breathtaking. So many people saved. Of course, at the same time these discoveries were happening we had the successful public health movements that started in the 1800s and continued throughout the 1900s, helping to keep so many disease outbreaks at bay and mitigating damage to those afflictions that did break out. Public health programs were developed in Germany in the 1840s to deal with outbreaks of typhoid and typhus and later cholera. These public health programs spread to England and the U.S. They found poverty and crowded conditions produced large epidemics."

"So, Doc, the 1900s saw the understanding and cure for vitamin B deficiencies like pellagra, beriberi, and pernicious anemia. It makes me wonder what other nutrient-driven diseases that we might not be aware of."

"Great point, David. As you know, vitamin C was found to cure scurvy, which had killed hundreds of thousands, vitamin D deficiency caused rickets, and a lack of vitamin A causes a lot of blindness. So what else might we be ignorant of?"

"Doctor, with so many advances in medicine such as vaccines, antibiotics, the public health movement, quarantines and sanitariums, I can see why modern medicine looks so appealing."

"Right, all these advances certainly gave modern doctors the edge in healing. It explains why the gentler herbal healers were pushed aside."

"Can we discuss some more of the common deadly afflictions that came to pass?"

THE KILLERS

"Hmm, remember we had discussed syphilis at the beginning of our meeting and how many that killed over the centuries?"

"Right, Doctor, you referred to that as the 'The Great Pox.'"

"Right. So we had that pox plus the really big killer smallpox that was dealt with in the 1900s. During my years, I have seen bacterial pneumonia go from a huge killer to a much lesser role. Before bacterial pneumonia caused a great deal of misery and death, a huge amount of hospitals' resources were used to treat pneumonia, often without success. So antibiotics gave us a huge victory in this area. I lived this era and saw too many good people die this way. But, David, I did see an illness that took its toll on families to an even larger degree. This illness impacted some of my family members and strained us to the point of breaking. It may be responsible for over a billion deaths. Would you care to guess what that was, David?"

NATURE'S GREAT KILLER

"OK, Doc, let me guess. A number one killer for years was tuberculosis."

"Right you are, David."

"I'm curious, why did they call tuberculosis 'consumption?'"

"So many people who had TB not only coughed constantly and spit up blood, but they also lost lots of weight. It looks as if their affliction was consuming them. Hence, the term consumption."

"So, Doc, how common was it?"

"Was, David?"

"Well, yes, Doctor, was?"

"Let me say this, David. I know you are aware TB is still around, infecting millions and millions of people, and we will discuss that dilemma soon enough. However, in the U.S. in years past most people were exposed to TB but did not show any symptoms, but saying that, it was extremely common."

"So, how many of those would end up dying from it?"

"Hard to say. If a patient had active tuberculosis, they had about a 60% chance of dying from it. In the 1800s, probably 25% of all deaths were the result of TB. During the early 1900s, that may have reduced some, slowly disappearing as a major cause of death as the 1900s progressed. However, saying that, millions upon millions of people have died from TB. In many parts of the world, like India and Africa, they still do. I would estimate tuberculosis kills more people per year than malaria. So it's easily over a million deaths each year."

"Really? I mean I have to tell you, most young Americans don't know this. They only know what they see on television. Like Doc Holliday having TB in the movie *Tombstone*."

"I know, David, but so many have had TB and so many have suffered from it, including U.S. presidents Andrew Jackson and James Monroe, Henry David Thoreau, Vivien Leigh, and Eleanor Roosevelt."

"So what slowed it down here in the U.S.? Antibiotics?"

"Great question, David. Antibiotics are a great tool against TB, but rates started dropping a little even before they appeared on the scene."

"So what was causing the drop, Doc?"

"A combination of reasons. First and foremost was public health practices."

"Such as?"

"Well, identifying how TB was being transmitted helped a lot and isolating active TB patients was crucial."

"Are you talking about sanitariums?"

"Yes, so many people had TB that quarantining by itself would have been too harsh. So active TB patients were strongly directed towards group-style institutions run by medical personnel, the sanitariums."

"So the sick people that were constantly coughing and sneezing were sent to these sanitariums, reducing the amount of healthier people being exposed."

"Yes, David, public health got involved and insisted spittoons be placed in taverns so people would quit spitting on the floor. And, yes, David, having less people coughing, sneezing and spitting up blood did help the TB from spreading."

"Sounds like a series of steps were happening to reduce TB spread."

"Yes, they were, David. Some small steps and some larger ones. Public health staff was crucial. A TB vaccine was developed in France around 1921 and used around the world. While not totally effective, it set the stage for a huge reduction in TB cases in the years to come. It's interesting to note that very few people vaccinate against TB in the United States. So vaccines are not always the answer."

"Tell me more."

"Just one small example. Health departments made the connection that many cows also had TB infections. It was a very similar strain and could infect humans. So health officials demanded their milk be heat-treated to kill the bacteria."

"We're talking about pasteurization, right?"

"Correct, and pasteurization killed the bovine form of TB along with other public health threats like listeria, cholera, and others. This saved thousands of children and helped dramatically to lower our infant mortality rates."

"So, Doctor, pasteurization is a good thing?"

"Yes, for stopping the spread of bovine TB, but no, from the standpoint that once milk has been heat-treated, it loses a lot of its nutrient power. However, with the sad state of dairy cows in the U.S., I would pasteurize. After all, pasteurization kills all bacteria at the source, which helped cut off an avenue of exposure to one of mankind's greatest killers."

"This made milk safer?"

"Much safer, David, but let me add that I'm not a believer in drinking another animal's milk in the first place."

"Understood, Doctor, now you were saying that TB was a major killer in the U.S. up until the 1950s and still is around the world. But you still sound very concerned."

CONCERNED

"Good observation, because unless the world gets its act together soon, we may see TB resume its ugly role as one of mankind's greatest killers."

"Really, Doc? I'm listening."

"First off, unless we get TB under control, it has the potential of raging back throughout the world. TB is quickly becoming resistant to antibiotics in many cases, which could leave us with a drug-resistant strain of TB taking the place of the current TB. So TB once again may rise as a major killer."

"Ouch. So the world should treat TB like smallpox and try to eliminate it from the planet?"

"Absolutely, David. We need to do it now, before it gets ahead of us. Saying that, David, I wanted to add that the BCG vaccine against TB was first used in 1921. It took years to be accepted around the world, as the makers of the vaccine had some missteps, which caused the loss of life, especially in infants. Nowadays, the vaccine is considered extremely safe, with infants being inoculated in several large countries like Brazil, Korea, India and Pakistan. The vaccine is not perfect, and in my view governments need to be working on better vaccines. Here in the U.S. we don't routinely give TB vaccines but instead rely on testing patients to see if they may have it."

"Doc, I've made some notes here, let me just ask a few questions regarding animals and TB."

"Go ahead."

"You are saying that cows may have been the cause of TB starting amongst humans."

"I don't know. I do know researchers have found the TB germs in buffalo, cows, and other animals. Perhaps humans domesticating cows allowed us to have more direct exposure."

"Any other observations, Doc?"

"Several, David. Here in Virginia, TB was really epidemic. Virginia had many sanitariums to keep TB patients in and I can't help but notice all the dairy cows throughout the Shenandoah Valley. Before the age of pasteurization, I would think this helped fuel Virginia's epidemic of TB. I want to put this in perspective, David, I've lived with this on a daily basis. I had several relatives that went to sanitariums and never recovered. For far too many, sanitariums became waiting rooms for death. So when people tell you that the 1800s and 1900s were the good old days, don't believe them! Of course, with the advent of antibiotics, many patients were then being treated at their local doctor's office or clinic. This was the wonder of streptomycin. Injections of this antibiotic saved countless people."

"So when did this drug come out?"

"The late 40s, David, but really they didn't widely use it until the 50s. Thank God for the research done at Rutgers University by Albert Schatz in 1943. Streptomycin was just the start, other antibiotics soon were developed, which helped countless patients. But, David, as I started telling you, the 1900s were the golden era for modern medicine. The medical community saw more changes and more cures than the previous entire history of medicine. This allowed for many common diseases and illnesses to fade from memory."

"So how does all this information pertain to longevity now?"

"Good question. We must not forget history. We, as a society, have lowered our collective guard."

LOWERED OUR GUARD

"How so?"

"Several ways, David. We have forgotten the importance of keeping strong local health departments in place that have the authority and power to nip epidemics in the bud. Our current health departments are pushing too many vaccines like hepatitis B when really we need to be working on major killers like TB. Also, these health departments accept subpar vaccines, which may damage our children. With their resources and power they could insist on cleaner and better vaccines. We have lowered our guard and become complacent. We are not taking seriously enough the many antibiotic resistant strains of bacteria that are showing up in our hospitals and, worse, we are leaving the door wide open for one of mankind's biggest killers, TB, to come back into our lives in a big way."

"So stay aware, huh, Doc?"

"Absolutely, David. Until hospitals clean up their act, be on your guard for contracting antibiotic resistant germs from them. And the whole world needs to double down on its efforts to stop TB. So far we are not doing either."

LOOKING TOWARD THE HORIZON

"Ok, Doc, It sounds like most people are not taking this stuff seriously enough. Anything else they remain ignorant on?"

"Most people remain clueless on what's been taking place in the world of anti-aging," said the doctor.

"How's that?"

"We are on the cusp of the greatest gains for adding quality years to peoples' lives since the great public health campaigns started back in the 1800s."

"What campaigns were those?"

"David, tremendous gains were added to the average human life span when local governments and health officials started reacting to the large amounts of epidemics and the huge infant mortality rates of the 1800s. It was reported in London, England, that more than half of the children born at that time into working families would die before reaching their fifth birthday. Crowded living conditions and poor sanitation led to huge outbreaks of diseases. This was also impacting wealthier families who could no longer avoid the repercussions of so much filth and diseased conditions."

"So what did society do to alleviate this situation?"

"They cleaned up their act. It started in Germany and quickly spread to England. Medical personnel and governments realized they had to clean up living conditions and take care of the sick. Otherwise, disease was just going to spread continually. In 1849, John Snow figured out that contaminated water from various wells were causing the spread of cholera. That was their eureka moment. They started implementing clean water sites, got serious about waste disposal and open garbage on the streets, and instituted a series of practical steps to limit contagions. In short, they cleaned up the cities, and people started living a lot longer."

"Did that include the dirty air of London?"

"Right, the cleaning of London's air came later when they figured out that the dirty coal air was killing the poor and the rich equally. The expression 'London Fog' is not because of normal fog forming over the city, but, in reality, it was a description of London's constant dirty air in prior years. I recall London's dirty air killing thousands of people as late as 1952. So to answer your question, David, London did clean up a lot of its dirty air but not quickly enough. Luckily, the other major steps to protect lives done through public health steps were implemented much sooner."

"So, all those steps taken led to huge increases in life expectancy. Is that what you see happening again now?"

"Absolutely, David, we are at the start of a new leap in longevity. That is why everyone should take care of themselves now, so they can take advantage of the many new and numerous anti-aging strategies, teachings, and advances that are coming our way."

"So, tell me more, Doc."

"The base to build on starts with prevention, yet that can only take you so far. Other theories of anti-aging need to be followed hand-in-glove with prevention."

"Yet, Doctor, wouldn't you say the vast majority of Americans are ignorant of what's going on?"

"Yes, you are right. The world is on the verge of one of the greatest social changes imaginable, but few are really aware of this. Tucked away in the corners of the world are researchers, scientists, and doctors who are keenly aware of the developments and discoveries that will be impacting us soon. Will these discoveries be shared with all of humanity? Only time will tell. However, for now, make sure you stay aware of what the possibilities of anti-aging medicine can mean to you and your loved ones. Lots more time to enjoy the things you like to do, more time to enjoy your family or to work on your interests. These added years will be quality years. Remember, David, God gives you just one body, one soul, and one life. Use it wisely."

They spoke for awhile longer before making arrangements to meet the next day.

KEY POINTS

- Diseases have plagued humankind throughout history. Great discoveries and research have allowed humankind to overcome many killer ailments. However, apathy and a loss of respect for some of these diseases may cause a virulent resurgence.

- Our medical community may be focusing on the wrong vaccines to be given and ignoring the real threats.

Part II

12 Theories of Aging

7
The Prevention Theory
Theory I

DAVID ARRIVED AT the doctor's home the next afternoon. He had researched most of what the doctor had discussed previously. He could not find fault with what the doctor had told him. So David knew he was getting some good information. He hoped it would continue, but he also worried that if he quoted the doctor correctly, many people, including the drug companies, medical associations, and other doctors may have a problem with his views. So he would make sure to get the complete story before putting anything in print.

Esmeralda showed David to the study once again. After they all enjoyed a small serving of fresh cut fruit and a fish spread on whole grain crackers, the conversation started up in earnest. The doctor continued, "So, David, as I said yesterday, the first step would be 'First, do no harm.'"

"Yes, I have that duly noted from our meeting yesterday. Sounds too simple, Doc."

"Can you think of a better first step?" said the doctor. "So David, first, do no harm. This means do not ingest things that have no business being in your body in the first place. No processed food, no artificial food coloring, no artificial preservatives or natural ones like sodium nitrates, or heavily salted foods, for that matter. No fake foods made by gene splicing, no pesticides, no fungicides, no coal tars, no unnecessary prescriptions, and no hydrogenated oils or fake fats. Try your best to avoid mass-produced agriculture products that were made by employing the lowest cost methods possible, such as growing genetically modified food in dead soil. Also, no fluoride in your water, no chloride in your water, no bug sprays on your lawn or in your home, etc."

David responded with a sly smile. "Jeez, Doc, I am a little confused, is that your short list or long list?" And before the doctor could respond, David added, "Doc, this list is no easy task for the average consumer to do is it?"

Now the doctor was smiling. "Right, David, I never thought of having a short list versus a long list of these items, as if you leave even one item off, it could impact your health. Since you asked, let's just call this the medium list, just in case we left off some items, which I am sure I did. And by the way, David, I disagree with your contention of not doing these things as being difficult. I mean, it really isn't hard if you think differently. If someone told you that you could not eat white bread as it would kill you instantly, then you would not eat it, ever! But because the body can handle garbage carbs so well, for awhile at least, then people continue to consume such stuff like white bread, sugar, bad oils, and such. What I feel you first must do is get it straight in your mind that certain items are off limits. Once you really treat items that way it will get much easier to deal with such stuff. For instance, in our house we do not allow any overly processed oil or trans fatty oil-slash-hydrogenated oil at all, ever. As far as I am concerned, scientists have known for years that it has been undermining our health and causing harm for decades. They didn't know how much harm, but now they link this stuff to something called inflammation."

Which, by the way, the doctor assured David may be the real reason so many Americans are dying before their time. A diet of processed foods rich in sugar, junk flour, additives, and poor food choices causes the body to inflame itself through a series of chemical and hormonal actions. But he promised David they would cover inflammation in much more detail later.

David smiled, "OK, Doctor, but I need a whole lot more convincing at this time. So tell me more on how this first step works."

THE FIRST STEP

"Right, David, keep in mind that what I tell you is just the start of an overall life-prolonging routine. This first step is the base or the foundation for what follows. I mean, if you don't stop harming your body in the first place, then most of the other steps will prove meaningless. Does that make sense, David?"

"Of course," said David grinning. "So the first step turns into the first steps."

Smiling back, the doctor responded, "OK, David, here it is. First, do no harm. Forget all the claims of advertisers and their marketing. Ignore the paid spokespeople or actors who have been pushing things on you your whole life. Review with suspicion anybody who tells you to take a certain medicine, supplement, or food product. Ditto for cleaning products. Always ask yourself first, does this really make sense? Do I really benefit? A great second question to ask yourself is will this be health-promoting or could it damage me now or down the road. Also, think about what you are about to eat or drink. Did our ancestors consume this thousands of years ago; if not, think hard before you do."

"Got it, Doctor. So first, do no harm to myself, don't believe the claims of others, watch what I eat and drink, and don't take drugs or supplements unless I really need them."

"Yes, David. That's a lot of it, but regarding the supplements, you will in fact be forced to become knowledgeable about them because they will help you with some of the other steps to achieve a maximum life, full of energy. But we will cover that in much more detail later."

THE SECOND STEP

"OK, Doctor, so what else?"

"Well you must think differently than your friends, co-workers, neighbors, and even your family. Once you understand the importance of the first step of doing no harm, then you truly have the responsibility of doing something proactive about it."

"Like how, Doctor?"

"First off, I told you to do no harm. It is amazing how many of us inflict damage to ourselves. Society makes it easy and masks the consequences, but ultimately we are the ones who do ourselves in. So after the main statement of 'do no harm,' commit to the following strategy, from this day forward: I will simply choose the right food selections over the bad ones. This is easily remembered by eating only good fats, good carbs, and good protein sources and not consuming the bad ones."

"OK," said David, "so do no harm, only eat good food and not bad food, and my health will change. Really, Doctor, those are your first two steps?"

"Yes, it is that simple, as the truth usually is. You first must do these steps so the other steps will work. It's like driving a car; you first need gas in the tank and wheels on the car to get anywhere. Miss the basics, and you are stuck in your driveway. You won't see much of the world that way. But let me share some information with you that will give some perspective of where us doctors have been and where we are coming form nutritionally speaking. We have learned so much over the years yet also we have failed to observe the obvious."

"What do you mean, Doc?"

NEWS FROM THE PAST

The doctor said, "In the 1950s an amazing study was done. JAMA, which stands for the Journal of the American Medical Association, reported on a medical study done on the autopsies of 300 soldiers killed in action while serving in Korea. Even though the average age of these deceased young men was 22, over 75% of them showed evidence of coronary heart disease. This served as a wake-up call to all Americans that something was wrong with our diet.

Yes, young men had consumed lots of milkshakes in their hometowns, eaten standard American fare like hamburgers, French fries, etc. However, to find over 75% with various stages of heart disease was stunning. Furthermore, it was reported that one in 20 of them had such severe clogging of their arteries that 90% of at least one artery was blocked with plaque deposit, a waxy substance made from cholesterol.

"The scary point is that hardening of the arteries and heart disease cause most heart attacks. Of those folks suffering a heart attack, only two out of three will live to tell about it. So for many of us, it will be too late to change our ways or change our diets. Also, this tells me that if you want a longer life, assume you have some degree of heart disease and start doing something proactive about it. Young men dying of heart attacks are not so uncommon in our country anymore. Middle aged folks dying of heart attacks are so common that we no longer are surprised to hear of a neighbor or friend dying from one."

"That's right," David said, "I mean I have seen several people close to me die this way. I guess that is why everybody is trying to lower their cholesterol levels, right?"

"Yes, David, but let me give you a more detailed history where us older doctors are coming from, as we lived those times and recall clearly how many people have died before their time. I mean heart disease is a great robber of life for many and a great burden to so many people's vitality. "

THE STUDY

David nodded in understanding.

The doctor continued, "Slowly a picture was developing on heart disease and how common it truly was. Fortunately, a study that began years ago in 1948, in Framingham, Massachusetts, had started but needed years to track its results. This study tracked a large group of over 5,000 people and reviewed many of their lifestyle factors. They measured various things like blood pressure readings, exercise levels, weight readings, habits like smoking and drinking, etc. These measurements soon were seen as risk factors and or as biomarkers.

The things that seem to increase heart disease were seen as risk factors. The measurements of body's chemistry, cholesterol, sugar levels, blood pressure readings, etc, were classified as biomarkers or measurements of the body status. So biomarkers are items that can be measured that will indicate the probability of disease or health status in the future. These risk factors and biomarkers could indicate to a great accuracy who would suffer heart disease or a heart attack.

"This was so important because, up to then, we thought heart disease came with age and was normal. Doctors just assumed it was the heart and blood vessels wearing out. This study was monumental since it illustrated that there are known risk factors for heart disease and that heart disease was influenced by these risk factors. This study clearly showed the chances of having heart disease increased if you had more risk factors. It also may be the first real study to show a correlation between a persons cholesterol levels and their probability of heart disease. This study eventually identified that certain types of cholesterol could be good for you like, high density lipoproteins referred to as HDL versus the bad stuff called low density lipoprotein, or LDL."

"So Doctor, I understand what you are saying and where we are coming from as a country. You are saying that this is study brought some of the medical terms we use today into common language and conversations. Also, I think you are trying to show me where some of the common things we talk about in preventative medicine come from, right?"

"Right, this study gave the average American something they could follow in the pursuit of making their health better. But most Americans remain ignorant of several of the study's findings."

"Such as?"

"Well, they failed to see that there are a host of biomarkers that they can use to monitor their current state of health. Using these biomarkers, you can measure whether you are moving toward a state of disease or toward a state of health. A big difference, if you ask me, and one worth knowing. Sometimes if we do enough things right, we can avoid many of the diseases and disorders that we find so common here in this country. And like the Framingham study showed us, a lot of ill health is cause and effect, not just a mile marker as we grow older. There is a direct link between our diet/lifestyle and our health."

"What else, Doctor?"

"A major point of the study was the link between cholesterol and heart health. What most Americans still fail to recognize is that the consumption of all the animal products, which include dairy as well, have been injurious to our heart's health. Furthermore, the high consumption of animal products in the group of people studied leads to high blood pressure, which leads to strokes. So while the evidence is staring most Americans in the face, they do not see what is so plain to see."

David responded, "Don't eat meat and don't eat dairy, is that what the study is showing us Doctor?"

"Almost," said the doctor, "In essence, if you are living in America with American food choices, you should limit your intake of all animal products, as they contain too many things that our bodies seem to have a hard time dealing with. We can still use this food group for its high vitamin B-12 content, but certainly not every day. Everything in moderation. Too many Americans consume animal products three times a day, if not more often. That is a lot of saturated fat, which also causes us to consume less in other needed nutrients."

"Yeah," said David, "But why is it that the latest diet fads like Atkins, the Paleolithic diet, and even the Zone diet seem to be working for people. I mean, I'm hearing great success stories from people that follow those protocols."

The doctor nodded. "I agree David, and those diets are giving some very nice results. But those diets also all restrict the many modern food choices that most Americans consume way too much of, things like sugar, white flour, processed carbohydrates, and bad oils and fats."

"So it is the avoidance of those items that have been giving good results, right Doctor? But my point is that they still are eating a lot of animal products."

"Agreed," said the doctor, before adding, "In our country, and around the world, simple carbs, bad oils and fats, and animal products, in general, lead to illness. Now, it is true that if you avoid the simple carbs, processed foods as we call them, and the bad fats, then you may get away with eating animal products. My view on this is, yes, it is possible to have good health for a long time if you are avoiding bad food choices. Regarding animal products, you may be able to live on them long term, especially if they are high quality and natural, but how will that sustain health in the long run? We do not know, but there is a more sure way of proceeding."

"I'm all ears, Doctor," David said with a grin.

Likewise, the doctor responded with a smile, "Eat your vegetables."

EAT YOUR VEGETABLES

They both laughed as the doctor continued. "Seriously, the conclusion many doctors came to as a result of these studies and several other large population studies, is that the more a society consumes animal products, which contain lots of saturated fats, the more they suffer from heart disease. This heart disease can manifest itself in many ways. Over the years we have learned that your arteries don't even have to be fully clogged to suffer a heart attack. Plaque and its attending inflammation can eventually cause the cholesterol laden plaque to rupture, closing the artery and killing the patient. So anything we can do to lower this problem needs to be addressed.

"Now here's the real big news. Those countries that consume more plant based foods had far less heart disease and far less cancer. Now this is not to say that animal products and saturated fats are the sole cause of heart disease because we know that when you consume hydrogenated oils that they can behave similar to saturated fats in your body by causing mischief. When you add to this mixture the high sugar levels caused by high sugar intake or by consuming too many simple carbs, then you are adding fuel to the fire of something we now call inflammation.

"Doctor, you keep talking about inflammation. We need the body to produce inflammation, don't we? I mean that is how our bodies deal with infections or cuts and such, right?"

"Yes, it reacts to infections, wounds, and other things but many of those situations could be short term. That would be a healthy inflammation response not an unhealthy one. Inflammation can get out of control however. I am also including things that irritate our bodies over the long term causing immense damage from the inside out. Damage to our arteries for one, our brain for another, and even our DNA, along with damaging our energy factories inside our cells which we refer to as our mitochondria."

"That sounds horrible, Doctor. I mean we expect inflammation when our bodies are trying to heal us from a cut, puncture, or wound, but to have it raging within our bodies all the time would be horrible. That is what you are saying, right? That we have this long term inflammation going on?"

OWNER'S MANUAL

The doctor nodded, "Yes, that is right. A bad diet of processed food, bad fats, and too much saturated fat seems to do exactly that, cause a steady state of irritation, which we know as inflammation. We need to turn down the heat of this fire. The answer seems clear if you keep an open mind."

"How's that?"

"Just read the most comprehensive study ever done on food and health and make up your own mind. For a complete revelation on the connection between consuming animal products and health, one needs to review the most detailed book on the subject I have ever seen published, called *The China Study* by Campbell and Campbell." The doctor paused as David made notes.

"But in fairness, David, remember what I said: Eat only good fats, good carbs, and good protein sources. That alone can be life changing. But how can you do this if you don't know what they are? By reading the book *The China Study*, you can see for yourself what the right fats, carbs, and proteins are to begin with.

After all, none of us were given an owner's manual for what we should eat. This book comes as close to that owner's manual as anything I have ever seen. This alone can be life changing. Ignore what most everybody else in this country is doing as they really are clueless or have grown tired of thinking for themselves."

"So give me some examples of what an anti-inflammatory diet might be?

The doctor readily said, "Eat naturally and just make the right choices as often as possible. We all need to just stop with all the processed food already."

THE CHOICE

The doctor continued, "Look at food as your friend, it is the fuel your body needs for a good life. Good food in the right amount will lead to a good life. Also, if you choose bad food, the opposite effect will occur. Bad food, especially in the wrong amounts, will lead to a life of disease, misery, and missed opportunities for a fulfilling life. So choose good, ignore bad."

"Ouch, Doctor; when you say it that way, you get my attention. Good foods equal a good life, and bad foods equal a bad life. Did I get that right?"

"Yes, David, that's it in a nutshell. Once you realize the importance of consuming only real food that is fresh and full of good fats, carbs and or proteins, your eating pattern will change. For instance, David, tell me what you ate yesterday so I can see how much work we have ahead of us."

"Hmm," David paused. "I cannot say that I really remember everything I ate, Doctor, but let me see. I had oatmeal yesterday morning with toast, then for lunch I stopped at Taco Bell, where I had three tacos, and then for dinner, my wife and I had chicken, potatoes and corn."

"OK, David, now what did you have to drink, and by the way, tell me about any snacks that usually sneak their way into your day."

"Oh yeah, Doc, I forgot about those."

"I thought so. That's why everyone should keep a food journal for one week. It keeps you honest and is an eye opener. We're living in a time where we have forgotten our natural environment and lifestyle. Look at what chimps and their cousins' bonobos eat. Their diets are heavy in berries, fruit, roots, green leaves, and sources of protein like insect larvae, small animals, and even small amounts of dirt. It's long been known that various microorganisms exist in that dirt, and even vitamin B-12 can be found on roots, assuming those roots are in real soil, nurtured by natural fertilizer. Not to mention the benefits of moderate amounts of sunshine, as it filters through the jungle canopy. That steady source of vitamin D may go a long way in preventing premature aging. Add to this the exercise a primate group gets moving from location to location and the tremendous social interaction. We need to be aware of how our ancestors really lived. No stress of getting to work on time, paying taxes, or picking up kids from school. In short, a simpler time. Their stress was usually more short-lived, like when they had to deal with a predator or when dealing with their social hierarchy."

"Yeah, Doctor, but what about all the negatives to their lifestyle, like dying from falls, diseases, and being eaten by a leopard?"

"Fair enough, David, but what I suggest is that we have the intelligence and wherewithal to 'take the best and leave the rest.'"

"Right Doc, I think that makes sense."

"Keep in mind that healthy aging is a lot about preventing bad things in the first place. But let's take a break and resume our conversation tomorrow."

They headed out of the room and approached the front door. David could see a few people waiting for the doctor. Several appeared as patients, but he couldn't help notice a gentleman dressed in a suit holding a leather valise-type briefcase. David made his way down the front porch and walked to his car. Parked in front of him was a car with a state seal on the door. He put two and two together. The gentleman in the waiting room was from the government. David hoped that the doctor had paid his taxes.

CHECKING HIS PROGRESS

In a few days, the doctor and David got together again.

"Good to see you, David. How goes it?" the doctor inquired.

"Well, Doc, as you know, I needed over a week of trying your advice before sensing its effects. It makes me realize that I haven't been doing enough of the right things. In fact, I now realize that I wasn't really living a healthy lifestyle."

"Tell me more, David."

"Well, I read a lot, do research, talk with medical professionals all the time, so I thought I was doing what you're supposed to do."

"Like?" asked the doctor.

"You know, Doc, eat less fat, trim the fat from my meat, skip the mayo, don't eat too many hotdogs, all that stuff."

"Hmm, David, you hit on a key point. In my view, most people really do think they are trying to eat healthy. In their mind, French fries are a viable vegetable selection. But it doesn't work like that. Adding a tomato slice and a leaf of lettuce to a greasy, double patty cheeseburger is not going to save you. Many parents think if their children are eating commercial breakfast cereal in the morning that this equates to their children eating whole grains, but you have to look at the ingredients, which are mostly sugar. Look in the restaurants and grocery stores, and you still see tons of margarine being sold and hydrogenated oil peddled. They present the product like there is nothing wrong with it. They give the impression you are buying something healthy for your family. It's an epidemic."

David replied, "Right Doctor. I see what you are saying now. I can't go by advertisers, but I need to look at buying and eating food in its more natural state." David thought a little and then said, "You know, Doctor, maybe these so called health nuts are not really nuts. Everybody else is for eating the way they do."

The doctor replied, "You have a real point there."

David added, "I mean the way most people eat is not natural. We need to eat more simple foods in their more natural state, just as the rest of the world's animals do."

KEEP IT SIMPLE

"That's right, David. Keep it simple. Simplicity works for several reasons. One is that you can focus on what foods are really good for you like fresh vegetables, fruit, berries, legumes, some whole grains, etc. Then you can find choice protein sources like cage-free chicken, Alaskan cod, non-farmed salmon, or even sardines. Two, you will find you are spending less in the long run when you purchase wholesome food. Even if it's organic, the savings from buying fresh, unprocessed food usually is enough to offset the higher costs of highly processed frozen entrees, high sodium canned stuff, or processed boxed goods. Why do I say it's cheaper? Because, when it comes to organic food, you can either pay a little more now in price or pay much more later if you don't use organic. Paying now means a little more money but a whole lot more of good health down the road. Eating non-organic or the traditional American way may cost your health much more than money can repair."

"Doc, when you said to eat simpler and more close to the earth, were you saying I should follow a caveman diet? I've seen books on the Paleolithic diet. Is that what you are talking about?"

"David, the paleo diet can work for many people and is certainly better than the average modern diet most North Americans follow. I think it would work just fine. Our ancestors followed such a diet for thousands of years and did very well. The proponents of paleo state that people do very well on this diet. They see their weight go down, their cholesterol plummets, and other age-markers or biomarkers, as we call them, improve as well. Biomarkers are ways we can measure what is going on in our bodies. Use these types of markers to see if a certain lifestyle or diet is influencing your body positively or negatively. After all, we need a way to keep score. For instance, I have personally seen patients on such a diet see their blood-work improve dramatically. What I mean by that is their triglycerides drop, their C-reactive protein levels drop, their bad cholesterol drops, and their insulin levels improve, often dramatically. Yet, I feel that it is not the paleo diet doing this as much as avoiding the garbage in the modern American diet."

David said, "OK, I see where you're going with this; tell me more."

"Well, David, eating fresh food close to the earth along with lean sources of protein and the right fats is the way I would go. Avoid most processed foods and the adulterated food they keep selling to us. Consume only ocean fish that have been found to be much lower in heavy toxins, such as those found in Arctic waters, not farm-raised fish. Consume only real poultry that feed in the wild or on a more natural diet and not strictly on a grain or corn-based feed diet, which will only result in high omega-6 content anyways. So what I am saying is a paleo diet will work just as any diet that avoids modern junk food would as long as it is diversified and something we are meant to eat. The paleo diet stresses too much meat for my taste. I've seen many healthy people who don't consume meat at all for me to be convinced that we need to eat a lot of meat. If consuming meat, remember not to fall into the trap of eating meat three times a day as many Americans do. Humans are omnivores, similar to bears, we are able to eat a varied diet and seem to thrive on it. However, saying that, I would urge any meat eater to cut down their meat consumption to five times a week. That would mean that only five meals would contain meat within the week instead of 21 meals. That could go a long way in improving their heart health. When I talk about meat, I don't mean just red meat like beef, pork and lamb; I include chicken, turkey and fish in that category too.

GOOD VERSUS GREAT

"Back to your diet, David, I note the observation that 'Good is the enemy of great!' So when people think they are eating a diet that is good enough, they often really are fooling themselves. So keep your diet clean and close to what our ancestors ate for hundreds of thousands of years, not just what we may have started eating when our recent ancestors discovered fire. Remember, man was eating for many more years without the benefit of using fire than he has been with using fire."

"Well, Doctor, I guess it can get confusing if you read too much into it. I mean, you did say to focus on eating real food with good fat, good carbs, and good protein. It's funny, because many years ago, most Americans never heard of the difference between good fats and bad fats or especially a good carb versus a bad carb."

"That's true, David. When we ate a more natural diet, we didn't have to know the differences between good and bad. Our fats were mostly natural without the trans fats or hydrogenated fat we have now adapted. Even beef, pork, or lamb meat was wild or grazed their way into our food chain. So we didn't need to monitor the good from the bad as it was mostly good. In fact, grass-fed or range-fed meat has more omega-3 content than grain-fed animals, which have higher omega-6. Too much omega-6 is inflammatory, leading to a cascade of bad things going on in your body. The same goes for carbs, since we have consumed mostly good carbs for our entire history. By good, I mean primitive people would consume root vegetables, greens, nuts, and berries. All things that held vast nutrients within their own natural container complete with wholesome vitamins, fiber, phytonutrients, antioxidants and minerals. Not the sugary garbage we are forced fed today."

BORDERLINE DEFICIENCIES

"You just mentioned minerals, Doctor. What common minerals are usually too low in our diets?"

"While most people think it is calcium, magnesium is often too low. But speaking of minerals, we sometimes miss the micronutrients our body needs."

"Such as?"

"Iodine deficiency is very common. It is crucial to have enough iodine within your body so your thyroid functions properly."

"Right, Doctor, I've heard we used to have a lot of goiter in this country, especially in the Great Lakes area."

"Right, that area was known as the goiter belt and, sad to say, also the cancer belt."

"Really, Doctor? So they are all connected?"

"Seems so, I always tell my patients to consume natural forms of iodine several times a week, usually from kelp tablets. Try to get at least 100% of the recommended daily allowance. Also, I tell them to avoid things that interfere with iodine absorption."

"Such as?"

"Fluoride and bromine. Fluoride can be found in medicines, toothpaste, water, etc. Bromine is found in flour products. It is listed as an ingredient on the package, avoid it completely."

"So is a lack of iodine causing the cancer?"

"I think it could be a factor, especially in the Great Lakes region, along with a lack of selenium in the soil there too. A lack of either could lead to higher cancer rates."

"So make sure you are getting enough iodine and selenium?"

"Both, David, but never take too much of any mineral, especially selenium."

"How common is iodine deficiency?"

"The World Health Organization, known as the WHO, estimates about two billion people are lacking in proper iodine amounts."

"That's sure a lot of people. Do you have some suggested doses for iodine and selenium?"

"I would take 100% of the recommended daily allowance several times a week, just to make sure I wasn't running a shortage. Do not take most mineral supplements every day. I would not overthink this situation. Just make sure you have enough, but not too much as that would prove to be most counter-productive."

"So take your vitamins?"

"Right, David, and your minerals. We have talked about the negative effects of being low in just one vitamin and how that alone could foster disease and an early death. Well, making sure your body has all of its proper micronutrients could go a long way in getting you to your full life expectancy, assuming you avoid other bad things. I note that the celebrity Bob Hope took a quality vitamin supplement his entire life and lived to be 100. His wife Dolores lived to be 102. Is this by chance? I don't think so. Of course, Bob Hope was also told by his doctor, in his middle aged years, to switch to a breakfast of stewed fruit, as he was eating a mostly unhealthy typical American breakfast."

"So Doc, is that why so many doctors tell their patients to take a multiple vitamin and mineral supplement as insurance?"

"That's right, David. They may not have any hard evidence to support that advice but their gut feeling tells them to recommend this."

"Do you agree?"

"Yes, I think you should take a quality multiple vitamin and mineral supplement several times a week, but not every day. Be careful, David, a lot of supplement manufacturers produce an inferior product made with synthetic vitamins and junk minerals. The tip off is when the vitamin label reads synthetic vitamin E, called dl-alpha-tocopheryl. Note the difference, real vitamin E is labeled with a simple 'd' not 'dl.' So a label that has d-alpha-tocopherol would be a much better buy."

"Really, Doc, what else?"

"Then, if you really looking for a quality product it should have on the label not only d-alpha-tocopherol but also have mixed tocopherols and/or gamma-tocopherol. In short, a real vitamin E product that is balanced, not a junk, synthetic product that was cheap to manufacture. The supplements we are talking about need to be quality supplements."

"Wow, Doctor, do consumers know how to read these labels?"

"Not really, David, they shop by price and they will almost always buy a junk product. Something with the wrong form of folic acid, the wrong amounts of B vitamins, the wrong mixture of minerals, and on and on."

"So making sure you have all of your proper and quality micro-nutrients could be crucial to living a long life. Right, Doc?"

"Yes, a major part of prevention theory would have to include another theory that fits into the prevention theory like a hand into a glove."

"What's that theory called and, by the way, Doctor, can you give me some research that backs that claim?"

TRIAGE THEORY

"David, I could give you examples of many different current research programs going on but let me share just one simple example. I've pointed out how being deficient in one vitamin or mineral can negatively affect your health. Dr. Bruce Ames developed a theory of aging called The Triage Theory. Most people know our bodies need the macronutrients like protein, fat, and carbohydrates. Dr. Ames theory states something along the line, that our body also needs micronutrients such as vitamins, minerals, and essential fatty acids. We require a certain amount of these for optimal health and if we run even a small deficiency it could cause us to age prematurely. Therefore he stresses that we should strive to make sure we are getting what our body needs on a consistent basis."

"Well, Doctor, I do know our bodies need at least 15 vitamins and 15 minerals and at least two essential fatty acids for survival. So what do you think of his theory?"

"It makes sense, David. Dr. Ames believes that our body has its priorities. Triage is a medical term for the process of determining the priority of treatment for patients based on the severity of their condition. In a war zone, those that can't be saved are placed in one group while those that can be saved are placed into two groups, those who need the treatment immediately and those that can wait."

"I'm a little confused, how does this make it a theory of aging?"

"David, Dr. Ames believes our body has its own triage system. If it only has a little of a micronutrient such as a vitamin or mineral, it may use that in the best manner for the body at that time. Perhaps a substance that is needed might be directed to a critical body function like reproduction. The body may be focused on what may be most important for our species not our life span. Or our body may sense one function needs to be serviced before it will release the micronutrient to another part of the body. Numerous other examples could be given but let me just say the body has its priorities based perhaps on evolutionary survival. So it may appear we are doing well when we are short of a vital nutrient, but damage may be going on that we don't see. The body may be taking care of body functions short term but ignoring critical repairs or allowing damage to occur that will impact us dramatically in the future."

Smiling, David responded, "So could you wrap that up in a sentence or two?

With a light chuckle, the doctor added, "That's easy; a lack of any critical nutrient may be causing aging. So make sure you have an optimal diet. Of course, the hard part is to pin down what the optimal diet for anti-aging really is."

"That does make sense, and goes along with what you were talking about earlier."

"It sure does, David, but also we must also keep our digestive systems healthy so we can utilize the nutrients we do consume, especially as we get older. Lack of a strong digestive system may be the start of our biological downfall."

"How do we do that, Doc?"

"David, we could spend an entire week on that topic but let me say there are proven ways to do so. Eating smaller meals, proper food combining, eating the right foods in the right amount, preparing our food properly, not drinking too much liquid with all of our meals and using digestive supplements like betaine, hydrochloride, pepsin and digestive enzymes and such."

UNIFICATION

"So, Doc, is prevention a viable method for extending your life expectancy?"

"Absolutely. While it is not held to be a theory of aging or in the pursuit of anti-aging, it is the platform you must start with to allow the other theories of aging to work or to truly take advantage of what we are learning. Prevention is the main tool we have been using to reach our natural life span."

"How's that, Doc?"

"Most theories of aging want to address the extension of an animal's life expectancy. Prevention Theory simply seeks to allow an animal to live a full and healthy life up to its life expectancy before it dies off, hopefully in its sleep. One must practice prevention first and foremost to allow time for the other anti-aging methods to work."

"Hmm," David replied. "So is it a real theory on longevity?"

"Good observation, David, and yes, it is," said the doctor. "What we refer to as diseases and sickness for most people, are really bad lifestyle choices."

"Really, you think we make that many bad decisions?"

"David, look at all the misery and death that smoking has caused. There is a clear cause and effect between smoking anything and your health. If you want to prevent 60% of lung cancer, simply avoid smoking or a smoke-filled environment. Eliminate factory fumes, diesel exhaust, radon, asbestos, and radiation sources, and you would eliminate another 30%. There you go, 90% of lung cancer is caused by environmental factors. A simple case of cause and effect. Prevention in this case would help many people live their full life period, if – and this is a big if – they also avoid the other big no-no's like drinking excessive alcohol, eating the wrong diet, and undue stress. I mean, pollution, bad diets, and stress cause 80% of all the heart disease and probably half of all cancers."

David was quick to respond, "So, prevention is the key?"

The doctor responded, "A key, but not the only key, as there are many doors to aging and good health. But to make prevention really work you need to practice all aspects of it and combine it with some other methods of anti-aging medicine. As valuable as it is, prevention only gets you to your full life expectancy. You need to follow another protocol called caloric restriction, which I will share with you next. These two protocols combined with some other theories of aging or anti-aging in our case, will give you the complete method to handle aging in this era. It will be your unified foundation for going as far as you can in life expectancy based on current data. It's what I have used in my personal life and with my patients. But as new discoveries are made we add those protocols as soon as we can judge their true value and safety. I will cover other methods that all appear very powerful in the battle against premature or accelerated aging as we know it. You see, aging for most people should not be occurring at the fast rate it is. Most people, however, are ignorant of what the human body is really capable of when taken care of properly. This will change quickly, however, and soon we will have more and better tools to assist. But for now we can do a lot, as long as you group all of these methods as one unified body of knowledge and apply it to your life as soon as possible."

The doctor and David wrote out together the main points of their conversation. To summarize the Prevention Theory of Aging, they were as follows:

KEY POINTS
PREVENTION THEORY

- First, do no harm.

- Eat real foods, which consist of good fats, good carbs, and good sources of protein.

• Eat close to the earth, which means avoiding most processed food.

• Never forget where we as a species came from. That alone should lead you to enjoying real food and not the processed stuff they want you to believe is food.

• Food is supposed to be free of preservatives, pesticides, fungicides and other harmful ingredients.

• Health nuts may not be nuts but everyone else truly is for eating the horrible way they do. It simply is not natural nor is it healthy.

• Keep in mind, what is your vibrant health really worth to you?

• Drink pure water, free of chlorine, fluoride, arsenic and other contaminants.

• Don't assume anything when it comes to medical care or treatment. The cure may kill you even if the initial medical condition does not.

• Never forget cause and effect.

• Think differently than your friends, family and community.

• Make your own lifestyle decisions.

• Allow time each day to commune with nature, such as walking outside.

• We all have lead in our systems. Why? Leaded gas was used for years around the world (it allowed gasoline engines to run smoother), along with lead-based paints used in homes. Many of us have been overexposed to these harmful lead products and have accumulated lead in our systems. Keep your current exposure to lead to a minimum by not using lead products and not removing harmful lead paint found in older homes. Also, consider ways of getting lead out of your system, such as chelation. People that have used chelation therapy have far less cancer.

• Trace minerals are important. Kelp tablets are an excellent source of iodine. Iodine and selenium, in small amounts, can be protective. Large amounts, however, can be toxic.

• Take a quality vitamin and mineral supplement several times a week.

• Observe your digestion and digestive track and take steps to improve digestion, assimilation and elimination.

• Do not overconsume the preformed source of vitamin A that is contained in most supplements, as too much may cause more harm than good. Too much vitamin A, often listed as retinyl acetate or retinyl palmitate, may interfere with proper vitamin D utilization. This reason alone should cause you to limit your intake of multiple vitamins on a daily basis. Natural vitamin A, also called retinol, can be found in fatty fish, fish liver oil, eggs, and liver. Heat, air, and light readily destroy vitamin A. Plant sources contain beta carotene, which the body can convert to vitamin A. Stating this, you should get vitamin A from both sources: fish, eggs, liver, and plants.

• Get your own blood work done before seeing doctors. Life Extension (www.lef.org) offers the ability to do so.

8
Caloric Restriction Theory
Theory II

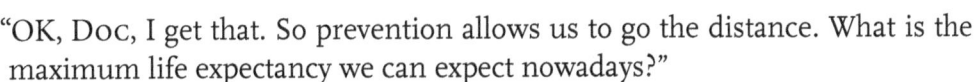

"OK, Doc, I get that. So prevention allows us to go the distance. What is the maximum life expectancy we can expect nowadays?"

"Comedian George Burns, who lived to age 100, wrote a book called *How to Live to Be 100*. In this book he writes about eating a light diet. Heavy only in variety, but not heavy in calories. Very insightful. The oldest person on record was a French woman named Jeanne Calment. She made it to over 122 years. She passed away in 1997, and many articles were written about her. She exercised most of her entire life, even riding a bicycle past age 100. She did most things in moderation, like having a glass of port wine each day and a bit of dark chocolate. She even smoked a little, which might explain losing her vision to blindness late in life.

"But, David, I am convinced that many people have lived to that age in centuries past. There are countless stories of centenarians living well beyond that age in isolated regions of China, Japan, and other places. Given the right environment, our life expectancy might be 125 years. The problem is that most of us are our own worst enemy."

BIOMARKERS

After several more hours of discussions concerning the importance of first not harming ourselves, the doctor interjected more on the most significant and important major theory of anti-aging.

"David, I know you've heard of caloric restriction and its effects on aging. Am I correct?"

David replied, "Of course, most people have heard a little but few follow it, right?"

"Yes, that's true, David, because most people haven't taken time to explore easy ways to approach this. After using methods of prevention, or self-preservation as I call it, the greatest thing each of us can do is caloric restriction. Before you grimace, David, keep in mind that if you are eating correctly, caloric restriction is easy. If, however, you are eating incorrectly, then caloric restriction is nearly impossible."

"How's that, Doctor? I mean, how can one way be so easy and the other so difficult?"

"If you stick to a natural diet, a regimen our ancestors would have followed because of their environment not out of choice, then your total caloric intake on most days would be restricted. How's that you might ask? If you were a primitive man, you would forage for food. So not only were you getting sufficient exercise but you were mostly grazing for food, not sitting down to a large table and eating fried chicken, potatoes and gravy, biscuits, and mom's apple pie, which by the way would be a whole lot of calories.

"So our natural state is to forage like other primates searching for such things as tubers, which are a root-like plant. There are many types, but when I tell people that potatoes are tubers, they understand much quicker. These can be loaded with carbs or fibrous starches, a great energy snack. Our ancestors would eat leaves, nuts, seeds, berries, flowers, green shoots from plants and even parts of water grass, cattails, and other such stuff."

"Well, Doc, I guess that makes sense. When you look at it, lettuce and cabbage are leaves, cauliflower and broccoli are plants, and I know some ethnic groups eat their flowers. But what about protein sources?"

"Good question. Plants have protein, as do nuts and seeds. Where the mistaken belief that they do not contain much protein comes from, I don't know; perhaps from the dairy industry. But keep in mind that our ancestors had no problem eating grubs, insects, insect larvae, caterpillars, small animals, crayfish, clams, and fish, all excellent sources of protein. In fact, David, I think the reason humans have such good memories is because we needed to remember what foods were edible and at what time of the year we could safely eat them. For instance, baboons and chimps have a tendency to eat different plants at different times of the year. Also, they favor quick growing plants perhaps because they may know that those plants have not built up too many toxic protective agents that discourage insects and animals from eating them."

"I see, Doctor; so you're saying that nature really has given us a lot of food choices in the wild."

"Absolutely. We see animals existing in nature without the benefit of grocery stores or restaurants yet think we are helpless in these matters."

PLANTS ARE BEST

"So, Doc, you're saying a plant-based diet, low on calories, along with some lean sources of protein gave us an automatic way of restricting our calories? Does that about sum it up?"

The doctor smiled as he said, "David, not only did that diet automatically reduce our caloric intake but that diet would have included the healthy fats found naturally in nature via seeds, nuts, and fish, not the toxic fats they are trying to feed us in our grocery stores and bakeries nowadays. Thankfully, nature gave us strong livers, which help detoxify some of our modern food, just as it did with many of the toxic plants we tried eating in the wild."

"So, no fat cavemen, right, Doctor?"

Laughing, the doctor responded, "Not as far as we know, but anything is possible. I mean bears get fat for the winter, and gorillas get extra weight eating mostly a plant diet, but all in all, we would have been thinner then. A lot thinner. And based on a grazing diet, often we would have gone several days in a row without eating any food since sometimes it simply could not be found."

David responded, "What about getting proper nutrition back then, Doctor?"

"Well, its speculation, but many think grazing for food would allow us to have more variety of food, not less, since most modern people eat the same group of foods over and over. Add to this that humans are one of the few animals that cannot produce their own vitamin C. That tells me we have a long history of grazing for plants, berries and fruit. Eating such a diet naturally reduces your risk of dying from cancer, diabetes, and heart disease."

"So being in a modern world, how do we eat that way today?"

FRIEND OR FOE

"Great question and one deserving much thought. My best answer is to never forget where you came from. Eat close to the earth and eat a variety of fresh wholesome goods." The doctor paused briefly.

David added, "And?"

"And it's a given that we should eat organic since our livers and bodies cannot handle the toxic stuff they apply to our food. Also, avoid most processed foods. If you do that David, you are avoiding most of the unnatural sugar they put in our food and all the other empty calories found in white rice, white flour, corn flour, and all the useless oil that seems to have found its way into our diets."

"So, Doc, give me a path to follow. How do I incorporate caloric restriction these days living in a modern world?"

"Well, David, first I recommend looking at the modern world as your friend, not a foe..."

David smirked a little before replying, "How's that, Doc? I mean it is the modern world which is making it so hard to eat right, isn't it?"

The doctor nodded. "I know, David, at first it seems a contradiction but remember I said it's all how you look at things. You can look at eating healthy as a hardship, which many do, or look at eating healthy as a pleasure. For instance, in years past, people living in North America had to work long hours just to feed themselves. Nowadays, many people work very hard not for food, but for houses, cars, gadgets, insurance premiums, credit card debt, student loans, cable television, and other stuff. However, what they spend for food is actually far less than prior years. I look at the variety of food available in our supermarkets, farmers markets, and specialty shops and I am in awe. I remember when getting a simple orange out of season was a novelty. Now, it is so common we don't give it a second thought."

"Wow, Doctor, I guess I didn't think of it that way. I mean things like oranges, bananas and grapes seem to have been available year round for years. I guess they just import them from South America, right?"

"Right," the doctor added, "and from South Africa, Asia, and Australia. It really is amazing."

"So," David added, "What you're saying is given the free market, we really do have a lot of food choices?"

"Right, we have a lot more food choices, especially if you put some thought into it. You can buy most whole grains like brown rice, millet, or beans anywhere, things like potatoes and other root vegetables can also be bought in bulk and stored in a cool place. You can buy grass-fed beef, farm-raised chickens, eggs, and turkeys from specialty vendors. Search out a real farm that allows their animals to graze on a natural diet of what they are supposed to eat, not a factory farm diet of corn, soy, and other inflammatory stuff."

"OK, Doctor, when you say it like that, it almost sounds fun. I mean searching out the best food sources and such."

"It is. David, it only takes a small amount of effort to garner large benefits. You can mail order a lot of specialty products like range-fed buffalo meat, wild salmon from Alaska, and organic products of all types. Many folks will join a buyers club or buyers circle through their contacts at a health food store or food co-op. There are hundreds of these groups all around the U.S. and Canada. I've made excellent contacts at farmers markets, which lead me from one seller of products to another. An endless chain of food opportunities, if you ask me."

GROW YOUR OWN

David responded, "OK, I see where you're going with this line of reasoning. Any other tips then?"

"Of course, don't forget to grow some of your own fruits and vegetables. I remember in years past when almost every family had a garden. It just made sense. Nowadays people forget how rewarding these really were. Even as a busy doctor, I grow several vegetables. In the fall, I have so much surplus that I swap with neighbors. I give them tomatoes, squash and green beans at harvest time in exchange for them having given me blueberries, strawberries and apples during the year. Not a bad deal. People don't jar their produce like they used to, but you can still store a lot of stuff in a root cellar or in a large freezer. There simply is no excuse for not doing so."

DIET ADVICE

"But Doctor, how would you put a diet together that anyone could follow?"

"I would recommend looking at a real Mediterranean diet for anyone, as it favors unprocessed food, along with fresh vegetables, whole grains, fruit, fish and a small amount of eggs. Red meat is consumed only once or twice a month. Also when it is, it is varied, ranging from lamb to pork to beef. They use virgin olive oil, which many times is unfiltered, allowing it to retain much more of its beneficial traits. Even so, they used it in moderation, as fat is fat. This oil is more neutral in the body than heart clogging saturated fat, or worse trans fat that is made originally from supposedly healthy polyunsaturated oils like safflower, sesame, soybean, corn, or the worst of the bunch, cottonseed oil. While these types of oils might be OK in moderation, they are not acceptable at all if they have been processed using hydrogenation. This process extends their shelf life but kills any nutrient value. Also that process takes an omega-6 fat source, which we need in moderation and turns it into a toxic ingestion of fats that the body doesn't know what to do with. If you want a healthier polyunsaturated fat, then eat sardines twice a week. Fish contains mostly omega-3 oil, which our bodies like, especially when we are consuming too much omega-6 to begin with."

"Doc, when you talk about the Mediterranean diet, which country or countries are you referring to?

"Good question, David. Dr. Ancel Keys, creator of the infamous K-rations that were fed to American soldiers during World War II, also helped author an historically imporant nutrional study called 'The Seven Country Study,' and from that study introduced to the rest of the world a diet that we now call the Mediterranean diet. He based that diet primarily on the eating habits of the people of Crete. This is when the people of Crete were extremely healthy. However, like many other countries these days, they are also consuming too much modern processed food and more dairy and meat. So their health is trending downwards, just like so many other modern countries."

"Well, Doc, that's disheartening to hear. So what other guidelines should we consider."

"Along those lines, I've noticed the latest editions of the South Beach Diet seem to be stressing a better arrangement of fats found in fish than its earlier edition but I would go more with the Sonoma Diet plan by Connie Guttersen. Her recipes are following the Mediterranean diet protocol almost perfectly, but she adds some local flavors more familiar to Americans. So I'd be comfortable seeing a patient follow that diet initially as well, until many of their cravings for processed food fades. Like I said, David, eat the right fats, proteins, and the right carbs, not the bad ones."

"Wow, This stuff gets overwhelming, doesn't it, Doc?"

With a chuckle, the doctor said, "It doesn't have to be, David. We make it far harder than it has to be. I mean society gives us a lot of false choices when it comes to food for one real reason."

"Why's that?"

"Profit for the food companies," said the doctor. "Just keep it simple, David. Most fats actually contain all three main categories of fat, such as saturated, monounsaturated, and polyunsaturated, just in different proportions. As always, variety is nice but just make sure it's mostly heart healthy and not inflammatory. Do some basic research and by all means, avoid all processed oil and shortening that has been hydrogenated or heat-treated, as this can make almost any oil toxic to the body when consumed long term. The natural shelf life of oil that has not been hydrogenated is about six months. So why hydrogenate it in the first place?"

CUTTING CALORIES

"So," said David, "use a Mediterranean diet or the latest Sonoma diet – is that the simplest advice for controlling your appetite and lowering the overall amount of calories?"

The doctor paused before responding, "Well, David, I read several books years ago by an expert in caloric restriction, a Dr. Roy Walford. He gave a regimen and recipes to follow, but I found his approach inadequate for me. He had great recipes, but he would prepare a dish one night and freeze several servings for future lunches and dinners. I found that hard to follow as I believe food should be eaten as fresh as possible, when available. Heating, freezing and reheating destroy nutrients, especially folic acid. However, having said that, I read and reread his book at least ten times. His book, *The 120 Year Diet*, was full of useful information. I note that he stresses that one should not lose weight too quickly as that seems to eliminate the life extension benefit of the caloric restricted diet. In fact, he recommends you work toward a much lower body weight over a period of at least two years. My own thoughts on this would be in full agreement. You need to give your body time to detoxify, especially after having eaten poorly for a lifetime. Many toxins are stored in your body fat, and to lose weight too quickly could cause those harmful agents to overwhelm your body's natural detoxification pathways. Many of us have been exposed to lead, mercury, cadmium, nickel and perhaps too much iron.

"Now it's interesting to note that Dr. Roy Walford started his own caloric restriction diet in his mid-50s. He did this after seeing the astounding results of several animal studies. In most species of animals, caloric restriction, if used along with adequate nutrition, prolonged the average life of that animal species. The good doctor knew this and started himself on the diet. However, I can't help but feel that he was too good at following this diet and lost weight too quickly. He had a healthy life until he tragically developed ALS, or Lou Gehrig's disease as it's called, in his 70s. I think he died around age 75."

David interjected, "So, Doctor, caloric restriction works if you start slowly?"

"Right," the doctor responded, "It works best when implemented slowly and also when started earlier in life. One should wait until they are a young adult, let's say age 22, before starting a serious caloric restricted diet. Reducing your calories by 20% to 30% would be the maximum goal. So limit your daily intake to less than 1,800 calories for a woman and less than 2,000 for a man, as a start. Then start your reduction from there. I would only reduce by 10 or 20% That being said, each calorie has to count. One should select real food only, not processed food. Variety would be crucial and in my opinion, plenty of raw, organic food."

David could see that the doctor knew his stuff and had done a lot of research. What surprised him, however, was what the doctor said next.

NOT THE FIRST

"While Dr. Walford wrote about these findings and did much to bring this information to the public, he was not the first. It seems like another lifetime ago, but back in the 1930s, the researcher Dr. Clive McCay announced to the world his surprising research on caloric restriction. So caloric restriction is not a new concept. In fact, I, and several of my associates, immediately understood the concept and put that protocol to use."

David laughed, "Doctor, it seems like the 1930s was a lifetime ago, because it was!" David saw a surprised expression on the doctor's face. He could not tell if the doctor had misspoken or was contemplating his next response.

"Of course, David, that was long ago, but what I am saying is that this whole caloric restriction business is not new. Scientists have had decades to research it. In fact, I recall that Dr. McCay used a rather primitive diet in his experiments. He focused on supplying rudimentary macronutrients and didn't focus on optimized nutrients such as micronutrients."

"You mean micronutrients like flavonoids and trace minerals?"

"Exactly," said the doctor. "In fact, at first, Dr. McCay only gave the minimum to animals studied and did not focus on all the micronutrients that may have added even more health and years to those animals' lives."

"Yet the animals lived longer on the most basic of diets?"

"Yes, David, that is what is so surprising. All the animals lived a longer life collectively speaking, even with a bad diet. Of course, you couldn't say that to Dr. McCay, as he went on to develop a food biscuit that he later tried selling as probably the world's first nutrition bar. It was primitive, in my opinion. It consisted of protein, carbs, corn oil for fat, etc. Of course, the good doctor later added soy protein, wheat germ, and dried milk to improve its nutrient content."

PALEOLITHIC DIET

The conversation between David and the doctor continued for hours, only to be interrupted by the doctor's wife as she served a robust red tea in the afternoon along with some snacks of small round pieces of coarse bread and nut butter. David noted the small size of this snack along with a small side of blueberries. He then realized that both the doctor and his wife most certainly were practicing a lifestyle of caloric restriction. Either that or they just plain didn't have appetites that day. During the snack the doctor brought up another story he had read from a book called *The Buccaneers of America*, first published in 1678.

"David, do you recall us talking about the Paleolithic diet?"

"Of course, I've interviewed several practitioners of this diet, and they all seem pleased with the results. Just a little boring they say."

The doctor sat back deep in thought and said, "I would think so. I would like to relate a story of interest, but it relates to a Paleolithic diet and boredom you spoke of. A servant had been left behind with one of the hunting dogs. His cruel master assumed him lost forever during a hunting foray." The doctor walked over to his bookcase and returned with a book, *The Buccaneers of America*, which depicts the lives of pirates during the 17th century. He proceeded to read out loud the exact excerpt regarding this servant as follows:

THE SERVANT

"'A servant along with a dog were left abandoned. The servant found other wild dogs and led them as their pack leader. They survived by eating wild pigs for over fourteen months. They ate the meat raw. When found by other hunters they noted his good health.' The author of the book noted, 'I happened to be at the place when they brought him back, and stared at him with amazement, for he was fat and sleek and far healthier than when he had depended on his master. He was so used to raw flesh he would not willingly eat cooked meat, nor could his digestion tolerate it. As soon as he had eaten any, he would be groaning the next hour or so with stomach-ache, and would spew the meat up again as whole as when he'd eaten it. But when he ate raw meat, all went well. We tried to keep raw flesh from him as much as we could, but he managed to get at it when we weren't looking. I have noticed the same thing with wild dogs: after they are a month or two old, they don't fancy cooked meat. I have told this story to show the cruelty of these hunters to their indentured servants, and also to show how a man can accustom himself to all kinds of food. In fact, I believe a man could live on grass just as well as animals do.'"

"Wow," said, David, "so, are you saying humans can live on raw meat if they need to?"

111

"Apparently so. Various native tribes of Indians and Eskimos also tell of existing on raw meat for very long periods of time. As long as it is not really lean meat like rabbit, they actually seem to do well."

"I don't understand, Doc. Doesn't eating meat cause cancer?"

"Not necessarily, David. You will hear studies about processed meat causing cancer and perhaps too much red meat, especially if grain fed, increasing cancer rates, but the news media misses a huge point."

"Like what?" .

"Cancer cells lover sugar. They thrive on glucose. Our cells can either use glucose as fuel or they can use fat. When you consume a low carb diet, which many Eskimos were consuming, your body's cells are using fat as a fuel instead of carbohydrates. This is known as ketosis. Since the body is burning fat instead of carbs, cancer cells would starve themselves into oblivion."

"A ketosis diet? Did doctors know this back then?"

"For cancer? No, not really, David. It's only now, looking back, does it make sense. Eskimos ate a diet of all protein and fat, very low in carbs. The end result, almost no cancer. But, David, I can say one surprising thing about the ketogenic diet."

"Such as?"

"It was used in the 1920s and 30s to control epilepsy in children."

"Really?"

"Really. It worked well for about half of the people trying it."

REAL FOOD

"Doctor, I have heard that each group of raw food contains their own enzymes to help digest them. Can we cover that?"

"Of course David, I want to cover that in much more detail but not quite yet. I will say this – in fact, enzymes may be one of the simplest remedies for cancer. This information is very important, so I want to really cover it later, David."

"Well," said David, "This certainly gives credence to the caveman diet, doesn't it?"

"David, speaking on the Paleolithic diet, it's interesting to note that many Native American tribes followed that diet instinctively, as they lived off their environment. The tribes that existed mostly on hunting seem to have the best health. They were the tallest, best built, and had excellent teeth. History tells us that almost all Native Americans could run all day if necessary. Most tribes also practiced periodic fasting. Even today, the Tarahumara tribe in Mexico will have members cover 200 miles over a two-day period, outrunning history's most famous runners, the Greeks. The most famous runner of ancient Greece, Pheidippides, ran from Athens to Sparta on behalf of the Athenians. If this wasn't enough, he soon after ran from Marathon to Athens, about 25 miles, then back again where he supposedly dropped dead from exhaustion. However, I believe he really died from dehydration not exhaustion. Hence, to be on the safe side, modern marathons are just over 26 miles long. However, remember the Greeks had a very healthy diet at that time. It's well known that Dr. Ancel Keys wrote his best selling book *How to Eat Well and Stay Well the Mediterranean Way* in 1975. That diet was based mostly on the Greek diet, especially Crete. Keep in mind that Dr. Keys lived to be 101, so his advice seems to work."

MY REAL POINT

The doctor continued, "But, David, my real point is that scores of Indian dispatchers would run 125 miles straight with mail bags. In Mexico, Indian mail carriers years ago would run over 60 miles a day, seven days a week. Now, while the North American Indians ate a lot of meat, the Mexican tribes ate mostly whole grains like corn, beans and vegetables. Real food seems to give the body the energy and ability to run, but modern junk food does not."

"Wow," David responded. "So, why is there so much ill health with Native Americans today?"

The doctor let out his breath. "Contamination with the white man's food and his ways. David, if you look at much of the food shipped to Indian reservations, you will find white flour, sugar, canned food, and other garbage. Not their traditional healthy diet."

"Gotcha," said David, "It makes sense to me. I mean look at all the diabetes that Native Americans are suffering from today."

"Exactly. Good food equals good energy, bad food, bad energy."

WE NEED FAT

"So, eat real, natural food and you will be working on getting great health and not consuming too many excess calories."

"Right," replied the doctor.

They sat and discussed this topic in detail. The doctor made a point of showing David his research via articles on this topic. He showed David the value of using olive oil, which seemed to prevent the strong inflammatory responses that hydrogenated oils caused. The doctor explained that he knew that Dr. Keys felt one of the main reasons the Mediterranean diets seem to confer good health was that most meals included a lot of greens. The people would use olive oil with these green salads or cooked greens and now scientists have noted that the right oil with various plant foods can increase their bioavailability of various nutrients. Olive oil is mostly monounsaturated fatty oil with high amounts of oleic acid. Dr. Keys believed that saturated fats were the chief cause of heart disease, so his diet guidelines in his book and the observations of many people in the Mediterranean area show low intake of saturated fats. So low meat and dairy consumption is normal.

An important point the doctor stressed over and over again to David, it is not necessary to consume a lot of omega-3 oils, but more important is the ratio of consumption between omega-3 oils and omega-6 oils. Too much omega-6 is found to cause inflammation in the body. The more omega-6 you consume, then the more omega-3 you need to counter-balance its effects. Olive oil is rich in omega-9, which appears to be much more neutral in the body. This is not considered an essential fatty acid. Having said that, however, these fats appear to be good for our cardiovascular system when consumed in moderation.

The doctor explained that we actually require omega-6 fatty acids because they contain linoleic acid, which is considered an essential fatty acid. It's one we need to produce various chemical and hormonal reactions in our body and for wound healing, along with omega-3s, which contain the essential fatty acid alpha-linolenic acid that is considered essential for long-term human health. Both omega-3 acids and omega-6 acids are considered polyunsaturated fatty acids.

The doctor made an important point of telling David that we still need saturated fats in moderation, as they provide important fatty acids like lauric acid, myristic acid, and caprylic acid. These saturated fats help with the making of various hormones. Our bodies perform in an optimal range when we get some saturated fats from natural sources like coconut oil or animal products, especially when they are not overly processed.

ANY SURPRISES?

"So, Doctor, being that you studied caloric restriction, what surprises did you find?"

"Great question. Let's take a short walk while I explain."

They both left their seats in the library, and the doctor directed them through the back door of that room to a beautiful garden. The doctor's yard gently sloped down a rolling hill of green grass surrounded by rosebushes, raised boxes full of vegetables growing, and past what appeared to be an herb garden. They stopped at a long bench just in front of a water fountain that filled the air with its rhythmic sound of water as it cascaded from the upper levels of the fountain downwards.

"David, one of my greatest surprises is how young Dr. Clive McCay was when he passed away and another surprise was the food he used in several of his experiments."

"How's that?"

The doctor shifted his posture. "Well Dr. McCay was only 69 when he passed away. What is really surprising to me is how long many of the animals lived on the diets he designed. Quite a bit longer than one would expect. Dr. McCay developed and perfected a bread that was often called 'Cornell Bread' after the university where he taught. This bread consisted of many ingredients, and Dr. McCay kept improving it over the years by adding soybean products, dry milk, and even wheat germ. This was a vast improvement over his first bread or biscuit product, but it never really caught on nationwide. Dr. McCay used the full fat soy flour to add the amino acids that were missing in the wheat flour, thereby making it a complete protein. Now, I feel that Dr. McCay was in love with using soy products. Actually, I think this may have been a mistake. I note that while fermented soy may be good for you, too much soy in other forms may not be so good."

"How so, Doc?"

"Well, Dr. McCay consumed a lot of soy, and I dare say he suffered several strokes before passing away at age 69. I note this because another advocate and consumer of soy products, Henry Ford, also passed away from a cerebral hemorrhage, considered a form of stroke as well. I note both were thin and considered in excellent shape for their age group. I think too few people realize that soy contains a high amount of phytic acid. This acid can bind to minerals thereby blocking absorption of necessary minerals like calcium, magnesium, copper, iron and zinc. Studies have shown that thyroid functions can be suppressed by over consuming soy products as well because it interferes with the proper uptake of iodine. Also, overconsumption of soy mimics the effect of consuming estrogen. They are called phytoestrogens, and too many can cause negative effects. I also note what a veterinarian told me years ago about chickens."

"Chickens?" said David. "How's that related to soy?"

"Well David, the vet told me of several farmers who were losing their chickens to aneurysms, a weakening of the aorta artery or other arteries. His answer? Add a nickel's worth of copper to the feed."

"Did it work?"

"Yup," said the doctor, "After a month of using the mineral-enhanced feed, the chickens stopped dying. This was confirmed when Dr. Joel Wallach reported on a project dealing with nutrition and 250,000 turkeys. Half of the turkeys died, mostly from a ruptured aortic aneurysm. In the next batch of raising 500,000 turkeys, they doubled the amount of copper within the feed. The results? No turkeys lost to ruptured aortic aneurysms. So copper, like most minerals, can be a cure, or if in excess, a poison. In this case, the chickens needed more copper not less. My concern is that too much soy in your diet may block the ability of your body to absorb needed minerals."

"Any other surprises, Doc?"

The doctor walked a little further through the garden and stopped close to the raised herb garden before responding, "David, I have seen a lot of things and heard of even more. One of the strangest pieces of information was regarding one of the longest lived individuals in U.S. history."

"Who was that, Doctor, and what is strange about him?"

The doctor continued, "Well, it could be just a random coincidence or a real important point to remember. There was a man who lived out most of his 114 years in the Deep South. During an interview, he mentioned how much he liked sardines and crackers. Now with what we have learned lately about omega-3s in fish and their anti-inflammatory effects, that might have been what kept him healthy. Like I said, it is a random observation, but one that may be important to those that want a long life."

David replied, "Doc, you might be missing the real piece of the puzzle here."

"What's that, David?"

"Well, Doc, you said he liked sardines with crackers. Maybe it was the crackers that kept him going."

They both laughed. The doctor added, "That's right, let us discuss that topic in detail as it may be the only real known method that we have for extending our lives."

BIOMARKERS

The doctor started, "Remember we started talking about biomarkers? Well, manage your biomarkers and you will manage your life. For longevity that is."

"So," asked David, "what are some other biomarkers we should be looking at?"

The doctor proceeded to explain more to David, "I have to say that the person that brought many of the biomarkers to my attention was Roy Walford, MD, in his book *The Anti-Aging Plan*. In this book he writes about a biomarker test for lung function called the vital capacity test, which measures the strength and integrity of your whole respiratory system. Using an instrument called a spirometer, doctors can measure if you are above or below normal for your age. You want to be above average as it shows you may have a longer life ahead of you. Dr. Walford said this test was being used on many people, and it did not matter if they were athletes or not. It seems to accurately indicate if an individual was aging ahead of normal or below normal.

"One of the easiest tests to find out how you might be doing on a lower calorie diet is the fasting blood sugar test. You want to have a lower fasting blood sugar level than normal, as this shows that you are heading in the right direction. If you levels are higher than normal, then you have been given a wake-up call. So biomarkers are not tests you do once and forget about. You can repeat them often to make sure you are heading towards better health and more longevity, not less.

"Interestingly, another simple test is for your white blood count. Lower is better, so try to not be in the normal range for this test. Lower than normal is better from the standpoint of living longer, that is, if you are bringing your levels down by restricting your food intake. Too low of a white cell blood level brought on by sickness or disease is not good. Dr. Walford warns his readers that after a long time on a caloric restricted diet that your white blood cell count should drop and not to be concerned about it. You may not worry, but your doctor may, so make sure that you let them know what may be causing your low white blood cell count when that situation comes up."

HOME TEST

The doctor explained, "Now a test that anyone can do at home is the static balance test. It is done by closing your eyes and standing on one leg at a time. Simply lift one foot up off the hard surface of a wood or tiled floor at about a 45 degree angle. If you can hold this position for ten seconds then you are functionally 50 years old or less. Now if you can hold this position for 25 seconds or more then you are functionally age 30 or less. Perhaps this is why you see older people that seem to have no balance. They may, in fact, not have much. It would not be uncommon to see a 70 year old who can only hold this position for 3 or 4 seconds. If they can hold it much longer then they may be doing something right with their lifestyle. Don't be hard on yourself at first. Try doing this test at least three times and then average your actual time."

OTHER BIOMARKERS

Dr. Tessler continued, "Now the other biomarkers you are familiar with – as they are used to measure known risk factors such as high blood pressure and high cholesterol, triglycerides, and high LDL levels – you need to get these items tested. If you are following a low calorie diet of nutrient-dense food that is prepared properly, then all your biomarkers will start looking good. It gives you confirmation that you are going in the right direction."

A QUICK EXAMPLE OF
CALORIC RESTRICTION IN ACTION

"I will give my own example for practicing caloric restriction as I understood it from reading Dr. Walford's work on the subject," the doctor said. "Dr. Walford recommended using a set-point weight target before starting a caloric restricted diet in earnest. Why? He felt that you should have a target weight in mind to start with so you could track your progress. This target weight would usually be what you weighed in your early 20s, assuming you were not overweight then.

Say you are a male weighing 200 pounds today. If you weighed 160 pounds at age 24 then you want to go back to 160 pounds over the next year or two. Once there, at 160 pounds, you want to slowly reduce your caloric intake so that your weight is 10% to 20% below that number. So if you need 2000 calories a day to maintain a weight of 160 pounds, you would aim for a caloric intake of 1800 calories a day for a 10% reduction or 1600 a day for a 20% reduction. That's if you are really seeking a much longer life potential. Keep in mind that if you are at a lower body weight, you then consistently use fewer calories since you need fewer calories to maintain that weight. Since people are different; perhaps you would need more calories or less. There is no one answer for everybody. You first must get to your ideal target weight then decide how much caloric restriction you wish to live on. Less calories means less metabolic waste, less usage of enzymes by your system, less waste elimination, less iron accumulation, and a host of other positive things. As long as your restricted caloric intake is from good nutrition you will start seeing tremendous health benefits. These benefits would be slower aging, better health, less infections, less illness, better skin, delay of graying hair, more endurance, far less heart disease, much less type II diabetes, and according to all the animal studies, far less cancer."

"How much longer life expectancy could one expect?"

LIVE TO 100

"Based on animal studies including monkeys, if you started a caloric restricted diet at age 25 and practice a caloric restriction of say, 20%, I would assume you would live quite a bit longer than those that did not follow such a regime. You would have a huge chance of reaching age 100 in good shape and not crippled over with the ailments of older people. At least that is what the animals' studies show. Now, from my view and mine only, since most scientists do not want to give false hope to anybody, especially when an actual study has not been done on humans for obvious reasons, it would take too long. If you did a 40% reduction at an early age, it is conceivable you could reach age 120 or more. It's almost too much to think about. I have to tell you that you would look very thin at that amount of caloric restriction. But you did ask what was possible. You would also have to make sure you did not accidently starve to death, since your calorie status would be so low each day."

"So, Doctor, would you suggest someone follow such a regime?"

"A 40% reduction? Goodness, no, but we would all benefit from some caloric restriction on an ongoing basis."

David asked, "But how do you acclimate to this lower caloric intake without feeling hungry?"

ENJOY THE JOURNEY

The doctor replied, "It has been shown that you can reduce your caloric intake by up to 20% with no major cravings. Just make sure you are eating real food, which usually includes a lot of fiber. Since your caloric intake will be more limited, cut out eating so much fat. This chops off a lot of calories that won't be missed after following such a diet for several months. Fats can creep into your diet way too easily, as they are used to enhance the taste of so many dishes and recipes. Once you lessen your exposure, or avoid most of them, your taste buds will change. You will start tasting the other flavors of wholesome food. Of course, you still need fats, but not as many as you think or as often as you want them now. A few nuts, a little avocado, some olive oil, an egg, or a piece of fish, all of these will give you some fat. After all, you don't need the extra butter, ice cream, doughnuts, or spare ribs that so many Americans eat."

AN EXAMPLE

The doctor continued, "For many years I would only eat starting at two in the afternoon when I would have a little fruit, a salad, and perhaps some soup. Then around eight at night, I would enjoy a moderate dinner of mostly raw vegetables in a large salad format along with a protein dish. I was only eating about 60% of what most everybody else was consuming, and I had tremendous energy all the time. I felt great and did not miss three meals a day plus snacks. I also don't drink a lot of my calories as many people do. Most people can follow my regimen quite easily as you know you are only several hours away from having a meal. Drink herbal teas in the morning or green teas. Even a cup of coffee is OK. After about two to three weeks, you won't even miss your old routine."

David and the doctor made their way back to the house while the doctor continued, "As we discussed, follow caloric restriction and you most likely will enjoy a long life, free of the many diseases we assume are normal, especially for the elderly. You will also enjoy mobility, clear thinking, and good energy. Unfortunately, most people in our society think small and can't conceive of living to age 100. If enough people followed a well-balanced, caloric-restricted regimen, either through a reduced weekly caloric-intake diet or through periodic fasting, I predict we would experience a paradigm shift – that shift being the realization that we can live a long healthy life, and most surprisingly that opportunity has always been with us. It just took someone like Dr. McCay to bring it to our attention."

RESVERATROL

"Doctor, do you suggest resveratrol to your patients?" David said. "I mean do you think it is of value?"

"Good questions. I will suggest that as one small step that all of us could benefit from is adding a small amount of quality resveratrol to our diets. It may act on the body the same way caloric restriction does. Note, more of this supplement is not better; you simply want some exposure to it each day or every other day. As you may know, it is found naturally in grapes, Japanese knotweed, and even peanut butter. Note that while organic grapes, organic grape juice, or red wine can be a good source, you would need to consume over a hundred glasses per day to equal what a good supplement would give you. Pomegranates and peanuts contain some resveratrol but not enough to prove helpful for mimicking caloric restriction."

"Peanut butter, Doctor, really?"

"Yes, complement your diet with natural food products that contain resveratrol, such as grapes and peanut butter. After all, peanut butter is good as a snack as long as it does not contain hydrogenated oils, which most brands do. And also make sure the brand is tested for aflatoxin, which is a powerful cancer producer, especially within the liver. Most American companies supposedly test their peanuts for this before they proceed with the processing of it into peanut butter. This is usually only a problem in a Third World country and has been reported in the Philippines, where mold-covered peanuts are sold since farmers don't want to lose their entire crop just because of some mold. The problem occurs if someone eats this aflatoxin contaminated product daily or weekly for a prolonged period. The FDA does sample testing, just as most companies do. It has not been a problem here in the United States; however, just to be safe, one brand that does test quite often is Arrowhead Mills."

"Sounds good, Doc. So what brand do you use?"

The doctor smiles and said, "Of peanut butter or resveratrol?"

Smiling back, David said, "Both."

"Arrowhead Mills for peanut butter, and regarding resveratrol supplements, there are so many brands nowadays. Just don't buy a cheap supplement. Make sure it is well prepared and nitrogen packaged to keep its strength. Many such supplements have added supplements such as quercetin, polyphenols, catechins, coca, or IP6. Liquid forms may make sense, as do the products used in prior university and medical studies. A supplement from a company called Longevinex appears to give you the right amount of resveratrol in addition to several other helpful supplements, so that is the product I use."

"So eat real food and not too much. Sounds simple, Doc. What else do you have for me?

WHAT ELSE WOULD YOU RECOMMEND?

"David, in my opinion if you practice moderate caloric restriction your diet should consist of mostly fresh, unprocessed food. Every calorie should count plus you want a feeling of fullness when you eat. Also, don't consume too much protein. Keep protein at no more than 20% of your diet. Keep fat to 20% and that leaves 60% for complex carbs."

"So, when you say fresh, unprocessed food, are you saying raw food?

123

"That's right. Have food as you would have had it thousands of years ago, food in its natural state. All the world's animals consume food this way yet humans insist on cooking, boiling, microwaving, or barbecuing their food."

"That's right, Doctor, when you say it that way it does sound kind of crazy."

"Kind of? David, our society is so turned around that they call raw food practitioners food faddists or worse. I suppose a lot of businesses would stand to lose billions upon billions of dollars if people started insisting that food be served in its more natural state. The sad part is that science has known for over a hundred years that raw food was much healthier for the body. People consuming a diversified mostly raw food diet remain thin and they have so few health problems."

"Wait a moment, you said science knew this? Where is your proof on this, I mean I read all the time and I never heard of these findings."

"Interesting, David, I suppose it's a case of information overload or maybe something deliberate going on called misdirection."

"Misdirection? Really, Doctor, what do you mean by that?"

"Well David, the studies have been done, the reports published but people are not getting the real message. If they really knew what processed food was doing to them, their families, their babies, they would change their ways. At least I hope they would."

ENZYME BANKRUPTCY

"OK, Doctor, but give me some examples."

"OK, David. Remember I said that many good and original studies were done in the 1920s and 1930s? We knew so much then and modern medicine seems to ignore these studies. Truth can be ignored but not changed. A diet of processed food will lead to weight gain, brain shrinkage, and enlargement of our pancreas. None of these three things are healthy in the least. This was known back in 1924. The study was done on albino mice, but the results are the same for humans and other animals. Food for thought: Wild animals have larger and heavier brains than their domesticated counterparts. The reason? Their counterparts, called pets or livestock, are given dead processed food devoid of its enzyme potential. Some scientists feel that our bodies are only capable of producing so many enzymes in one lifetime. If we use these up, trying to process and assimilate processed food, then we use up our precious enzyme reserves and die early of enzyme bankruptcy."

"But, Doctor, I was taught that the body needs very little in enzymes and produces what it really needs."

"David, that is my point. Doing as you say is what causes the pancreas to enlarge as it tries to keep up its enzyme production to deal with eating processed dead food. It will peter out sooner or later, and you will find yourself old, close to death, and enzyme deficient."

"So how do we incorporate this into caloric restriction in an easy fashion?"

"You could take enzyme supplements I suppose, but just by eating food in its natural state you would be getting the right enzymes that naturally come with it, as long as it's fresh and you don't destroy those enzymes by cooking it. Of course, meat should be cooked especially nowadays with most livestock coming from industrial farms."

David stared at the doctor and asked in a sincere voice, "So this is easy to follow?"

"As I have laid out, absolutely. Many years ago, I used caloric restriction to reduce my own weight to an ideal level that was much lower than today's weights and measurements. As I told you, I only ate two meals a day instead of eating three meals a day and snacks. Later on, once my wife and I got to our ideal weight, we then would fast four times a year, counting off the seasonal changes that Mother Nature gives us. It was easy each season to go without food for five to seven days. It wasn't a long fast, but we derived a lot of benefit from them. We broke bad habits, found strength, gained confidence, and felt more energetic than ever. We actually got below our ideal weight, and I feel that has given us the benefit of great health and a long life. Some scientists feel this intermittent fasting is one of the most beneficial ways to practice caloric restriction. It mimics what we faced in nature going back thousands of years. It seems to activate various parts of our bodies to go into survival mode."

ONE LAST THING

"So, Doctor, I am a little confused about this whole process of caloric restriction. Are you saying to restrict the types of foods I am eating or just the amounts?"

"Great point, David. No, I am not saying that you cannot eat what you like or what you are used to eating. However, and as you may know, the word however, often negates what someone has just said. So let me put it this way, I would recommend that you form a different relationship with food to make caloric restriction easier."

"How's that, Doctor?"

"For starters, I mentioned that you will be eating more of your food in its natural state: raw. Of course, you still can consume cooked food, but when you do, it will mostly consist of vegetables, grains, and such. Some staple foods like beans and many grains have to be cooked or else they don't get absorbed properly in your body. But let me be clear on one point, many people that practice caloric restriction will state that they are eating more food each day, not less."

"How can that be, Doctor?"

"David, you will be eating more volume of food, as it takes more fruit, vegetables, and salads to fill you up. Often people who follow a caloric restricted lifestyle will mention that they chew a lot, and that is the point. You should be eating more like our ancestors and chewing wholesome food instead of eating heavily processed foods. Many of today's processed foods dissolve quickly in your mouth, being absorbed by your body too quickly, raising blood sugar levels and turning to fat within your system."

"So, Doctor, you would be consuming a lot of broth-based vegetable soups, salads and such, right?"

"Right, David, a lot of broth-based soups containing a lot of nutrition and not empty calories that a lot of processed foods contain. You can consume a large amount of vegetable soup, cabbage soup, pea soup, miso soup, not to mention soups like pumpkin, squash, beans, and on and on. And it goes without saying that salads are a great choice as you can mix different types of greens and add small amounts of many other types of vegetables and fruit. Also, many people add almond slices or walnuts, not to mention some cheese or lean meat source. Keep in mind that when you are on a caloric restricted diet, you need to focus on food that gives you the most nutritional bang for the buck."

"Such as?"

"I may start to sound like a broken record, David, but focus on fresh vegetables, fruit, wholesome grains that are not overly processed, beans of all kinds which are usually best when cooked, lean sources of protein and nuts and seeds."

"What lean sources of protein do you use, Doctor?"

"Well, David, my wife and I both decided a long time ago that we love animals. So we gave up beef, pork, and poultry. I am not saying that you should give those up, but you should think about your food and what those animals went through before they ended up on your dinner table. When my wife and I saw first-hand how these animals were treated and killed off so early in their lives we decided to stop eating them."

"What are you saying, Doctor? What did you see?"

"We saw cattle being killed as soon as they reached a certain weight. Their lives cut way too short in the name of profits. We saw pigs butchered the same as cattle, being carted off way too young to the slaughterhouses or food processing plants, as they are called."

"Doctor, are you saying people should be vegetarians because of the cruelty shown to farm raised animals? I mean that is why they are farmed raised, so we can consume them right?"

"David, I do not want to get into a deep discussion on this topic. I am just telling you, since you asked how my wife and I look at food. We cannot come to terms with how people can be nice to some animals like their dogs and cats, yet turn around and eat a beautiful cow, pig, lamb, or chicken. It just doesn't sit well with us. By the way, David, these animals did nothing wrong to deserve such a short existence. Also, David, we were shocked when we found out how cruelly dairy cows are treated. The only way a female cow can give milk is if it becomes pregnant. When it does, they have their young babies ripped from them and then are just used for their milk-giving ability. As long as you keep stimulating these cows they will continue to give milk, even though their babies are long gone. When their milk generating ability diminishes, they are sent off to the meat packing plant. Also, the baby cows they had, if female, are slated for the same lifestyle, while the poor males are mostly escorted directly to the slaughterhouse while still babies since they have no milk-giving ability. It just doesn't sit right with me or my wife."

"Are you saying you don't ever eat meat or drink dairy?"

"David, my wife and I do use goat cheese because we know the source. It is from goats that are treated in a humane manner, are left to graze on a natural diet, and free of growth hormones and antibiotics. Most people don't know that there are more people on this planet consuming goat's milk than cow's milk. Goat milk is superior in many ways as it is easier to digest, containing less lactose, and goat's milk is higher in minerals such as calcium, phosphorous, potassium, magnesium and such. So we don't have a problem with cheese made from this milk. We also eat eggs that come from these same farms where the hens are allowed to roam and consume a natural diet and, as you may have guessed, my wife and I consume seafood. So, all in all, we get plenty of protein between the grains, vegetables, nuts, seeds, and the lean sources of protein I just mentioned."

"I see, Doctor, I am just curious, that's all. How much protein should you be consuming on a caloric restricted diet? I would imagine it would be higher, right?"

"Great point, David. First off, most Americans have a poor understanding of protein and what foods really contain it. Most Americans consume too much protein thinking it is required. If most Americans eat a diet of about 15% lean protein, along with healthy carbohydrate choices, and proper fat choices, they would see their energy levels soar. High protein diets will fatigue most people."

"So are you saying to consume just 15% of your calories from protein on a caloric restricted diet?"

"No, not if you are on a caloric restricted diet. Remember, David, your body does require protein for many of its needed functions. What I am saying is not to overdue protein consumption. Keep in mind that many vegetables and grains also contain large amounts of protein. So you don't need a lot of protein from other sources anyways. Most people overdue protein from animal sources thinking somehow it's better for them. Not true. However, if you are on a restricted diet, you still need adequate protein, so in that case, if you are consuming less than 2000 calories a day, you should up your protein percentage to at least 20%. Otherwise leave it at 15%.

THINK QUALITY AND QUANTITY

The doctor continued, "For optimal nutrition think quality and quantity, not just taste. For instance, a tablespoon of butter or peanut butter might taste good but both contain 200 calories. Based on eating quality calories and optimal nutrition, you could instead eat an apple, three stalks of celery, and two slices of turkey. So what would you eat after knowing this? The butter and/or peanut butter? Or the complete snack of fruit, vegetable, and lean protein source?"

"When you say it like that I get the picture. Eat purposefully to get the most nutrition for the calories consumed, right?"

"Right, David. With my clients I use the example of a small bag of potato chips. That is the typical side dish given in many sandwich shops as they hand you your lunch. Think long and hard before eating that snack. Do you want a small personal bag of chips at 400 calories, void of any real nutrition, or in its place for the same amount of calories you could have two pieces of whole grain bread, one egg, a small side of plain yogurt, and a few grapes? It all comes down to eating food in its more natural state. The more natural state of a food, usually the less calories, especially when dealing with carbohydrates and proteins."

"What about fat choices?"

"We all know that fat is different. As the saying goes, 'fat is fat.' It's hard, if not impossible, to get a low caloric form of fat; all you can do is try to get the best form of fat into your diet. Use natural sources found in nuts, avocados, olives, and fish. Avoid all the processed forms if possible, such as heavy saturated meats, dairy, most liquid vegetable oils, and worst of the bunch, hydrogenated shortening."

KEY POINTS
CALORIC RESTRICTION THEORY

- Follow the previous steps outlined for prevention as they apply to caloric restriction as well.

- Always undereat compared to the norm. Most people consume way too many calories each day.

- Only consume nutrient-dense food that contains wholesome ingredients and are known to be good for you.

- Avoid all processed food since it is health destroying. This includes most products that have added sugar, added fat, fried foods, processed meat, most flour products, and products with additional sodium added, etc. Avoid overly processed food found in a jar, prepackaged food, and canned food with some exceptions (sardines). Note many prepackaged soups only look healthy but in fact are laced with artificial taste enhancers and sodium. These taste enhancers damage the brain.

• Shop around the outer rim of the grocery store buying only fresh vegetables, frozen organic vegetables, fresh fruit, and low-fat meat products (if consuming meat). Frozen fish is good, but make sure it was caught in Alaska, Iceland, or other northern cold waters. Consume fish such as cod, salmon, sardines, etc.

• Avoid tuna, swordfish, battered fish (which usually contain flavor enhancers and trans fat oils), most farm raised seafood such as farm-raised salmon, tilapia, or shrimp. Consume lake fish rarely, as it usually is high in contaminants.

• Avoid using too much heavy cream, butter and fat containing sauces like cheese sauce, Alfredo sauce, etc.

• Avoid all processed oils, which mean that they have been hydroge-nated or heat-treated to last longer. These are also known as trans fatty acids or partially hydrogenated oils. Food companies like to sneak them into their products since it extends the shelf life of those products. Many bakeries continue to use these same cheap oils for the same reasons.

• Focus on using only good cold press oils for cooking or for adding to salads and recipes. Keep olive oil on hand for salads. Don't deep fry, as that will convert any healthy oil into unhealthy oil due to its high temperature. If stir frying, then consider non-hydrogenated nut oils like peanut oil or macadamia oil for that. Unprocessed coconut oil is good as a skin cream, on toast, and for baking as well. Also, real butter can be used for baking, as can non-hydrogenated palm shortening.

• Even when consuming healthy oils, do not consume more than 2 to 3 tablespoons total per day. Afterall, fat is fat and always higher in calories than carbohydrates and proteins.

• Shop for organic goods to reduce your toxic exposure to so many heavily sprayed food items. Food companies have convinced people that the abnormal act of spraying pesticides, fungicides and other toxins is normal.

• Load up on wholesome food such as salads, homemade coleslaws, fresh fruit platters, avocados, nut spreads, lightly steamed vegetables, interesting side dishes such as hummus, tabouli, lentils, bean dishes, brown rice, wild rice, and root vegetables of all types.

• Avoid packaged products entirely that are promoted as low fat, no cholesterol, etc. Notice that many of them are cheap carbohydrate products mixed with cheap oils, lots of flour, lots of sodium, and dangerous flavoring agents known as MSG, yeast extract, spices, autolyzed plant protein, hydrolyzed plant protein, textured protein extract, etc., which damage the brain.

• Do use small plates and bowls to serve food. Many people do not know that plates used today are far larger than dishes that were used even forty years ago.

• Avoid using processed food or heavily laden restaurant food in a social setting or as a personal reward. Instead, focus on having a good cup of herbal tea, green tea, oolong tea, or black tea. Coffee is good in moderation but avoid overconsuming as it then drives up cortisol levels mitigating its good effects such as clearing the liver, initiating bowel movements, and helping blood sugar.

• Consider using a supplement called trans-resveratrol. Many studies point to it as a supplement that may mimic caloric restriction by activating some of the same genes such as the SIRT1 gene and the SIRT3 gene. It also seems to positively affect sugar levels, reducing the risk of diabetes, and it may even help reduce beta amyloid plaque, which may lead to Alzheimer's disease, along with protecting against other neuro-degeneration diseases in the brain. Note that more of this supplement is not better; you simply want some exposure to this each day or every other day.

• Commune with nature by taking daily outside walks. Caloric restriction works best when doing a moderate amount of physical activity and consuming real food in its natural state.

• Saturated fats are derived from three sources: animal products, coconuts, and vegetables oils that have been hydrogenated. These hydrogenated vegetable oils are called partially hydrogenated oils, or trans fatty oils. The body can handle a fair amount of saturated fat from animal products and coconuts, but it cannot handle hydrogenated or heat-treated oils that are created by the hydrogenation of normal vegetable oils. While normally most vegetable oils are considered unsaturated or monounsaturated, once you hydrogenated them they can become a very harmful type of saturated oil. The human body has a hard time processing these oils. Likewise, coconut oil is normally a healthy saturated oil, but is turned into an unhealthy saturated oil when hydrogenated. Avoid all hydrogenated oils for this reason.

• Eat a wide variety of food. Most people only consume about 20 different foods, month in and month out.

• Eating eggs and meat, especially fish, several times a week is OK. Your body will need the protein and vitamin B-12. Most people only need 15% to 20% of their diet to consist of protein. However, on a caloric restriction diet, you will need to increase your protein levels since you are consuming less calories overall. Your body stills need enough protein to repair itself. To make sure you have enough protein on a caloric restricted diet, consider moving your protein percentage up from 15% to 20%, to around 25%.

9
Alternative Treatments

David and the doctor had agreed to meet outside the doctor's office at a small coffee shop in downtown Lexington. David entered the coffee shop and was surprised to see how full it was. He stood motionless scanning the room looking for the doctor. Seeing this, the cashier directed David to the doctor who was in the back room.

David made his way across the old wooden floor to an adjacent room that held fewer people. In the corner by a window, he spotted the doctor speaking with an elderly man. Approaching the table, David could hear parts of the conversation. The doctor appeared to be concluding his talk and was discussing what supplement the man might want to consider. The advice was more consultative than instructional.

The doctor was suggesting two brands of enzymes that may aid this man's condition. David overheard the doctor telling the man to take these enzymes six times a day. David waited for the man to depart before closing the distance to the now vacated chair across from the doctor.

The doctor spoke first, "Good morning, David. How's the day treating you?"

Smiling, David responded, "Great, Doc, and I see that you just can't get away from seeing patients."

Smiling back, "Not really a patient, David, just someone seeking free advice."

"Wow, I didn't think doctors gave free advice."

"All the time, David. Every doctor I know is always being approached either outright or in a more subtle fashion for their take on a person's condition."

"So, is that what was happening here?"

"Sure, this man's wife had passed away from pancreatic cancer several years ago. Seems she went through the standard treatment of surgery followed by heavy duty chemo."

"Ouch," replied David, "I hope she didn't suffer too badly."

The doctor hesitated, "She held up pretty well until the end, or so he told me. It seems the chemo was making her very tired but she was not in a lot of pain. Thank God for that at least."

David wanted to know more, "Doc, if you don't mind me asking, why were you discussing enzymes with this man?"

"Sure, I wasn't around to treat this man's wife but I did have a few conversations with him after arriving here. He wanted my opinion on the treatment plan his wife had gone through. He wanted to know my thoughts."

"And...?"

"And, I told him as gently as possible, that with most pancreatic cancer, the surgery procedure called the Whipple procedure, which may be very helpful, must be done as soon as possible. If done without delay, you may actually have a good outcome. But even waiting a few weeks could make a sad difference. After that procedure, many doctors want to do chemo or even radiation, which I find too harsh. People need to look to the alternative world of medicine for a better chance with this cancer."

"Are you saying people are having success against this type of cancer?"

"More than traditional doctors are having. I mean surgery may work if done soon enough, otherwise the treatments doctors are offering only extend the patient's life by a nominal amount and often makes the patient sick. I have seen people being treated by a Dr. Nicholas Gonzalez from New York, who uses enzyme therapy and a clean diet and the results are better than traditional treatments."

"If chemo and radiation treatments don't work so great, why would people do them?"

"Often, people want to turn their case, their cause, their hope for cure, over to a doctor or a team of doctors. Most people want to believe that chemo, radiation, and surgery will eliminate their cancer. Many forms of cancer just don't respond significantly to these treatments. I have to deal with those issues and try to wake them up to other possibilities. Perhaps we would recommend Dr. Gonzalez or Dr. Stanislaw Burzynski out of Texas."

"OK, Doc, what you are saying? Are there other ways to treat cancer than what you have mentioned?"

"Absolutely, the last thing you want to do is completely hand over your treatment to someone else. I mean your life means everything to you, but unfortunately, not as much as it should to others. Many oncologists will give you treatments that they would never take themselves or give to a family member. So my question is why are they giving that treatment to you? Not only are there many viable alternative treatments available, but people need to wake up to the fact that they should have a second and third alternative plan of treatment ready to go."

"Go where, Doc? What do you mean?"

"I am saying that just because a doctor tells you he cut out your cancer, say from your prostate or breast, doesn't mean it is over. While surgery makes a lot of sense and can lead immediately to a good outcome, especially if the cancer is localized, in many cases it does not always get all of the cancer. After surgery, they may want to radiate you or give you chemo, which in itself may cause your demise. What I am saying is that there are also many natural treatments you can do that provide positive aspects to your healing process without harming you. These treatments and protocols are seldom, if ever, discussed by American oncologists. They state they want to follow evidence-based medicine where they can look at studies and results. Well, if that is their yardstick, then have them show you their results and be very careful how they state things. Saying that one study found a response rate to treatment means nothing. Forget the response, was the cancer cured? Worse, are studies that show a small, 4% higher survival rate where the people that did not survive were no longer counted. Amazing but true, these studies are slanted so far to a drug company's advantage that many times no one can say for sure if the drug really provides any benefit."

"Doc, you're saying that you don't like chemo or radiation? That you wouldn't go that route?"

David, "I would use chemo and radiation for some types of cancer but not many. It has a very good outcome for some cancers but not the major killers like colon, lung, brain, stomach, pancreatic cancer or mesothelioma or breast cancer that has spread. By placing the patient on chemo or radiation treatments, the person involved is missing out on some much gentler alternative healing plans."

"Give me an example. Like what would you do for breast cancer?"

AN EXAMPLE PLEASE

"I should note that surgery is not always the best course of action, but with breast cancer, if the cancer is small enough, surgery may be all that is required.

After surgery to remove as much cancer as possible, I would urge that a person start using all the tools they could. I would use selective minerals like selenium, iodine, small amounts of zinc, selective vitamins like a natural vitamin D, spices and herbs such as turmeric extract with ginger, a natural plant-based diet based on the Gerson therapy, digestive enzymes as outlined by Dr. Gonzalez, clean water, a quality omega-3 supplement along with a German treatment called the Budwig treatment that helps rejuvenate your cell membranes and allows for better oxygen utilization. It uses flax seed oil along with organic cottage cheese. It works by restoring cell membrane permeability, which allows for better oxygen utilization and waste removal. To allow this to work, however, you must swear off of all processed oils. No amount of trans fatty oils, hydrogenated oils, or partially hydrogenated oils can be used. Keep in mind that even if a food label states that it has zero grams of trans fats, it still could contain up to one half of one gram. Incredible isn't it? Check your label for the tip off words, partially hydrogenated oil. Most all cooking oils are of this type. Dr. Budwig felt that these dead oils derived from corn, cottonseed, etc. by using extreme heat and chemicals in their processing causes much illness. She felt they changed the electrical charge of our bodies' cell membranes."

David replied, "Dairy, Doctor? For cancer? That sounds like an odd and possibly an old treatment."

"Yes, David, old, not really but odd, that is for sure. Now I would add, while she recommended organic cottage cheese produced without added hormones or growth factors, I note that non-dairy consuming nations like China and Japan have dramatically less breast and prostate cancer to begin with. So my advice is to give up drinking milk and consumption of all cheeses now or if you are fighting breast or prostate cancer. It may activate a growth hormone within our bodies' tissues, especially within our breast and prostate cells. If a non-dairy diet, along with clean eating, does not clear up your cancer then by all means I would implement the Budwig treatment, which does utilize a small amount of dairy. Dr. Budwig felt the cottage cheese was necessary to get the other ingredients into your cells' membranes. So I tell my patients unless you are following the Budwig protocol, consume no dairy. I will add that goat products are less inflammatory than cow's milk, due to its fat structure, particle size, digestibility, and lower sugar content. After all, what other animal consumes another animal's milk, especially when they are grown? If that is not crazy then I don't know what is."

"But, Doc, why would excess dairy fuel cancer?"

"Good question, David. Many breast and prostate cancers are fueled by excess estrogen. The body reacts to this and other chemicals contained within dairy such as pesticides and hormones. These other substances are often referred to as xeno-estrogens. Dairy also increases a form of estrogen called estradiol. Now estrogen can be found in many foods, but with dairy you are getting a high dose of an animal's milk, which is loaded with estrogen and potent growth factors. After all, the mother cow is doing what nature has evolved her to do: help her baby cow grow as quick as possible so it doesn't fall victim to a predator. These growth factors impact humans' reproductive organs such as the breast glands and the prostate gland. Furthermore, today's dairy milk may be too high in casein and lactose, both which may increase inflammation."

"If that's true, Doctor, we should all lower our intake of dairy. Are there any other steps we can do to lower our estrogen intake or estradiol?"

"Sure, David, skip eating so much meat and leave dairy where it belongs: to baby cows. We also have many clients reduce their alcohol intake, as that is a cause of increased estradiol for many. If further reduction is needed, we consider a dietary supplement called DIM."

"What's that stand for?"

"Well, DIM is derived from cruciferous vegetables like broccoli, cabbage, and Brussels sprouts. The full name is dindolylmethane or more properly Di-Indoly Methane, it helps metabolize estrogen."

Smiling, David, replied, "Oh, I see, Doctor, now I know why they just call it DIM. So, back to the Budwig diet, people actually eat this combination of cottage cheese and flax seed oil. What else do you tell them?"

"What is so bad about cottage cheese and flax seed oil anyways? I mean you get a healthy snack along with helping your body better defend itself. As I said, David, I would also tell a person to swear off of sugar, which makes the body acidic, a haven for illness. Excess sugar also dramatically lowers your immune system. It's nearly impossible to defeat cancer unless you dramatically lower your sugar load. I would even add periodic parasite purges to that routine based on the theory that parasites within our body take our needed nutrients and create their own growth hormone, which may stimulate cells into turning cancerous. All around the world, people practice periodic parasite purges, but here we ignore it."

"Really Doctor, many in the medical establishment around here must hate you. Aren't you taking people away from proven treatments that could cure their cancer? I mean parasite purges...you really tell people about this stuff?"

"Yes, I really tell them about all this stuff, but not all at once. It is too much to hear, too much to handle, especially when most people come from a traditional allopathic medical outlook. I mean people want to take a pill or do a procedure and in doing so feel they will solve the problem. Sorry, David, life doesn't always work that way. Really, there is not one way of getting cancer nor should you depend on just one way to treat it. If you look at the track record of most chemo treatments and radiation treatments they are very injurious to the body, spirit, and have poor outcomes in most cases. They do not really cure or delay most major cancers. Now, special chemo agents are a godsend in many blood cancers and rare cancers like testicular cancer, but in many cases, chemo will destroy your health and the very immune system you need to fight cancer. We need to wake up to all of the possibilities as people are fighting back against cancer every day and winning. Of course, you don't want to criticize or judge what others do, especially when dealing with such a scary condition such as cancer."

"But?" said David, trying to draw the doctor out more.

"But is correct, David. I feel that most people approach the cancer dilemma incorrectly."

"How's that, Doc?"

141

"Well, I always ask the patients, 'Why do you think you got the cancer in the first place?' Almost all of them tell me they don't know. So I usually just talk with them for a while, asking exploratory questions as we go."

"And where does that lead you?"

The doctor quickly answered, "As I said, most people have no clue what caused their cancer."

"Why would they? I mean most people are too busy living life, paying bills, taking care of kids, pets, or relatives. So where does that take the conversation?"

"Well, David, most people never stop to examine the effect of their habits, environment, or lifestyle on their health, especially as it relates to getting cancer or avoiding cancer. My role is to get them to stop and identify what they might be doing that allowed cancer to come into their lives. Often people determine when they were exposed to some chemical, usually at work or on the farm. Perhaps they remember many X-rays that they had taken or some other exposures like the summer job they had working around heavily sprayed lawns."

David was quick to state, "But, Doctor, you're not saying that people are to blame for getting cancer are you? I mean, they don't need a guilt trip on top of the illness, do they?"

"No, David, no one needs a guilt trip on top of such a serious illness as cancer, but people need to wake up to the fact of 'cause and effect.' I simply try to make them aware that advanced cancer almost always develops after we have inflicted some type of insult to our body."

LOOKING FOR THE CAUSE

"OK," replied David. "But, even if you could track down what may have caused their cancer, what use is that? I mean they already have the cancer, right?"

"That's correct, David. However, when one identifies what may be causing the harm and removes the harmful agent, then one can, many times, help resolve the issue. Of course, some insults can't be removed, and those cancers need to be dealt with differently. Often, however, I feel it is their personal terrain. That terrain being their own body's environment that has been compromised from a harmful diet."

"Doc, doesn't that go against current cancer research? I mean I have always read that cancer is brought on by something that causes harm to the cells or tissue then progresses to cancer. You know, damage to our genes can lead to cancer. I mean once it starts, you have to get rid of it, right?"

The doctor interrupted, "David, what I have to say may sound unconventional, to say the least, but hear me out. What I try to make clear to people is that something they have been doing led them to this point in their life. That something could be as simple as not filtering out the chlorine in their water supply as they took showers or perhaps a host of other things like a high estrogen diet, pesticides in their food, or bad habits like smoking and drinking. Also, possibly very harmful is consuming a diet of yeast- and fungus-forming food – which can result from, you guessed it, a diet of processed food, high sugar foods, acid-forming foods, too much alcohol, and hydrogenated fats. Now other secondary factors could be at play as well, such as a lack of digestive enzymes in their food supply or your body's pH levels."

David interjected, "Doc, I hear you, but removing what caused your cancer doesn't equate to stopping or removing your current cancer, does it?"

"It makes little sense to me to treat a current cancer if the offending agents are still there, so first I would remove those offending agents, if possible. Second, I would build up the body to have it fight the cancer, as it was your body that allowed cancer to take hold in the first place. As you know, we all get cancer every day on a very small scale, but the body deals with it on an ongoing basis. As scary as this sounds, take comfort that a truly healthy body does in fact know how to deal with this process. Just as our hearts beat constantly, your body deals with abnormal cells all the time."

"OK, Doc," replied David, "But I have to tell you that in my study of the cancer process, I learned that typically a carcinogen damages a cell's chromosomes

143

and causes that cell to malfunction and starts an endless growth progression of that cell. That growth, once started, needs to be dealt with."

"David, you are making my point. Why do Americans get so much more breast, prostate, and colon cancer? Is our DNA more prone to being damaged than a typical Japanese person. I don't think so. However, accepting your view on cancer and its progression, then what you would want to do is to protect that cell from genetic damage and the mutation process in the first place, correct?"

"Of course," said David, "keep it from initiating into cancer."

"Well," responded the doctor, "Let's deal with that aspect first, as it just makes sense. But note, later I want to address how your body can be prompted to deal with this genetic damage as it does millions of times a day and the other support mechanisms the body has in dealing with cancer, including the power of enzymes and our cell's metabolism, two crucial items often overlooked by cancer specialists to the loss of their patients. But, David, using the common belief that we should prevent the genetic damage from occurring in the first place, we should look at another level of anti-aging that naturally follows prevention and caloric restriction. Just as those two main methods unified to establish a good health foundation, the next step aids the body and sets up all the other steps to work much better."

"OK," said David, "Let's discuss that."

KEY POINTS

- Prevention is much better than needing a cure.

- Always have a back up plan. Too many cancer patients wait and rely on conventional doctors to cure them. What happens if their treatments fail or are deemed ineffective for your type of cancer? Have several alternative plans of action ready to go. Do your own research as well, as the life you may save could be your own.

10
Free Radical Theory
Theory III

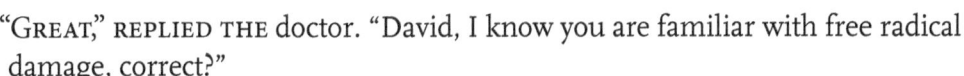

"GREAT," REPLIED THE doctor. "David, I know you are familiar with free radical damage, correct?"

"Of course, Doctor. Free radicals are just atoms with unpaired electrons. Since they are missing some of their electrons, they want to borrow those missing electrons from another atom. So this creates instability amongst the atoms, because if an atom takes an electron from one atom then that atom will want to take an electron from another atom, and it starts a destructive chain reaction. That chain reaction is called oxidative stress or free radical damage. To counter this, we need to consume antioxidants, since antioxidants are molecules that inhibit the oxidization of other molecules." David chuckled. "I will never forget that topic because of an example my college professor used with our class back in the 1970s when we had high gas prices. People were actually stealing other people's gasoline from their cars. Now it only took a few bad apples to do this, but it seemed that when they stole the gas, they many times never replaced the gas caps. So adding insult to injury, people found themselves minus a tank of gas and their gas cap missing. Now most people are pretty honest and wouldn't steal someone else's gas, but when it came to gas caps, that was a different matter. After all, they only cost a couple of bucks back then and you really shouldn't drive your car without a gas cap. So even honest people, finding themselves in a bind, would borrow someone else's gas cap. When that someone else noticed their gas cap gone they would do likewise, starting off a chain event that went across the country. Is that about right, Doc?"

"Yes, David, but it sounds like you are explaining cap and trade theory," said the doctor with his own heartfelt chuckle. "Really, you give a good description of Free Radical Theory, but let me add that while Denham Harman first proposed this theory in the 1950s, he was first in stating that free radicals could be a problem in biological life, free radicals were well known in chemistry. Moses Gomberg discovered this reactionary process back in 1900 at the University of Michigan. He found free radicals pertain to atoms and molecules. While many free radicals are short lived, others are not. This means both can create a lot of mischief in our bodies, causing diseases and aging. Many free radicals are produced by the combustion process. Since our bodies use oxygen for fuel and chemical reactions to produce energy in our bodies all the time, our bodies are constantly dealing with these highly reactive free radicals. Since being proposed, Free Radical Theory has grown to encompass and describe much of the destructive processes that occur in our bodies due to oxidative action. Many people are convinced that too many free radicals prematurely age us and diminish our health capacity."

"So, Doctor, you agree, don't you?"

"For the most part, but, I have to tell you that this oxidative story is still unfolding. In 1954, Dr. Rebecca Gerschman was one of the first to recognize that free radicals in excess are toxic, leading Denham Harman to propose the Oxidative Theory of Aging in Biological Systems, now called the Free Radical Theory. An additional reason for aging was theorized by Dr. Leslie E. Orgel. In the early 1960s, he theorized that aging may be brought on by damage to the DNA and impairing its ability to reproduce itself correctly after being damaged. Even small errors in this process could impede the cell's ability to function optimally. Of course, this theory led him to speculate the exact nature of the error, its mechanisms and pathways. Many scientists feel his theories do not hold up. However, they may be missing the point. What he was saying was oxidative damage was occurring probably in the DNA, but he couldn't be clear on the exact nature of that oxidative damage. We now know that damage may be undermining our cells energy factories, mitochondria, as well as shortening our DNA's telomeres, causing premature aging. You see, everything is related. It all flows like a pathway to health, one step on top of the other. If one step is missed you will stumble on the path. So this is why we need to practice prevention and caloric restriction along with supplying the body a constant stream of antioxidants. It helps deal with the oxidative damage that life brings us, especially the assaults from our environment that are certain to come our way."

ANTIOXIDANTS

"Excuse me, Doctor, I see your point and I agree it's all connected, but isn't that why people take their vitamins and antioxidants? To fight these free radicals?"

"Right, but, David, I can assure you that you must approach the oxidative part of living with care and use natural antioxidants in food when possible, as they usually come wrapped with other powerful synergistic compounds as well. Supplements are just what they are, supplements. For instance, our bodies produce their own natural antioxidants such as catalase, glutathione, and superoxide dismutase, which is usually abbreviated to SOD. These antioxidants are far stronger than ones found in pills and are made available to all the cells in our bodies. Many scientists now feel that it is ingesting natural foods that trigger these antioxidants within us that are really beneficial and not just taking an alphabet soup of antioxidants in pill form."

David added, "So how do we choose natural antioxidants then?"

"It's quite easy. Focus on getting the majority of your antioxidants from the food you eat. I note a healthy, mostly plant-based diet produces more of the antioxidant SOD in the body naturally. Don't rely on taking one or two handfuls of various supplements, as it just won't work. We really must focus on eating real food filled with antioxidants, not just a select amount of supplements, as we really don't know what may be helping our bodies."

David focused his gaze on the doctor, "Are you sure about that?"

"Very sure about that, David. I have seen too many people that eat poorly try making up for that bad habit by consuming a vast amount of supplements. Far better to focus in on good eating habits like avoiding bad fats, bad carbs, and the bad protein choices, like high-fat luncheon meats, fatty sausage, and greasy burgers and instead focus on eating a varied diet of green plants, berries, unprocessed nuts, grass-fed meat, high omega-3 wild fish, and seasonal fruit."

AN APPLE A DAY

"So, Doctor, you are saying to get most of your antioxidants naturally, if possible, and that your body likes them that way?"

"Yes, David, if you can ingest your antioxidants naturally, then your body does know what to do with them. It prefers them this way versus just taking a supplement. The problem with supplements is that will usually be missing synergistic ingredients."

"Give me an example."

"Its simple, David, like in, eat an apple a day."

"Really, how's that going to help?"

"Well, if you are eating an organic apple, it may help quite a bit. It has been known for years that eating an apple every day had many health benefits. They are loaded with polyphenols, which according to several studies extend life dramatically, reduce the signs of aging, and protect us from heart disease and cancer."

"All that protection in an apple?"

"Well, as you know, apples have soluble fiber along with polyphenols and catechins, which really seem to decrease visceral fat which is the type of fat that increases insulin resistance within our bodies. Just make sure you are eating organic apples, as commercial apples tend to have a high pesticide residual to them. I also recommend combining a green apple along with a red apple each day. Sour green apples may contain the most beneficial protection. Simply cut them up and eat these slices with a good snack such as peanut butter or nut spread. A great snack."

"So are you saying an apple itself is better than a supplement?"

Smiling, the doctor replied, "Right, David, I mean you can either take the apple by itself or take a supplement in its place or with it."

"Such a supplement would be what, Doctor?"

"Apple polyphenols is a supplement that can be taken along with apples or by themselves. It contains a high amount of polyphenols that seem to increase an enzyme in our bodies called catalase."

"So is this natural for us, I mean these polyphenols?"

"Yes, David, in our primitive environment we would forage for food, many of them containing polyphenols. This would have made them one of the largest antioxidants groups we would have consumed. Most people think we can simply just take a handful of antioxidants to protect us from oxidative stress, but it is more complicated than that. Remember, David, the body will create its own antioxidants if given the proper nutrients from our diet. Such a diet would allow our body to create natural antioxidants within like catalase, glutathione, superoxide dismutase, or SOD as we call it, and methionine reductase. That is why we need to eat fresh fruit, berries and such."

"So do you recommend supplements to your patients or not?"

"I do, but usually after they demonstrate that they are consuming a pretty healthy diet. Then we supplement with various supplements mostly depending on the results of their blood work."

"How's that, Doc; I mean, what tests?"

"We test for vitamin D levels, folic acid levels, vitamin B-12, total cholesterol, HDL, LDL, C-reactive protein, homocysteine levels, iron levels, estrogen, testosterone, creatine, and many others."

"Any surprises there? I mean as you view a person's blood work?"

VITAMIN D

"Absolutely, we often find that many people are low on vitamin D, which, if low, can impact your immunity, increase your chances of getting osteoporosis, and sadly, cancer as well."

David's voice rose an octave, "Cancer? Really, Doctor?"

"Yes, David, and another real surprise is I have observed high levels of iron as being very bad for people long term."

"But Doctor, I want to slow down and cover the vitamin D and cancer connection, but now that you mention it, why would iron be a problem?"

"OK, David, but be aware that the reason I mentioned high iron levels is because I have observed that high iron levels seem to increase cancer just as high levels of nickel, cadmium, lead or arsenic seem to do. That's why blood testing is so important. We, along with the patients, really need to see what is going on in their system before we can make any recommendations."

"Wow, Doc, no one seems to be talking about this stuff. I mean I have heard that high arsenic levels cause cancer and I know industrial contaminants like chromium or nickel and benzene can cause cancer, but iron?"

IRON

"Right David, the dose is the poison; even iron can kill you if the body takes in too much. But the real poison metals, as we know, are arsenic, beryllium, cadmium, hexavalent chromium, lead, mercury and such. However, saying this, know that too much iron can kill you as well. I learned a long time ago that dead is dead, regardless of how you got there. Now a lack of iron is the number one cause of anemia in this country and that has led to many people using iron supplements. Mostly iron-deficient anemia can be traced to losing blood or poor diet. Many people openly have these iron supplements sitting around in pill form, liquid form or in their daily vitamins, not to mention iron-fortified food. Too many children die each year because of an accidental iron overdose, mostly from supplements they find in the household. Now if you are getting too much iron in your diet, the symptoms are much more subtle, but high iron levels will certainly lead to premature aging. I note that people with a genetic disorder called hemochromatosis can quickly succumb to iron overload and die quite rapidly, usually from liver failure. At first, many of their symptoms mimic accelerated aging. Iron overload can easily damage the heart, kidneys, liver and cardiovascular system. Even if you do not die from liver failure, it can increase your chances of getting liver cancer and be a real factor in other cancers."

"But, Doctor, how many people really suffer from that disorder?"

"It's not common at all, but I'm just saying high iron levels can lead to ill health. I test my patients and note about 10% have too high of levels of iron. About 1% of them have dangerous levels. It's a cheap blood test to find out if they are heading in the wrong direction."

"Do you note a difference between sexes?"

"Yes, mostly men suffer the ill effects. I think that is because women lose some iron when they menstruate. Also, men tend to eat more meat, which contains a highly absorbable type of iron called heme iron. As people get into their late 50s and beyond, then both sexes can equally get iron overload. It may be a reason why both men and woman start getting the same amount of heart disease at that age."

David responded, "So what does all this have to do with the Antioxidant and Free Radical Theory of Aging?"

"Good point, David. High amounts of metals causes oxidative damage, mainly through free radical damage. I have seen this when people consume too much iron or too much copper."

"OK, Doc, so what do you recommend?"

"Watch your metal intake! I don't like copper surfaced cookware, especially if you have copper water pipes, this can be a major problem if your water is acidic. I don't like to see people use iron cookware indiscriminately nor do I like to see them consume too much meat. Yes, we need enough iron if we are to live, but too much will cause you great harm. Know what you are doing before you run into problems. It helps if you see the connections."

CONNECTIONS

"The connections, Doc?"

"Keep in mind, David, that while we need iron, too much can cause oxidative damage. We will cover that later in much more detail. But for now I want to focus on oxidative damage and the power of antioxidants. The connections I am speaking of concern things we do; they really do impact us. One thing leads to another. For instance, drinking something like orange juice can accelerate the absorption of iron, while drinking black tea can inhibit it. Most people have no clue about these connections, and they can cause harm to their bodies by doing the same things over and over. So if you get a man who likes his steak, likes his orange juice, and also takes vitamin C with his meals, well, he could have potential high iron levels. Of course, if he is a moderate drinker of alcohol as well, then his iron levels could soar even higher. See, when I look at people I see these connections all the time. But most people are oblivious to it all. But for now let me say high mineral or metal intake can cause excessive aging. We will discuss this Mineral Overload Theory of Aging later, which may be the most overlooked theory of aging out there."

David inquired, "So too much iron can be oxidative and harm the body. What else do you mean by connections?"

"Fluoride is a huge insult to our bodies and too many people consume way too much."

"Fluoride, Doc? Harmful? Doc, first you tell me my dentist poisoned my kids with mercury fillings, now you're telling me they are hurting my children with fluoride. I mean my kids get fluoride treatments every year. You don't mean that fluoride, do you?"

PINK POISON

"Yup, that innocent looking pink gel or red colored rinse they put in your children's mouths is a poison. But, David, I want to deal with that later when we go into detail about minerals and your health. Just say no to fluoride treatments in the future. Your children are getting way too much now in their toothpaste and in city water."

"But, Doctor, you can't tell me something like this and expect me to wait for more information?"

"For now, let me say that fluoride causes mischief in several ways. It decreases antioxidant enzymes like catalase (CAT), superoxide dismutase (SOD), and phospholipid hydroperoxide glutathione peroxidase (GSH-PX). Worse than that may be its effect on the pineal gland and the thyroid gland. These glands control our metabolism and almost all of our body functions. Women who consume too much fluoride or not enough iodine may gain weight quickly. So while I mention the negative effects of fluoride and oxidative stress, I also note that all the theories of aging and anti-aging are closely interrelated. Fluoride is one of many items that's a foe in the pursuit of good health. I point out the mischief it can do while discussing oxidative damage as we are now discussing and the Free Radical Theory of Aging, but I also discuss it with my patients when discussing the Mineral Overload Theory of Aging, the Endocrine Theory of Aging, and of course, when we first discuss the Prevention Theory of Aging. It all really does interact."

"But, Doctor, why don't we hear more about this connection?"

"David, I know that fluoride was used as a rat poison for many years. Now when physicians first spoke in favor of fluoride they were speaking of the small amount found naturally in several Southwestern states. That naturally occurring element, in small amounts, seems to help prevent cavities. Even that type can still cause problems. Keep in mind, even the natural fluoride can damage your teeth by causing pitting and a mottled and stained appearance. Now for a reality check concerning natural fluoride, around the world it has been estimated that over 50 million people have been negatively impacted by naturally occurring fluoride found in their water supply, mostly around granite rock areas. It causes severe damage to their bone structure. This fluorosis cripples and disfigures people. Their limbs become bowed and appear rubber-like, not to mention useless. It's a horrible, life-crippling condition, something you would not wish upon your worst enemy. This condition occurs a lot in India, China and other countries. As bad as this natural fluoride is, however, and as much misery had it has had on people, it is not as poisonous as the type of fluoride they are adding to our water or toothpaste. The stuff they are adding is far worse. The stuff they add is pure poison, and if it appears to work at all I can't help but speculate it's because this poison may impact the bacteria in your mouth, as many poisons might do."

"This is incredible, Doctor. Tell me more."

The doctor continued, "Five to ten grams of sodium fluoride is all that is needed to kill someone. Remember, this is the same type of fluoride that was used in many insecticides and rodenticides before companies began changing many of their formulas to something less toxic. They now use blood thinners in rat poison. Most public water systems use fluorosilicic acid or sodium fluorosilicate. This stuff is pure poison and probably worse than what they first started using in our water supplies to fluorinate it. I remember a quote from a noted scientist, Dean Burk, Ph.D., former head of the National Cancer Institute's Cytochemistry Sector, 'In point of fact, fluoride causes more cancer death, and causes it faster, than any other chemical.' And, David, fluoride particles are very small and very negative. They interfere with enzyme function on every level. So this toxic mineral also is negatively involved in the Enzyme Theory of Aging as well."

"Doc, as I've said before, how can they be allowing this stuff in our lives?"

"Great question, check out fluoride on any search engine and you will get the answer: profits."

"I will check it out, Doctor. Back to antioxidants, we were discussing their impact on longevity. I've been writing about many things that seem to confer antioxidants. For instance, I've written about antioxidants and their direct impact in maintaining good health. I also read Jean Carper's books on antioxidants and her food book. She made the case along the lines that just a carrot a day could lower your stroke risk by two thirds. Do you attribute that to its antioxidant content?"

"Could be, David. Carrots have good fiber, beta carotene, and potassium as well. But as you mentioned Jean Carper has written several bestsellers, and I feel that she does a great job in explaining what antioxidants are readily available in our foods. And while you are reading her books, note the studies she quotes on tea drinkers."

"Refresh my memory, Doc."

"She wrote about studies in Japan that show green tea greatly reduces the chance of getting lung cancer, even in smokers."

"Doc, that's great because I love tea, but I've also heard that our black tea here is not as heavy in antioxidants."

"True, David, black tea has been heated up, which destroys many of its antioxidants. While it still has other good things in it, green tea would certainly be better. Another good choice is using oolong tea. That's what many Chinese use, and it is processed more than green tea but not as much as black tea."

"So drinking tea is a great way to get antioxidants then."

"Sure, but it's ironic that we are discussing tea, David; just be aware most tea, especially instant tea, contains a large amount of naturally occurring fluoride. So make sure you don't use fluoride water to brew it with or you will be getting a larger dose of fluoride than you were expecting."

"Really, Doc? I've not heard of that before, and it seems we just can't get away from this stuff."

"David, there's lots of quirky things out there. You research science all the time, so you know that most people have no real knowledge of what you know, is that correct?"

"Right, Doc. My wife thinks I'm making stuff up all the time. I mean when I tell her about the studies for cervical cancer and such, she finds it hard to believe that we can take so many steps to prevent it."

FOLIC ACID

"Yes, I read your article on that topic," the doctor said. "You covered the benefit of having sufficient folic acid in your system to help prevent cervical cancer. I think your article covered a lot of bases, including how folic acid is also necessary for the repair of our DNA."

"Thanks, Doc, I just was reporting on the work done by Dr. Charles Butterworth. That doctor had written about the benefit of eating a little broccoli every day."

"I am glad he said to get your folic acid or real folate as it is from real vegetables, since the folic acid found in supplements is not the same as the naturally occurring folate you find in food."

"Huh? Run that by me again, Doc."

"The folic acid you get in most vitamin supplements is derived from folate but in an over-oxidized form, negating much of its good benefits. You should focus on a good diet containing folate, like the doctor indicated, from natural stuff like real food."

"So, Doctor, the folic acid we all are taking in our vitamins isn't really the real thing?"

"I guess you could say that. Most manufacturers use a cheaper form of synthetic folic acid, not real folate. Lately, some better vitamin companies are using a better form, called 5-MTHF or L-methylfolate, which is much more bioavailable, but nothing beats the real stuff found in green leafy vegetables. Some companies also offer these good folate supplements under the name of folinic acid or simply refer to it as a bioactive form of folate, which is much better than a regular folic acid supplement. We don't recommend that most people go heavy on a folic acid supplement but instead just tell them to eat a good leafy salad everyday along with several servings of vegetables, as you want real folate. Besides, too much of a folic acid supplement may hinder a proper diagnosis of a vitamin B-12 deficiency or anemia, which I know you are aware of. There are many forms of anemia, but they all share one common trait, they cause the red blood cells to be lacking or not correctly developed. Is the anemia caused from lack of iron, lack of stomach acid causing B-12 not to be absorbed, lack of enough folic acid, or some other cause? That's why we need to test a patient's blood. With our older patients we always test their levels of vitamin B-12 to make sure they are not deficient, especially if we think they have been taking a folic acid supplement on their own. A lack of good vitamin B-12 levels may lead to mental disorientation in these older people."

"So, it really does make a lot of sense to test your blood. What do you think about the studies that show too little or too much folic acid can lead to cancer?"

"Good question, David. Most people, including doctors, have not heard of any connection but as you mention it may be a problem with people taking high doses of synthetic folic acid. That question really concerns the supplement folic acid and not the real eating of folate heavy foods. There are several studies that show consuming too much synthetic folic acid may increase cancer. It seems the body can only handle a small amount of this synthetic type of folic acid at a time and the rest pours into the body causing mischief. Dr. Joel Fuhrman writes about this danger on his website. I read a lot of his articles, as I feel he is an original thinker. He reported on a meta-analysis concerning folic acid supplementation, which found that it may indeed increase cancer risk both in men and women. He also cited several studies, which I followed up on and found to be very credible. So like most things in life, proceed with caution when using synthetic supplements instead of real food. For instance, I don't think anybody really believes eating a lot of salad bars is going to cause an increase in cancer unless you're ingesting a lot of pesticides. Do you?"

157

EAT YOUR SPINACH

David responded, "I don't think so either, Doc, but you never know. So, what I am hearing from you, is that you think too much of the supplement folic acid is not the same as getting the real stuff from spinach or other salad greens, eggs, and such."

"Right, David. I still remember when researchers at the Lederle Labs developed this stuff. They created a crystalline substance. That supplement was a fully oxidized synthetic chemical compound. While helpful for many people who do not have access to real food, it is no substitute for the real thing. The same thing goes for antioxidants like vitamin A, vitamins C, E, and minerals that can assist antioxidants systems in the body like selenium and magnesium. You should get them from real foods not supplements, whenever possible."

"So do you use vitamin supplements, Doc?"

"Absolutely. I use a balanced vitamin E that includes gamma-Tocopherol, R-lipoic acid, resveratrol, magnesium, yeast produced selenium, melatonin at night, and others, but not everyday. I prefer to get most of my antioxidants from fruit like grapes, blueberries and various green leafy vegetables like spinach, kale, and lettuce. That way I'm getting a wide variety of vitamins, flavonoids, polyphenols, lycopene, carotenes, lutein and lignans. I also feel we are getting positive stuff from real food that we are not even aware of as it has not all been researched enough."

"Doc, do you take coenzyme Q-10?"

"Yes I do, but not every day."

VITAMIN E

"What about vitamin E?"

"Well, what about it?"

"You know," said David, "How a major study of other studies on vitamin E showed it to be ineffective. That study compared it to the beta-carotene study showing that taking it in a supplement form may actually hurt your health."

The doctor shrugged, "Oh those studies. Honestly, I don't think much of many meta-studies because they can be designed to come up with almost any answer they are looking for. A meta-study is a lot like data mining, you can input various questions and end up with the answers you were looking for. So to put it simply, the meta-study on vitamin E that showed it to be ineffective did not start with the right set of questions."

"Like?"

"Well, David, they looked at people taking vitamin E but didn't note the difference between those folks who took natural vitamin E from those that took a synthetic form, which I believe to be a garbage product. Furthermore, they did not note that even people that took natural vitamin E supplements mostly used alpha-tocopherol, ignoring the crucial gamma-tocopherol, which our bodies seem to like better. Vitamin E, which is useful to protect our DNA from damage and it allows for reproduction ability in animals including humans, is actually a family of eight types of vitamin E. So just taking one form may not get the job done and taking a synthetic form may not work at all."

David chuckled, "Doc, that's a mouthful. I mean you really have thought about those studies, haven't you?"

"Of course, David. I mean I have not only thought about them, I lived the history of it. I have seen vitamin E discovered, used, built up, abused, put down, and now ignored. Knowing all the details, it's hard for me to not get incensed about all the nonsense some people are writing about."

"Tell me more, Doc."

"During the 1920s and 1930s lots of nutritional discoveries were made. Around 1922, Herbert Evans along with Katharine Bishop from the University of California, Berkeley, uncovered the need of a substance in our diet which helped with reproduction. That substance was vitamin E. They found it in green leafy vegetables and grains. It made sense, as they tested various diets on animals and noted major problems in the ability to reproduce and looked at the diet they were feeding these test animals. That diet was loaded with animal fats and they concluded that animal fats tend to oxidize leaving little essential vitamin E left over for needed reproduction ability as the animals were not producing live babies. Based on their research, I believe a high animal fat diet uses up a lot of our antioxidants and it makes sense to add selective antioxidants like vitamin E to our diets."

"So what conditions would vitamin E help with?"

"It's hard to prove, but many studies show many conditions benefit from vitamin E supplementation. I would expect brain function to improve, protection from Alzheimer's, Parkinson's, dementia, strokes, heart disease, DNA damage, and possibly cancer."

"Wow, that's a long impressive list..."

"David, for years, stating in the 1940s, two medical doctors in Canada helped thousands of patients. Doctors Wilfrid Shute and Evan Shute, believed that vitamin E offered numerous health benefits. My recollection is that they felt vitamin E helped break down blood clots within our circulatory system and allowed for better overall circulation. This would also help our heart rhythm. They treated scores of heart patients."

"Tell me more about them."

"The Shutes used vitamin E therapy for decades and treated thousands of people with cardio problems with good results, a real success story at the time. That generated a lot of controversial comments from the medical community but positive press from the community at large. They found vitamin E helpful for a host of conditions like angina, fibroids, endometriosis, atherosclerosis, wound healing, skin ulcers and heart ailments."

"Any conditions you would recommend vitamin E for?"

"I would add that proper vitamin E supplementation helps protect brain neurons from damage by free radicals, so using it may delay brain disorders. I note that when I use vitamin E, my immune function seems to improve. You need to purchase a quality product, however, and make sure it is fresh and not near its expiration date. Ironically, David, new studies show taking a full spectrum vitamin E supplement that contains all eight forms can really increase the thickness of your hair. I think that recent finding will encourage people to start using vitamin E again."

"Any others that you use?"

"Well yes, David, I use several like vitamin C and N-acetyl-L-cysteine together before I fly on airplanes to protect my hearing."

"Does it work?"

"What?"

Dave, speaking louder, "Does it work?" Then he hesitated before smiling. "Oh, I get the joke, Doc."

"Sorry, David, but you set yourself up for that one."

They both laughed.

David made several notes and both of them made their way from the back room of the coffee shop to the front section. The doctor wanted to buy them both lunch. David was anticipating a good solid sandwich as he had only eaten a small piece of toast that morning with a mouthful of eggs. He had taken a small portion of his wife's breakfast instead of getting his own.

David's anticipation turned to disappointment however when the doctor only ordered two cups of the vegetable soup. Caloric restriction be damned thought David. They sat back down at a different table. This time they were by the street observing traffic flow. The bright daylight was pouring through the windows and its heat felt good, especially with the coffee shop's air conditioner running full speed. The doctor put on his sunglasses and directed the conversation further.

SUNGLASSES

"David, do you protect your eyes?"

"Sometimes, Doc, I know that the sun can damage your eyes and cause cataracts. Of course, most people know that now so I suppose more people are wearing sunglasses."

"Right, and we think macular degeneration may be caused by too much sun over the years as well."

"Right, Doc, I have heard of that, and many healthcare people feel that an antioxidant cocktail of different supplements can help delay that effect."

"I would think so. I mean the eyes use several antioxidants for protection. Otherwise the integrity of the macula is compromised with devastating effects. A good amount of the right antioxidants really seems to delay the progression of this. I like using fresh blended vegetable and fruit juice for our patients. We have them take two glasses of fresh prepared juice a day using carrots, greens, blueberries, etc. To be sure we are doing everything possible, we also will recommend a balanced antioxidant supplement."

"I've heard of that. Does yours contain vitamins A, C and E?"

"Yes, but we use two forms of A, and a mixed vitamin E along with some zinc, a very small amount of copper along with lutein, zeaxanthin, bilberry, grape seed extract, and several other ingredients depending on the patient's profile."

"Wow, that's a lot to take every day."

"Not every day, but often. It's easier than you think, we use a general liquid vitamin mix then we supplement around that with high quality R-lipoic acid, but some people do fine with the cheaper alpha-lipoic acid. We don't go overboard as you want most of your supplements from natural sources like food. I mean even a supplement like lutein can cause side effects if given in too large of a dose."

"With lutein, do you mean side effects like yellowing of the skin?"

"That's right, just like carotenes found in plants and fruit that give them color, too much can turn you yellow. Besides, lutein by itself may not work effectively in older people as they need the ability of the body to convert that lutein into something else called Meso-Zeaxanthin, which seems harder for older people to do. However, too high of levels of Meso-Zeaxanthin from supplements may even make you dizzy. So we don't over do it. We normally only use a small amount of Meso-Zeaxanthin if the patient is already taking lutein and zeaxanthin."

"Doctor, have you heard about Super-Zeaxanthin?"

"I am impressed that you are aware of that formula, David. Yes, when a patient is diagnosed with macular degeneration, especially at the early stages, we use all the tools we can. We will have the client order up some super zeaxanthin from a company called Life Extension. We found their product to be pretty darn good. Their formula is the only one I know of that contains all three: lutein, zeaxanthin, and Meso-Zeaxanthin. They even include astaxanthin, a type of carotenoid found in krill and other sea creatures, and it is very powerful. It helps protect the eyes and your body. If you want the inside track on that, look up Dr. Mark Tso's research. He specializes in eye research so I would recommend that you see his latest papers. In short, astaxanthin may be one of the most powerful antioxidants known to help protect the eye from the sun's ultraviolet radiation. Since it is not normally in the average American's diet, I would periodically supplement with it. It is a very powerful antioxidant and is capable of crossing the blood-brain barrier, which many antioxidants cannot."

David replied, "I have heard conflicting reports on whether antioxidants can help prevent macular degeneration. It seems that you feel we really can do something preventive about it."

KRILL CAPSULES

"Absolutely," responded the doctor. "For protection, your eyes use carotenoids, like zeaxanthin found in colored vegetables such as kale, along with lutein, but make sure you are also either taking an astaxanthin supplement or consuming krill oil capsules for extra protection."

"How's that, Doc? I mean why krill capsules? I've seen them for sale, but they can be pricey."

"Right, but remember it's your health. Pay now or pay later. The reason I like krill oil is that it naturally contains astaxanthin and omega-3 oils. That makes it a good antioxidant plus a source for omega-3 oils, which help keep your arteries and heart healthier along with helping most cells in your body. But more on that later, David, when we talk about the Membrane Theory of Aging. Let me just say, I am a big believer in using omega-3 oils to keep your cell membranes healthy, which may make all the difference in your quest for good health. Saying this, if you are taking fish oil or krill oil, always take a taste test when you first get them. You need to bite into a capsule to make sure it is not rancid. Otherwise you will be doing more harm than good. As always, David it is buyer beware. If your supplement passes the taste test, store them in your refrigerator to help them from going rancid."

David responded, "Great advice, I've heard about the heart benefits but not the cell membrane part. Do you care to explain?"

"Sure. All of us benefit greatly from having healthy cell membranes. Many of us think of our bodies as machines. That is very inaccurate, as the body does more in a single day than all machines ever built have ever done. The amount of processes occurring in our bodies on a minute by minute basis is truly amazing. We have trillions of cells in our body performing functions like metabolizing, replicating, processing food, utilizing enzymes, converting energy, doing cellular respiration and getting rid of waste products. Anything we can do to allow the proper nutrients into our cells and to expedite the waste products out will be a real benefit. Good omega-3 fats do just that."

"Wow, Doc, so you get eye protection plus heart and cell protection all in one pill?"

"Right, David, all that and more. Omega-3 has been shown to reduce depression, maintain proper memory, turn down inflammation, improve your immunity, and in my opinion reduce the chances of getting skin cancer."

"Skin cancer?"

"Yes, David, our cell membrane structure is crucial for the cell's protection. When you give a cell the nutrients it needs to protect itself, it will better handle harmful things like UVB rays, which, after all, are a form of radiation."

"I know that well, Doc, as I wrote an article about UVA and UVB sunrays years ago. Those rays do cause cancer in more than 1 million Americans a year. That easily surpasses the amount of colon, lung, breast, and prostate cancers combined."

The doctor replied, "Shocking isn't it?"

"What's shocking is it's a cancer we can largely prevent."

"Most cancers are, once you understand what is causing them."

David stated, "People know now that they should not sunbathe or use tanning beds, but too many ignore all the warnings."

"Some do, but on the positive side, I've noticed a lot of people avoiding the intense afternoon sun. But I agree with you, David, too many people don't wear wide brim hats or protect their arms or hands from the sun. I see so much skin cancer on people's ears nowadays due to them wearing only baseball caps. They protect the top of their head but forget about their ears or back of their neck."

A LITTLE SUN, PLEASE

The doctor and David continued their conversation for hours. During that time the doctor reviewed with David the beneficial effects of sunshine in elevating mood and infusing the human body with beneficial hormones. The doctor pointed out that the vitamin D the body likes best is provided by sunshine. Some sunbathing before 10 am or after 4 pm can be beneficial. The doctor and David agreed that no one should experience sunburn or endeavor to get a dark tan.

The doctor went on to explain that vitamin D was both a hormone and a vitamin. The skin absorbs sunshine which it converts to vitamin D within the body. This natural form of vitamin D seems to prevent many forms of cancer, assists greatly with proper bone formation, and may even help with heart and mental health. The doctor told David that many doctors are concerned that people will overdose on vitamin D supplements, as they are a fat soluble vitamin and can accumulate in the body. Yet the doctor went on to tell David that he has never seen an overdose yet, however to be on the safe side, he tells his patients to take vitamin D only about three times a week.

He cautioned David that the only real problem he has seen with excessive vitamin D intake is if a person has a genetic tendency to not absorb vitamin D correctly, usually based on having too high of calcium levels, impaired kidney function, or a health condition like scleroderma or sarcoidosis. Then it can cause all kinds of havoc, as it will allow calcium to accumulate in the body, especially the soft tissues and the arteries including the aorta. To prevent this, the doctor told David to always eat lots of green leafy vegetables every day as they contain vitamin K, which is critical for handling this excess. Some manufacturers include vitamin K-2 with their vitamin D-3 supplements for this reason. He also felt that people that had a problem with D causing calcium to be stored incorrectly might be low in the mineral magnesium. He also recommended they get some genuine vitamin D by taking an early morning or early evening walk when the sun is not so strong and get their skin exposed a few days a week for 20 to 30 minutes at a time. Once you build up your skin to this exposure, you can venture out at later times with full sun, but never longer than 10 to 30 minutes, depending on skin type. Darker skinned people can tolerate afternoon sun and, in fact, may need more full sun exposure, as darker skin needs more sun to produce vitamin D. Natural ways of obtaining vitamin D, like sunshine, are actually the best way to go.

YEARS AGO

The doctor explained to David that, years ago, he saw many cases of rickets, a disease due to a lack of vitamin D which causes the bowing of a person's leg bones. He explained that is why our country started supplementing milk with vitamin D with the hope that that would impact the children directly in preventing rickets and it turned out to work. However, the doctor explained that while rickets might be an obvious sign of not having enough vitamin D, there are more subtle forms of deficiency that may actually affect a person's health just as much as rickets do. Weak bones, immunity problems, and increased cancer rates to name a few. David was surprised that the reason the doctor recommended only using vitamin D supplements a few times a week was because it could be toxic in larger doses especially for pregnant women and their unborn children. While overconsuming vitamin D can cause problems, it has not been seen when a person obtains their vitamin D via sunshine. It seems the body has a safety switch to keep too much from being produced or circulated within the body.

GETTING REAL D

The doctor continued about vitamin D. When getting your vitamin D from the sun, the doctor recommended that people should not shower or bathe for a while, especially with soap, since this cleans the surface of the skin where much of the vitamin D synthesis is taking place. The doctor told David that after sunshine exposure your skin may need 12 to 20 hours to do its thing.

The doctor even suggested that Americans may be taking too many baths and showers. He explained that years ago people did not bathe as often, which allowed the vitamin D to be absorbed. He mentioned to David that everybody should get their blood work checked at least once a year to see how their vitamin D levels were along with testing other biomarkers. He suggested that David do so by contacting a firm called Life Extension, which could arrange a blood testing facility along with a trained doctor to review the findings. He urged David to always get tested since either a low level or a very high level of vitamin D could prove life shortening. Optimal levels, however, could increase longevity. The doctor recommended his patients take at least an average of 1000 IUs a day with food containing some fat. He was aware that many people were taking 1000 to 5000 IUs a day. Most seemed OK with the higher doses, but to be on the safe side he insisted they get blood work done to confirm their levels. He also explained to David that you don't need to take it everyday as your body holds on to vitamin D, as it is a fat soluble vitamin not a water soluble one that may pass through your system relatively fast. He explained that vitamin D was also a good membrane antioxidant.

The doctor pointed out that almost none of us have a say in what the government is adding to our food and water. He noted out that in his opinion the government had no business adding fluoride, folic acid, iron or vitamin D to our food chain. He expressed concern that so far it appears that two of those four items – fluoride and iron – may be harming us a lot more then helping us. At this point in time, however, he felt that vitamin D in our food chain might be one right thing the government may be doing but he questioned the legality and wisdom of doing it.

David then asked about trace minerals and trace nutrients. "How many of these are really crucial to our diets?"

"Good question, David, we really don't know everything yet, but we suspect that many trace minerals may be very important indeed. Minerals like magnesium act as antioxidants within the body, iodine is needed to regulate the thyroid, zinc is good for enzyme functions, chromium is good for blood sugar regulation, and selenium may help prevent cancer." The doctor then proceeded to talk more about selenium.

SELENIUM & WHY MINERALS MATTER

Some supplements are not deemed to be powerful antioxidants by themselves but considered essential for good health. They work by allowing other antioxidants to be reused in the body. Such supplements as selenium, in moderation, can do wonders. Like many trace elements however, too much is toxic, but a small amount in our diets is essential, especially for immunity, thyroid function, initiating various enzyme processes, etc. He stressed that we should not exceed 200 micrograms per day. In fact, he would never take selenium every day, only twice a week. Enough, he said, to insure that you are not deficient, but not so much that there would be negative health consequences. The doctor mentioned that if you eat mostly organic, then you may only need to supplement once a week. Not only does a small dose of selenium help prevent damage to cells like other antioxidants, it allows some of the body's natural antioxidant mechanisms to increase their glutathione peroxidase function, which is a very important enzyme with antioxidant properties. Selenium protects against cardiomyopathy and cancer.

He stated to be sure you use the right type of supplement derived from yeast that contains the word selenomethionine, or better yet consume foods like garlic and broccoli. Better still, he added, simply consume two Brazil nuts per week to get a natural form of selenium in your diet. A warning to the wise, don't consume too much selenium, as this is the same stuff found in "loco weed" and too much "loco weed" consumption will poison and kill most animals. The dose makes the poison. Make sure your selenium supplement does not contain a majority of the cheap selenium selenite or selenium selenate. These forms will get into the system but seems to leave your system fast. While a small dose may improve immune function, the other natural forms of selenium may help prevent cancers, so it is worth paying a little more for. These two inorganic forms selenite and selenate are fed to animals due to their cheap price, but are not the ones you want to be consuming. While providing selenium in large doses, they are potentially more oxidative and toxic than organic forms. Manufacturers still place it in your supplements, as it is cheap and consumers don't know. It's a good indicator if your vitamin manufacturer really cares about you. You do not have to use selenium just by itself. It is contained in most multiple vitamin supplements, especially with a good vitamin E supplement.

BRAZIL NUTS

"Doctor, I've heard about Brazil nuts, but don't they say you should eat two per day? You said two per week."

"No, David, you heard me correctly. Most Brazil nuts are loaded with selenium. So high that two nuts will cover your selenium mineral needs for up to a week. The possible problems are that Brazil nuts are high in fat and their shells often contain high amounts of aflatoxin, which as you know can cause cancer of your liver if consumed on a constant basis. So don't get in the habit of eating them every day, especially in excess. You may end up getting too much selenium and other potential toxins."

169

"Really, Doc, I did not know that, any other possible hidden dangers with these nuts?"

"Interesting question, David. I have to tell you that there are two other possible problems with Brazil nuts, which at first seem unrelated but actually are. The tree is so tall, often reaching over 150 feet high, that the nut pods, or fruit, that carry the brazil nuts themselves are so heavy that people have been killed when those pods landed on their heads. Kind of like a huge coconut falling from the sky. But also, the height of the tree means that the roots go deep in the ground possibly explaining why these brazil nuts are high in radium."

"Radium, like in radioactive?"

"Yes, David. Now saying this, I still eat Brazil nuts, but not every day! I like them and they are high in a lot of other minerals as well. But like most things in life, everything in moderation."

A LITTLE ON OXIDATIVE STRESS

David initiated more talking points about antioxidants. "Doctor, I know that we humans are very sophisticated beings. Our bodies' organ systems work with each other in a very organized manner. Would it be fair to equate antioxidants as the oil the body needs to function correctly?"

"That's a good point," the doctor responded. "I would say that our bodies use antioxidants as one of the main ingredients to operate properly and that these antioxidants may help protect us from the constant steady exposure to oxidative stress, radiation, and a harmful environment. But so many things are important to the body such as hormones, micronutrients, proper fats, proteins, fiber, and proper carbohydrates, that equating antioxidants to oil might be over simplifying. Our bodies and that of every mammal are so sophisticated it is amazing to me that we are able to function or live at all. When animals started using glucose and oxygen within their cells to produce energy, it started us on the road to becoming more sophisticated than all the simple life forms that preceded us. We were able to evolve as more complex life forms because various body systems could specialize in one area. These successful parts helped create a successful whole, a much more sophisticated life form. In truth, it is a miracle that we operate as we do. Yet, the ability to create cellular respiration within our cells and the resulting free radical by-products of that utilization had to be accompanied by methods to keep those by-products from destroying us too quickly. This process produces so many free radicals that the body must deal with the resulting carnage quickly by providing its own antioxidants. If you are producing too many free radicals you can easily strip your body of the ability to keep up in neutralizing this threat. So your example of antioxidants being oil has a lot of merit. I mean, without oil, most engines would burn out fairly quickly."

"So, Doctor, are you saying the body can keep up with taking care of free radicals?"

YES AND NO

"Yes and no, David, since free radicals pose a constant threat to our bodies, especially our DNA, it will ultimately destroy us in the long run if given enough time. Perhaps we can call it a love-hate relationship. In fact, the body produces its own free radicals within white blood cells to kill off invaders or cells within the body that are worn out or worse, cancerous. So it has developed ways of dealing with the aftermath of those free radicals as well as with most of the free radical damage brought on by cellular respiration. While all mammals have advanced to being very sophisticated life forms, we are all still at the mercy of making sure we don't destroy our bodies with all the reactive oxygen our bodies generate within, during the process of cells converting glucose to adenosine diphosphate, or ADP, within our cells. As you know, this is called cellular respiration, and when glucose is converted it becomes oxidized. Our body has so many ways of dealing with this threat and we are just learning some of them. Some cells have better methods of dealing with this problem and, in fact, seem to never age as we know it. We don't fully understand how the body knows when it must deal with these free radicals but it uses many different methods to do so, including hormones. This DNA damage within our cells is the major downside of us exposing our bodies to too many free radicals or the wrong kinds of free radicals. I believe that this damage leads us to a few other methods of aging called the Mitochondria Theory and the Cell Membrane Theory. Also, it directly leads to us to another theory of aging called Inflammation Theory."

KEY POINTS
FREE RADICAL THEORY

- Follow the previous steps outlined for Prevention and Caloric Restriction as they apply to Free Radicals as well.

- Consume a diet rich in colorful vegetables and fruits. Use various grains and beans, along with nuts and berries. All of these contain natural antioxidants. Include daily vegetables from the mustard family which include cabbages, watercress, cauliflower, Brussels sprouts, broccoli, kale, and collard greens, to name a few.

- Do drink a small amount of real fruit juice that is made without added sugars, as it is a potent source of antioxidants. Fresh vegetable juice can be consumed more often as it tends to have less sugar. The need for such juices cannot be overstated. They flood your body with what it really needs: chlorophyll, antioxidants, flavonoids and minerals.

- Supplement wisely. Use supplements that have numerous antioxidants instead of those usually containing only one. That way you can get some synergy along with less filler material. This also saves you money. Buy on quality, not just on price.

- Vitamin C with quercetin and other bioflavonoids is good along with a full spectrum vitamin E supplement. The vitamin has to be natural not synthetic or else it may do more harm than good. For example, a good vitamin E would contain gamma-Tocopherol along with other mixed Tocopherol. The combination of vitamin C, which is a water soluble vitamin, is good along with a fat soluble vitamin E.

- Research has shown that many vitamin supplements are now available and affordable such as Q-10, lipoic acid, and vitamins D and K. Include trace minerals such as selenium.

- Don't overconsume overcooked food products, especially fried foods. They create glycation within the body.

- Don't consume foods with a high glycemic index. These include sugar, soda, fruit juices and drinks, and most snack products and junk food.

- Consume antioxidants along with a well rounded natural balanced diet. Consider a balanced B supplement every few days and make sure it contains real folate.

- Consider adding spices like turmeric to your diet. Turmeric is absorbed best when combined with ginger.

- If you are taking fish oil or krill oil, always take a taste test when you first get them. You need to bite into a capsule to make sure it is not rancid. Otherwise you will be doing more harm than good.

- Consider using a zinc supplement periodically.

    - Good forms of zinc:
        - zinc monomethionine
        - zinc picolinate
        - zinc orotate
        - zinc aspartate
        - zinc citrate

    - Forms of zinc to avoid:
        - zinc gluconate
        - zinc oxide
        - zinc sulfate

    - Don't overconsume zinc, as it displaces copper.

11
Other Theories of Aging

DAVID SAID WITH confidence, "Doc, I know we discussed prevention and caloric restriction, along with the Free Radical Theory, which focuses on antioxidants, but really, isn't only the free radical topic an accepted theory of aging? I mean the other two, Prevention and Caloric Restriction, only deal with longevity and staying in good health."

The doctor smiled. "But, David, doesn't longevity and good health have everything to do with aging?"

David immediately replied, "Of course, Doc."

"Then should they not be incorporated into theories of aging?"

"Well, when you say it that way, I guess it makes sense."

David paused before asking, "Doc, I thought I knew of all the theories of aging, but it sounds like you found a few more?"

The doctor laughed and added, "Good point, let's talk about a few, but first, David, what theories you feel that the public at large has heard about or that you would report on if writing an article?"

David replied, "Doc, I would mention five current theories of aging, which are: Free Radical Damage, Glycation, Methylation & DNA Damage, Inflammation Damage, and Wear & Tear."

Doc replied, "Very good, I suppose we could start with those, but it does not encompass all that is really going on in the body. Another way to look at it is to set up categories of the aging process that occurs in the human body and their direct effect on our cells, which I feel an expert in biogerontology named Aubrey de Grey did. He uses seven main reasons we age. They are easily remembered by me as the unlucky seven."

As the doctor spoke, David wrote down the list.

1. **Cell loss**
2. **Nuclear mutation and epimutations**
3. **Mitochondrial mutations**
4. **Cellular senescence**
5. **Extracellular cross links**
6. **Extracellular junk**
7. **Intracellular junk**

"He has identified these as the seven main ways we age. His hope and plan is for researchers to address each item and come up with remedies. So like an old car that is well taken care of, we may end up lasting indefinitely. If society changes their outlook on aging from that of accepting it to fighting it, we will see most, if not all, of these issues dealt with. That will take time, however. Until then, all we can do is follow simple steps now to avoid getting old too quickly."

"Wow," David replied, "How do you remember all of them?"

"It's easy, David; just think of what bad things can happen to your cells and visualize it. Then you will easily remember them. Similar to what you probably did when you told me of your five theories of aging. Now let me describe some other theories of aging. All of them may be related to the seven ways we age."

David smiled, "Go ahead, Doc, I've got my pen in hand. I'm ready for you."

HALF THE PROBLEM

The doctor then walked over to his bookshelf and removed a large binder. While opening the binder he said, "I only cover 12 theories of aging with my clients, as to discuss more would be overwhelming to them. So my clients and I go over the 12 theories I feel we can easily address in our lives. I have assembled a more extensive list, which by all means is not conclusive; in fact, half the problem is that we have not figured out all the reasons we age. Until we do, we will not be able to figure out the best methods for slowing down the aging process. But slow it down, we will. Even using a fraction of what we know, we can dramatically impact the course of aging as it occurs within our very bodies. That fact alone brings constant excitement to this field. I feel if more research dollars were pointed in this direction we could easily extend life 40% to 50% in the next two decades. While some people want to argue over why we would want to do so, I note that many scientists and concerned individuals are already taking many reasonable steps to do it. So while others remain as skeptics, many already are deriving great benefits by knowing more about the process of aging and what they can do about it. Saying that, I feel that we need to get the word out how many current theories of aging there are and work on finding others. I feel there are at least 25 theories of aging or living, if you will. I note the following theories but add that many folks will want to combine one or two of those in the same category, which is fine, but may not be accurate, to say the least. Each of these areas is so important that missing one link could accelerate the effect of aging on one's body. So in this case, ignorance really could cost you your life or lead to the lack of living your full life potential."

"But, Doc, most people are not aware of what our real life expectancy can be anyways."

"Right, David, what life may have been there to be lived will not be known. The loss of so many years by our generation due to this ignorance will be talked

177

about by future generations, that is for sure. Imagine the conversations sounding like, 'My poor Uncle Harold died at age 79, poor soul. To think of someone dying that early, when they are middle-aged, makes me sad. Especially when people are now living to 150 years of age!' Humph, they will think us stupid for not researching aging sooner."

Reading from his notebook the doctor continued. "My current Theories of Aging list is as follows:"

David wrote down the list while the doctor read outloud.

> The Prevention Theory
> The Caloric Restriction Theory
> The Free Radical Theory
> The Membrane Theory
> The Mitochondria Theory
> The Glycogen Cross Linking Theory
> The DNA Telomeres Theory
> The Inflammation Theory
> The Thymic-Stimulating Theory
> The Acidification Theory
> The Enzyme Theory
> The Mineral Overload Theory
> The Triage Theory
> The Calcification Theory
> The Pituitary Gland Theory
> The Neuroendocrine Theory
> The Autoimmune Theory
> The Death Hormone Theory
> The Errors and Repair Theory
> The Hayflick Limit Theory
> The Redundant DNA Theory
> The Wear and Tear Theory
> The Development Theory

"There are several other theories, which I don't bother getting into, such as **The Gene Mutation Theory, The Rate of Living Theory, The Cell Communication Theory** and **The Order to Disorder Theory**, as I don't sense there is much we can do about them, in a preventive sense, that is."

YOUR WHOLE LIFE

"Come on, Doc, how can any person follow all those theories? I mean you could devote your whole life to researching all these theories."

"Yes, trust me, I know. But what I've done is focused on the 12 theories I deem to be the most important and also the ones I feel we can easily do something about. For instance, the three theories we have discussed so far are simply the first three stepping stones along the path to anti-aging. There are several more we can follow with excellent results."

"That gives me hope, Doc. I mean I would not want to learn all those theories of aging just to live a little longer. I want my family and I to live a lot longer and especially to enjoy the journey. So what are the other stepping stones, Doc?"

"Well, David, funny you should mention that, as I was just about to discuss another one of them in some detail. I have what I call my daily dozen. Failure to pay attention to any of them will cut your potential life expectancy quite severely, I'm afraid. Just look at the three theories we just discussed; each of them are crucial."

HIS 12 THEORIES

"OK, Doc, since we already covered three of your 12 theories, I'm ready to discuss the remaining back nine theories."

Laughing, the doctor said, "Right, David, we will focus on the last nine of my daily dozen, which I consider the most important after the ones we just covered. You will start to see how they are related to the first three theories we spoke of: Prevention, Caloric Restriction, and Free Radicals. There is a real connection after all."

"OK, Doc, I get it, I think. Let me have your fourth theory. What is it called?"

"We will discuss that fourth theory in a moment. I just want you to understand that many of the other theories may be connected to each other instead of actually standing on their own merits."

"Such as?"

OTHER THEORIES OF AGING

The doctor went on to explain that many theories of aging are similar or related to each other. When examined one by one they can make a case for being a theory on to themselves, but in reality they are often connected in the sense that one theory may actually be the result of what happens from another theory. For instance, the doctor explained, "The Pituitary Gland Theory of Aging states that our pituitary gland, which is considered a main gland in our endocrine system, is a large part of aging. Scientists found that if they removed the pituitary gland of rats, but gave them the necessary hormones, the rats lived much longer. So the question is, and remains, is it the pituitary gland that sends out a message to age or to terminate our very life force?"

"So is that a theory, Doctor, or is it a result of something else going on?"

"Right, David, what is really happening? Part and parcel with the Pituitary Gland Theory we just discussed is one that gets more attention and perhaps is more accepted. The Neuroendocrine Theory of Aging. First proposed by the medical doctor and gerontologist Vladimir Dilman, published in 1954, aging may be caused by a progressive loss of various receptors in our hypothalamus gland causing aging and our eventual demise. The loss in sensitivity of these receptors may cause various feedback loops to be compromised, leading to diseases, aging, and death. They speculated that this Neuroendocrine Theory of Aging may contribute greatly to aging in our middle age and beyond."

"So, Doctor, which theory is correct? The Pituitary Gland Theory or the Aging Hypothalamus Gland Theory?"

"That's my point, they are related and it's left up to science to determine which theory is paramount and which theory may just be the result of the other theory in operation. Dilman's concept is that the endocrine system is indeed run by the pituitary gland but that gland is controlled by another part of the brain called the hypothalamus. Factors released from the hypothalamus go to the pituitary and activate the release of one or more of its hormones. These hormones stimulate other glands. Since the hypothalamus part of our brains relies on feedback from other glands it may start producing less or the wrong amounts of various hormones over time and this affects our aging cycle. It affects our homeostasis, which is the balance act our body follows to live. Aging is all about our body maintaining proper homeostasis, or the lack thereof. So, David, what theory is more important or correct? We don't know yet."

"Doctor, I am not going to pretend like I just understood everything you just said. It sounds like you were saying it could be one theory or the other. Having said that, I do see your point about why we need to explore all of these theories in depth. So why don't we just discuss that fourth theory you were going to tell me about?"

WHY DO WE AGE?

"Of course, David, but first let me say that the great mystery of aging is why do we have to age at all?"

"How's that?"

"It is believed that various life forms don't age until they are killed off by another animal or mishap. Hydras, sponges, various clams, certain fish like rockfish and sturgeons along with lobsters don't appear to die of old age. In many cases, they just keep growing. In fact, maybe it's when life stops growing that it starts dying."

"I see," said David, "But what about salmon? Why do they die off after mating?"

"Interestingly, David, in some species of salmon, chemical signals tell them to die off after reproducing. Perhaps that signal gave them some long term

181

biological edge during the last million years. However, other animals seem to develop other signals that tell them to keep growing, to keep living. Perhaps the cure for aging is to simply find those switches."

"So there is a chemical agent being sent?"

"Seems that way, David, we also need to know why germ cells found in our reproductive tract seem immortal, allowing life to go on generation after generation, perhaps stretching back millions of years, while our somatic cells found through out the rest of our body age and die off."

"Maybe, Doc, the answer is already in us, we just need to understand how to unlock it."

"Well said, David. We will find the answer some day, but I wish more scientists were looking for it. By the way, David, you wanted to know about my fourth theory. It's simple."

KEY POINTS

- Causes of aging have been ignored throughout history. However, many are waking up to the fact that something can really be done to delay its effects and impact.

- Only by shifting our attention from that of acceptance on aging to what can be done about it, will we see real progress being made.

- Take care of yourself and follow any steps you can to preserve what time you have left so you can also benefit from new or future breakthroughs.

12
The Membrane Theory
Theory IV

"It is called the Membrane Theory of Aging, and when you understand it you will see its direct impact to aging."

"Hmm," said David, "I think I already know a little about it. It's the theory that our cells' membranes need to be kept in good order or else the waste products that cells normally produce are kept inside too long. Not to mention, when cells' membranes lose their integrity, nutrients can't get in as easily?"

"Great description, David; you might well know then that it was first proposed by Professor Imre Zs.-Nagy of Debrecen University in Hungary."

"I didn't recall that part, Doc. So tell me more since I told you almost all I remember about this theory."

"Fine, David, Professor Zs.-Nagy proposed the theory that age and other factors impair our cell membranes in their ability to transfer nutrients properly into our cells and also impair their ability to expel waste products out. Along with those two major factors, the cell would find its ability to detoxify itself and to maintain its own metabolism impaired. It would be hard for our body's cells to maintain their homeostasis, which is so crucial to its proper function, its survival."

"Doc, I like that your description mentioned detoxify. I might add that many alternative health people talk about this theory and feel it is a crucial reason why all of us should detoxify our bodies periodically."

"Hmm, David, I hear you about detoxification, but you know that word has a negative reaction amongst many medical people."

"How's that, Doc? I mean detoxification makes sense, doesn't it?

"Of course, David, it makes sense but many medical people feel the term is too general. They want to know a single definition on it and feel the term is used too broadly to denote too many processes in the alternative health field. And also, they will point out that there are no proper studies showing the value of detoxification practices, even through most people figure out quickly that it just makes sense."

"So how in the world do you explain the Cell Membrane Theory to them?"

"Well," said the doctor, "We don't discuss detoxification at first, that is for sure. It would immediately set up a barrier against further conversation. Remember, since we are talking about the cell's membrane, I would first talk about what we do know. I mean, it was only in the last 40 to 50 years that we finally identified that cells, in fact, did have some kind of membrane at all. Many scientists thought before that there was some type of polarization holding the cells contents together or some other reason the cells kept their contents in place. So first I would focus on what we can all agree on. The cell's membrane is a type of fat substance that envelopes the cell's insides with a protective skin of some sort, called the membrane. After all, many doctors have had extensive biology courses and know a great deal about this topic to begin with. Start with that perspective and physicians get it."

"OK, Doc, I get it as well, so it's a type of fat, how does that help explain the Membrane Theory of Aging?"

"David, if our cells' membranes are made of mostly lipids, which are a form of fat, it makes sense that our bodies would create them from natural substances it finds within its body. So if you consume good fats, your cells membranes will be healthy membranes and in a much better position since they have use that good fat to do their job."

"So," David said, "The opposite would be true – the wrong fats would negatively impact our cells membranes...right?"

"You have no clue how correct that statement is, David. That is what the good Professor Zs.-Nagy was trying to tell us. It makes sense as the cells within our bodies find their cellular membranes becoming more resistant and less flexible as we age especially if consuming the wrong fats. High heat or frying of oil destroys fat's nutrient value. It also causes the oil to oxidize. Since it's oxidized, it will turn rancid much easier. Many restaurants and food manufacturers will use heated oil over and over again. This is a nutritional nightmare. Bad things happen when you do this. The oil loses any nutrient power and becomes free radical producing, which may lead to heart disease and cancer. Also, making matters worse, most manufacturers start with a cheaper hydrogenated oil. This really unhealthy oil is created by a process that involves infusing hydrogen through the oil using high pressure and a catalyst. This changes the chemical configuration. Since companies use this oil over and over again, it damages the oil even further making it hard for our bodies to handle. When our bodies do assimilate this oil it takes the place of a healthier fat that normally occupies a space where a good fat should be. This, of course, is very health destroying not health promoting. This damage slows down the transport of various substances in and out of the cell, especially with a lousy diet. In fact, with the wrong food, our cells may become more solid and less flexible as it were, which would impede the proper processes of letting in nutrients and getting out waste products, slowly killing our health, our vigor, and often dramatically shortening our life."

"But, Doctor, doesn't our stomach acid break all this fat down to its basic components? So it shouldn't matter what type of fat we consume, right?"

"Not really, David. You are thinking of proteins and carbohydrates, which get broken down by the digestion process, but fats are unique; they don't get di-

185

gested the same way as the other two macro nutrients – protein and carbohydrates. Instead, they get assimilated. All this means is they get emulsified by the liver and gallbladder. Then these broken-up fat particles get moved along to the small intestine, where they get absorbed into the blood stream and make their way to their place in our cells. What the body can use right away, it does, and what it can not use, it stores. So why store bad fats with the wrong chemical configuration? It will only lead to ill health."

CELL MEMBRANES

"Well, could it really be that simple?"

"Why not, David, I mean the loss of cells permeability leads, theoretically, to something we call lipofuscin damage. As we age, most people accumulate more and more of this lipofuscin. It manifests itself on the outside of our bodies as age spots. However, it also is accumulating on the inside of our bodies. It accumulates in our heart, lungs, brain and skin, just to name a few spots. The majority of our cells are surrounded by a double membrane of lipids with pores that allow material to move in and out. If that membrane gets less flexible through a bad diet, or if the cell faces insults from free radicals, there is an increased build up of toxic sludge known as lipofuscin. This lipid debris of sludge and pigment impairs our cells. Then it stands to reason our cells will not function well."

LIPOFUSCIN

"So, Doc, this lipofuscin impairs our cells' ability to function. I have to admit that most people have never heard of this stuff that you say is slowly accumulating in our bodies."

"I know, David, but it may be one of those things we can really do something about. During our lifetime we invariably will find most of our body's cells accumulating a residue of oxidized proteins and other junk like mineral deposits called lipofuscin. This residue is not healthy and serves only to impair our cell's ability to function properly. Too much lipofuscin in our cells causes premature aging. This lipofuscin damage causes our cells to become dysfunctional. We see it too often as we age, our cells accumulating too much lipofuscin impairing its ability to thrive."

"So, Doctor, are you saying that this excess lipofuscin is what may be aging us and it is not just a consequence of aging?"

"Absolutely, it has no positive benefit, so we must keep our lipofuscin levels as low as we can. An excess of this hinders proper nutrients from gaining easy entrance to our cells and allows waste products to accumulate. Often, this leads to the cell's inability to properly clean up its debris such as non-functional organelles and proteins. As you know organelles are the specialized areas in our cells that perform needed functions. If the cell fails at these tasks it will not function optimally and may even self destruct. We must maintain our cell's integrity, inside and out, so the cell can clean its house and replace worn parts. This is crucial to extending the health and life of the cell, other neighborly cells and ultimately our entire body."

"So the cleaning of the cell makes sense to me. I know if my wife and I fail to take out the trash, even for one week, there is a severe consequence!"

"Good point, David, indeed there is. Now imagine, your home filling up with trash and consider this, what if all of the doors and windows of your home were stuck closed so you could not breathe? How would you get fresh air into your home? Also, imagine if your water pipes become broken and water filled your home, how would you get water out of your home if all the openings are closed off? I think you get the mental image."

"Yes, I do, we would suffocate from our own waste. Can we actually reverse this damage?"

"Great question, it appears we can delay it in many cases and reverse it in some situations through a combination of supplements. I have heard of people using acetyl-L-carnitine, ginkgo biloba, DMAE, and some medical drugs like centrophenoxine and piracetam. The real story is how we have just recently become aware of how lipofuscin is damaging our bodies. That information has been a major step on the path to understanding aging and fighting aging.

For years we had no clue on why we seem to be aging or why we were accumulating damage to our bodies. Our body has methods of cleaning itself but we often interfere with this process by consuming too many calories and the wrong foods. The cleaning of our body's cells from within is called autophagy and may be the real key to extending the lifespan of most animals. It is a process where the cell cleans out debris and also where the cell renews old parts of the cell without killing off the cell. Kind of like remodeling an older home by making it much newer inside. We now know some of the questions that really matter and we need our science and medical community to really start working on the answers."

"So, Doc, what can we do about it?"

"Professor Zs.-Nagy himself became involved in research and development of nutraceuticals that assist in clearing up lipofuscin deposits within the body, which should allow the cell to better perform. This works by increasing a cell's ability to process nutrients much more efficiently, eliminate waste products, and communicate with other cells better. He helped create centrophenoxine, also called Lucidril, which helps tremendously with this clean up process and or prevention of lipofuscin deposits."

"I've heard of Lucidril being used for Alzheimer's patients. So, Doc, do you use these drugs to help clean up lipofuscin deposits?"

DMAE

"Well, yes, it does seem to help a lot with lipofuscin deposits and the build up of potassium in our brain cells and other cells. It seems to allow the cells to utilize oxygen much better as well. Poor cell membranes lead to a build up of potassium in our cells and a loss of water. It gets complicated, and we could discuss these aspects for hours. I might use these drugs on a much older patient if they were showing signs of dementia. However, for younger patients I recommend DMAE supplements of 75 mg per capsule twice a day, but not before bedtime. This does what a lot of these other drugs do but just takes longer. I also use vitamin C and a mixed natural vitamin E in synch with DMAE. Especially since vitamin E is also a good antioxidant for our cells' membranes.

I also instruct my people to drink lots of clean water each day since our cells seem to lose some of their moisture content as we age. Of course, I also like acetyl-L-carnitine, alpha-lipoic acid, and carnosine as well. I often use those three in unity for lipofuscin control and repair as well for the health of the body's main energy producing part of our cells, the mitochondria, which are involved in another theory of aging that we will cover later."

"I've heard of DMAE. What does DMAE stand for?"

"Dimethyl-amino-ethanol, David."

David grimaced, "Dimethyl-what?"

Laughing, the doctor replied, "Dimethylaminoethanol, David, and yes, it is a mouthful!"

"But, Doc, what about side effects of taking DMAE. I have heard people complain of anxiety and sleeplessness, even headaches?"

"Right you are, David, but I have only found that in a few people, especially those that took too much, took it late in the evening, or had existing problems like depression or were on meds. In my view, it is very safe, but like all supplements you should listen to your body. Of course, David, if you want to be really safe just eat salmon or those sardines I mentioned earlier. It is a safe way to get both your DMAE and omega-3 oils, or if you have the stomach, try anchovies."

David chuckled, "Thanks. I like sardines, but how many can one eat in a week? I mean every thing in moderation, right?"

Laughing, the doctor responded, "That's right, David, but really one needs only to set up some habits and in doing so, let the habits place you on autopilot. Some of those habits will involve taking certain nutrients and supplements on a weekly basis. I have found several products that combine several essential supplements in one package so that you are not spending your entire day swallowing pills or, as you mentioned, eating sardines."

"So, Doc, you are saying the Membrane Theory of Aging is really important to a body's cells?"

"Right David, and maybe in ways we have not identified. That is why I stated it is directly related to other theories of aging."

"How so?"

ENERGY FACTORIES

"Remember we talked about our cells' energy factories, the mitochondria? While this portion of our cells does an incredible amount of work, and they do not have enough protective defenses built into them like the rest of our cells. This is because many scientists believe that the mitochondria are not actually part of original cell material but inserted themselves eons ago. They may be involved in a symbiotic relation to our cells, giving our cells the ability to utilize oxygen and simple sugars for producing energy our cells use called ATP."

"Doc, I have heard about this theory before, but really what would the mitochondria in our cells get out of the deal?"

"Good point. What they get by supplying our cells with the ability to produce ATP and the resulting chemical energy we need to operate as total life forms is they get to live."

"Good point, Doc, but how does this relate to our cell membranes?"

"Our cells use their membranes for getting stuff into our cells via several methods including the more passive diffusion method that healthy membranes allow. These same body cells harbor the mitochondria, which need a steady supply of good nutrition, antioxidant protection, and waste product disposal. Healthy cell membranes can help the mitochondria while unhealthy membranes will hurt the mitochondria. The mitochondria are one of the most vulnerable parts of our cells, lacking the full defenses of the cell that they reside in."

"So, Doc, besides being one of our weakest links, since lacking the full spectrum of protection as the cell they live in and having to do an incredible amount of work, they are already at a disadvantage within the cell to begin with. Compound that with bad cell membranes, and you are setting yourself up for a problem. Does that about cover their dilemma?"

"That's right, David, possibly setting us up for cancers and aging disorders. Our body needs the mitochondria but does not give them the same defenses the rest of our cells enjoy. They are kind of like houseguests. They don't have the same double helix DNA but a single strand. They are very prone to mutation as we age. They continue as part of us by passing on from one human generation to another via the females of our species. If you are looking for a God part of our cells, then you need look no further."

David laughed. "Doc, don't you mean Mother Nature or God, since the females of our species allow this to pass on?"

Smiling the doctor added, "Touché, David, touché..."

"Now how does this relate to the other theories?"

"As I said, maybe more than we know. Quality cell membranes assist greatly and directly affect some of the other theories of aging such as Cross Linking, Hormone Theory, Neuroendocrine Theory, Pituitary Theory, Thymus Gland Theory, and the Telomeres Theory. I feel that our hormones also need good cell membrane quality in order to communicate correctly. I mean, look at what happens to insulin levels if our cells are not able to accept it into their cells at the proper rate."

"Come again?" responded David.

"If your cells' membranes become impaired, then hormones such as insulin have a harder time getting into the cells, thereby forcing your pancreas to produce more to try to regulate the sugar levels the body finds it requires. Bad permeability with cells directly impacts insulin levels, sugar levels, and how hard your pancreas will have to work. There is a direct connection. That is why a clean diet of good fats can diminish type II diabetes so quickly in most people while bad fats can lead people directly into type II diabetes."

"Doctor, besides these bad fats, what else really messes up our cell membranes?"

"Good question. Be warned that in our modern world bisphenol A, commonly called BPA, which can be found in many plastics, causes havoc within our cells."

"How so, Doc?"

"It blocks calcium channels in our cell membranes. Not to mention how BPA messes with our bodies' enzyme functions and even our hormones."

The doctor then sat down and reviewed with David steps that all of us should follow.

KEY POINTS
MEMBRANE THEORY

- Follow the previous steps outlined for Prevention, Caloric Restriction, and Free Radicals, as they apply to Membrane Theory as well.

- Consume a clean diet of healthy food.

- Consume good fats such as monosaturated fats like olive oil or avocado fat, a small amount of saturated fat from fish, lean meats, or coconuts, as long as they are not processed, and a small amount of polyunsaturated fats from fish and nuts.

- Consume non-contaminated fish like sardines or salmon.

- Use supplements that aid in protecting your cell membranes like natural vitamin E, alpha-lipoic acid or if available the better form called R-lipoic acid, acetyl-L-carnitine, carnosine & DMAE.

- Eat smaller meals and less often. Place food servings on plates and store the rest of the food away to avoid second servings.

- Stop eating when 80% full. To do this, eat slower.

- Fast periodically, as it helps your body cleans up its waste.

- Avoid too much sugar.

- Never ever consume processed oil. Oil processed through a hydrogenation process is referred to as partially hydrogenated trans fat. These are toxic, leading to cancer, heart disease and diabetes.

- Stop using plastic bottles or containers, especially those containing BPA.

- Drink clean water often.

13
Mitochondria Theory
Theory V

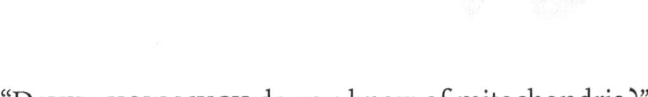

"DAVID, HOW MUCH do you know of mitochondria?"

"Well, Doc, as we discussed, they are the energy factories of our cells, with the exception of our red blood cells. There usually are many mitochondria contained within each cell, allowing that cell to utilize energy and process oxygen."

"Good, David. Recall that we discussed the theory that mitochondria are not really original to our lifeform but were added later?"

"Good grief, Doctor, we touched on that theory, but when you say it that way is sounds eerie or like some great mystery to be solved. I mean the theory is that mitochondria did not exist in many life forms eons ago but somehow, through a mutual symbiotic relationship, it became part of animal cells. Part of us."

"That's right, David, but the reason I bring this up is because so many people are ignorant of this theory and why it might be of major importance to all of us, especially concerning longevity. As you said, it could be reasoned that without the ability to utilize energy the way animals now do through the mitochondria, the animal kingdom would have remained a vastness of single cells or simple organisms. As without the ability to utilize energy, sophisticated life forms would have been impossible."

"Yes, Doctor, according to the evolution theory, which states that life constantly evolves and adapts, our cells have evolved because of the incorporation of mitochondria within them to utilize oxygen and sugars to produce energy efficiently. This has enabled animals to evolve into much more complex life forms. A major advance of this energy production and utilization ability is that life started to evolve from single organism to more advanced life forms. These life forms contained a multitude of cells acting in concert with each other, forming various body systems over time such as the lungs, stomach, digestive tract, brain, heart, immune system, etc."

The doctor thought for a moment and said, "So given time, life started simple and then through millions of years of evolution, life figured out how to make it work. As complex and as complicated as this would be, that does seem to be the belief of evolutionists."

"Yet when I learned of this in college biology, I felt it seemed as fantastic of a theory as creationism."

"I see, David. I don't want to get into a talk on religion, but I happen to agree with what you said. It seems to me that either way a miracle of enormous magnitude occurred, either through evolution, creation or something else yet to be figured out. Based on what you said, David, and what the science books state, our cells' ability to utilize oxygen, especially within the mitochondria, has allowed evolution to constantly create higher life forms. Along with this benefit, however, following step by step with it is something called oxidative damage. This damage is inflicted upon most life forms, especially within the mitochondria."

"How's that, Doc? I mean why do you specify the mitochondria?"

THE WEAK LINK

"Many of our cells have better defenses against toxic products created by the processing of energy than the mitochondria do. Of course, the mitochondria are the part of the cells that are actually producing the energy, so it stands to reason that they would be under more stress, especially from some toxic free radicals called reactive oxygen species, or ROS for short, such as hydrogen peroxide and other toxic ROS products naturally produced within our cells as we produce energy. Also, the body produces these ROS's to kill invading microbes. So the body does know how to deal with these reactive oxygen species on a certain level. However, our body can only deal with so many ROS products, before becoming overwhelmed. The sad consequence is that they are very damaging to our mitochondria that are busy producing energy. The body wants to maintain a balance between these ROS products which are free radical in nature and the body's antioxidants to counteract them. However, when damaged, most cells will allow themselves to die off so another healthy cell can take its place. So you end up with damage to your healthy cells at their weakest link, their mitochondria. In fact, as you get older, your cells have far less mitochondria, and the ones they do have are not as effective. This stuff killing off the mitochondria is called ROS. The defenses within our cells will strive to negate this oxidative stress but when they are unable to fully handle them, they will self destruct or are killed off during the process of negating the damage."

"You really make it sound like a war zone, Doctor."

Laughing, the doctor added, "I guess it is, especially if we are consuming the wrong food, too much food, or exposing our bodies to harmful chemicals or radiation. The body's normal defenses, especially mitochondria, can only deal with so much. The mitochondria do not have the same elaborate defenses contained in the rest of the cell, so they are more vulnerable."

"So," David added, "are we dealing with the Antioxidant Theory again?"

"Many theories, David, this whole process indicates that antioxidants are crucial to protect cells, that cell membrane health is crucial, that DNA damage can occur if things get out of control, and gives us a real good theory that we

197

are only as healthy as our cells' mitochondria. I note also that while most cells have lots of mitochondria organelles within their cells, some only have one. If the mitochondria fail, then the cell fails. It also explains and gives total credence to the Mitochondria Theory of Aging, along with the Membrane Theory, the Caloric Restriction Theory, the Prevention Theory, and illustrates that many diseases and disorders are related to these processes along with constant inflammation."

"OK, Doctor, then how does this Mitochondrial Theory of Aging directly affect us, and what can we do about it?"

"It affects us in a major way. Your cells will work in defending themselves and that is not easy, considering what we do to our bodies. However, the mitochondria are one of our weakest links. Even if your cells can defend themselves, they won't fully protect the mitochondria that are working so diligently within those cells. It's like having a smoke fire within a building. The building, which is the cell, can survive, but the occupants, in this case the mitochondria, may not. Knowing this, we must strive to keep the smoke very low within our cells. Hence, you can see the direct connection of the Mitochondria Theory of Aging to the DNA Theory of Aging, the Inflammation Theory of Aging, the Caloric Restriction Theory and others. Loss of mitochondria is a huge factor in aging."

Nodding, David added, "Sounds interesting and makes sense. Who came up with this theory anyways?"

ONE MAN, TWO THEORIES

"Believe it or not, the same person that came up with the Free Radical Theory of Aging, Denham Harman. It makes sense since he wanted to find out how free radicals were causing damage. He saw that the mitochondria were very vulnerable. Hence, the Mitochondria Theory of Aging. Now while Denham Harman proposed this theory, many people that came after him researched it and added greatly to what was going on, especially Jaime Miquel, who pointed out that different cells are affected differently, especially cells that don't reproduce over our lifetimes. Since each of our bodies generates its own antioxidants, we need to make sure that we don't interrupt that process, or better yet, we need to do things that will help the body produce the right amount of its own antioxidants like glutathione."

"OK, Doc, give me an example?"

"An easy one is to avoid Tylenol on a long-term basis. Use it for reducing an occasional fever but not for long term inflammatory suppression in situations like chronic pain or arthritis. Tylenol directly reduces the liver's ability to produce glutathione."

"Wow, that's a big one; is that why some people destroy their livers when they consume too much Tylenol?"

"Exactly, if you consume too much of this product at one time, or if you drink too much alcohol while using it, harm will occur."

"What supplements can we take to protect our mitochondria?" David asked.

"Great question and one that is getting easier to answer these days. Bruce Ames, Ph.D., at the University of California came up with an interesting combination of two substances that appear not only to protect the mitochondria but possibly rejuvenate it. He was able to bring zest back to the lives of lab rats simply by adding acetyl-L-carnitine and alpha-lipoic acid to their diets. Now I recommend his formula or similar formulas to all of my people. Note, scientists have found R-lipoic acid to be even more efficient. Of course, a winning formulation like this can't overcome a really bad lifestyle. So people need to help their bodies along by quitting smoking, stopping excessive drinking, eliminating junk food, reducing their intake of sugar drinks, etc. As do many environmental toxins, if something is harming the body, you must stop the damage. A hidden cause of much mitochondrial damage is mercury. Avoid it at all costs. If exposed, consider using the herb cilantro daily. Consume some every morning and use a soluble fiber supplement at night, like psyllium. Also, reduce your intake of meat, as their proteins cause ammonia to be produced during the digestion process. This overtaxes the liver and keeps the liver from the important task of neutralizing waste products.

"Saying this, for those that have developed impaired mitochondrial function and are seeing the symptoms such as impaired hearing, muscle weakness, or soreness, a newer supplement may prove beneficial. A nutrient called PQQ may be able to preserve brain function and, more importantly, produce mito-chondrial biogenesis, which is the actual renewal of mitochondria."

"Doctor, that means formation of new mitochondria?"

"That's correct. It's all new research, but for those suffering, it's worth looking into. After all, they may be too ill to use robust exercise or caloric restriction, which also works. As I said, stop doing the damage, use all the tools you can to maintain health, and use supplements wisely."

"So, Doc, sounds like you saying the prevention stuff all over again."

"Right you are, David. Eat well, consume plenty of fresh fruits, berries, nuts and vegetables, reduce inflammation by avoiding processed food like flour, sugar, and make sure to consume uncontaminated fish or fish oil. Take time to ex-ercise as well, as this aids the body's detoxification process and actually seems to increase the mitochondria's health, as long as you are not doing ultra-mar-athons. Don't forget about reducing your stress levels, and I almost forgot, get a good night's sleep. If you recall what I mentioned, this would help protect your cell membranes along with protecting your mitochondria. Remember the mitochondria part of your cells have their own membranes in addition to your cells having a membrane. So protecting all cell membranes is crucial."

KEY POINTS
MITOCHONDRIA THEORY

- Follow the previous steps outlined for Prevention, Caloric Restriction, Free Radicals, and Membrane Theory as they apply to Mitochondria Theory as well.

- Foremost for mitochondria protection and energy are R-lipoic acid and acetyl-L-carnitine. If R-lipoic acid is not available, use alpha-lipoic acid. R-lipoic acid is usually twice as strong as alpha-lipoic acid due to the chemical configuration. Lipoic acid is important, as it provides antioxidant protection both to water soluble parts of the body and fat soluble. Lipoic acid may aid in proper sugar metabolism. Using lipoic acid and acetyl-L-carnitine together gives it more synergy in providing mitochondria protection.

- Hint: Look for supplements that contain both of these ingredients together. For example, Life Extension Company offers a product that contains several ingredients such as R-lipoic acid, acetyl-L-carnitine, benfotiamine (a unique form of vitamin B1), and carnosine. All in all, a tremendous way to take all of these supplements together in a synergistic fashion and with a cost savings. Solaray also has a similar product which contains alpha-lipoic acid, acetyl-L-carnitine, resveratrol, and N-acetyl cysteine.

- N-acetyl cysteine and vitamin C may be a good second defense.

- Protect your liver since your liver produces so much of the bodies' glutathione. So what protects your liver? Healthy food along with various supplements like vitamin C, melatonin, turmeric extract, milk thistle, coenzyme Q10.

- Q10 also protects your mitochondria. Life Extension offers a synergistic supplement that includes PQQ.

- Avoid toxic food such as white flour, sugar, high fructose corn syrup, simple sugars added to processed foods, and preservatives. Avoid all processed meat products, and foods covered in pesticides. Weight gain can lead to a fatty liver, and that equates to a liver that cannot protect itself much longer or the body.

- Don't overeat.

- Do aerobic exercise at least four times a week for at least 30 minutes each session.

- Avoid taking Tylenol on a long term basis. When using Tylenol avoid alcohol.

- Avoid mercury.

14
Glycogen
Cross-Linking Theory
Theory VI

"DAVID, WE MENTIONED that oxidative damage is very harmful to the body, and that is why we must naturally consume a lot of antioxidants within our food products. In fact, most food comes loaded with its own antioxidants, if we just eat smart. Eat real food, not processed. Now, that we covered some main theories of aging, I know you see how they all work together."

"Yeah, Doc, but you also mentioned not eating so much helps to reduce oxidative damage but what about those folks that keep eating their average amount of food each day? Are they increasing oxidative damage even if they are consuming only healthy food?'

"Great point, David, the answer is yes, even if you are consuming only healthy food, if you are consuming an excess over what your body needs, you are increasing your oxidative load and should consider upping your intake of antioxidants, as your body is going to be experiencing more oxidative stress. So those that eat more need more antioxidants. Also, your body will be dealing with byproducts of those excess calories, the aftermath of metabolism, along with the added sugar that food naturally places within the body. When we have too much oxidative damage going on we could have a fusing of our protein structures within the body called cross-linking. This is not the natural structure of our cells, so cross-linking will make them less effective. It may even fuse proteins to our very DNA, a very bad thing to have happen. So once again it is better to eat less rather than more to reduce this damage. Experts are now saying that many conditions of aging are really excess cross-linking."

"Like what conditions?"

"On the outside of our body we see skin wrinkling and cataracts, and on the inside it's even worse with things like heart disease, Alzheimer's, kidney problems, bone loss, etc."

"Ouch, Doc, when you say something like that you really make me want to comply with an anti-aging program. So isn't this Cross-Linking Theory the same as the Glycation Theory of Aging?"

"Right, you are, David, of course you are familiar with the Glycation Theory of Aging as you have covered the health and science sections for years. The glycation theory is more formally known as the Glycosylation Theory but people just shorten it to Glycation Theory. Since you follow what is out there for the public on this topic, how much do you think people really know about this topic?"

"Like you said, Doc, we know cross-linking does some bad stuff to our bodies. Most people get it when I use the example of an apple that has been cut, it will quickly oxidize and start to brown almost in front of you. Also, if you mention the excess sugar levels, as you did, they connect it to increasing rates of Type II diabetes and the resulting damage that occurs. Likewise, when I mention that cells become less effective to high sugar levels they understand that, but the stuff about it causing DNA damage I have not heard."

"It is just a theory, David, but in addition to all the harm cross-linking does, it may indeed be causing proteins to be fused to our DNA and causing genetic havoc. Researchers tell us that high sugar levels in our body will induce the same damage to tissues as meat that is heated. In short, high sugar levels are very harmful and are to be avoided. Saying this, many Americans have turned to a high carb diet that is the same as a high sugar diet. Our food pyramid is a hoax. Following the government guidelines on many things will lead to subpar health results."

"Why's that?"

"As you may be aware, the government is leaned on quite heavily by special interest groups. You have dairy producers, corn, wheat, and soy farmers, the cattle industry, pig breeders, even soda pop and snack companies, contributing their input via lobbyists, direct campaign donations, and massive public advertising campaigns."

"Can we really stop it, Doctor?"

"The culprits or cross-linking?"

"Funny, Doctor. I meant the companies and industries that are feeding us both the products and the propaganda. But now that you mention it, can we reverse this cross-linking damage?"

"Sorry to inform you, David, that once the damage is done, it is probably permanent. There are some studies, however, of various new chemical agents that may be able to reverse this damage. It works in the test tube and it worked in small animals, but as of this date it is not working on humans. So, give the researchers some time and they may be able to come up with a drug that will reverse this glycogen cross-linking damage. When they do, say hello to nicer looking skin, an improved heart, better kidneys, and lower blood pressure. All these conditions may be caused by high glycogen cross-linking damage. Hence a lifetime of cross-linking damage will impair our body's ability to function. So the question remains, are we aging or are we glycating ourselves to death with high sugar levels?"

"I hear you, Doc, but we can take steps to lessen the damage, like avoid simple sugars and overcooked foods."

"Good point, David. I saw that advice in one of your articles, but I noted you did not mention taking any supplements. Why was that?"

"Well, Doc, I wasn't aware that the evidence was there for any supplement being available for fighting glycation, at least not ten years ago when I wrote the article. What are your thoughts, Doc?"

"Well, David, we have learned a lot in ten years. Quite a few researchers are recommending taking a supplement called L-carnosine. It helps with its anti-glycation properties plus it helps with other problems of aging like reduced lipid peroxidation. It works well with a supplement called DMAE. We also see people using a B-1 supplement called benfotiamine."

L-CARNOSINE / BENFOTIAMINE

"Doc, I've heard of L-carnosine. How do you see it benefiting us?"

"Well, it appears to have strong anti-aging benefits like being an antioxidant and, more importantly, helping to prevent the formation of advanced glycosylation end-products called AGEs."

"Right, AGEs being abnormal proteins in your body that are damaged and oxidized. Do you use L-carnosine?"

"Yes, I do, David. I take some most days as I believe it may delay many aspects of aging like cancer, inflammation, cell membrane lipofuscin, DNA damage, and more. So, for the money, it is an inexpensive supplement to take."

"How much do you take, Doc?"

"Most days, Dave, I just take 500 mg. However, two or three times a week I double that amount."

"How about benfotiamine, I hear a lot of people that are fighting aging use this supplement."

"Many people are using a form of vitamin B1, also known as thiamine, called benfotiamine. It is used for heavy drinkers of alcohol, side effects of nerve damage suffered by diabetics, and to decrease the effects of a high sugar diet. Natural sources of thiamine can be found in almonds, lentils, and beans. I use it but not in excess. Take it several times a week. Thiamine is needed by the body just like folic acid is. However, too much, especially in a synthetic form, may not be good for you."

CINNAMON

"Doc, since you brought up supplements for controlling sugar levels, do you recommend cinnamon? I've heard that helps mitigate sugar spikes."

"Great question, David. I do use cinnamon in moderation. It seems to lower sugar levels and using about one gram a day serves as a great antioxidant, but you really have to be careful not to take too much and really careful not to take too much of the wrong kind."

"Wrong kind?"

"Yes, if you are just using cinnamon once in a while, like spicing up a pumpkin pie, there is no problem. However, if you are using cinnamon quite often, then you should be aware of what's going on."

"How's that, Doc?"

"All cinnamon contains coumarin. This is both a blood thinner and irritant. Too much can be hard on the liver even causing damage. Coumarin is not the same thing as the blood thinner Coumadin."

"Really, Doctor? I guarantee you most people don't know that. I mean, I'm surprised to hear that myself. I use cinnamon all the time. Tell me more."

"Sorry to inform you, there are many types of cinnamon, but most of what Americans consume is *Cinnamomum cassia,* or common cinnamon, also called Chinese cinnamon, and is much higher in irritants. You can take it every day in small doses to help control blood sugar and is an antioxidant, but don't consume more than a teaspoon daily. It's dark red, has a strong flavor, and is used here because it's cheaper.

"Real cinnamon, or *Cinnamomum verum* (also known as *Cinnamomum zeylanicum*), is much lighter in color, almost a tan color, not a deep red. That cinnamon comes mostly from Ceylon, or Sir Lanka as it's now called. It is much lower in irritants like coumarin and cinnamaldehyde and is more expensive but worth it. This is the type of cinnamon my wife and I use in our coffee and for baking or when we will be consuming a lot of cinnamon in a short time frame. Having said this, while common cassia cinnamon is more of an irritant, it also seems to control blood sugar levels better than the more benign cinnamon from Ceylon. Some studies show a small amount really helps your liver, yet too much may hurt the liver. Go figure."

"I'm really surprised to hear that. So use real Ceylon cinnamon for baking as it contains less irritants, but the cheaper cinnamon may control blood sugar better, always a trade off. How do you tell the difference, Doc?"

"Read the labels on cinnamon spice and supplements, but expect the cheaper stuff to be in it. If buying real sticks of cinnamon, it is easier. Look for a lighter tan color and you can easily grind these up in your coffee grinder. The cheaper Chinese cinnamon, however, which is grown all through the Caribbean, is tough to grind. Cheap cassia cinnamon is real smooth, while Ceylon cinnamon has a little scraggy look in comparison."

CHROMIUM

"Doc, I've got to tell you, I have been using a cinnamon supplement that also contains chromium picolinate. It is marketed as helping to control blood sugar. Have I been hurting myself?"

"Maybe so, David. I mean it may contain cinnamon for helping control blood sugar levels, but the wrong form of chromium."

"OK, you've got me concerned now. Tell me more."

"David, studies have been done and they show two things. One, most Americans are slightly deficient in chromium, and two, chromium seems to help regulate sugar levels and may even increase longevity."

"Right, Doc, that's why I've been using a cinnamon supplement with chromium."

"Right, David, but supplement manufacturers are sometimes behind the times, ignorant, or just producing an inexpensive supplement for the masses."

"OK, Doc, so what should I be using?"

"While cinnamon and chromium in moderation may help your sugar levels and may extend longevity, I would suggest three things. One, using the better form of cinnamon from Ceylon for all cooking recipes, two, only use a very small amount of the cheaper cassia variety for blood sugar levels at a very small dose, and third, use a form of chromium called polynicotinate. It is a niacin-bound chromium and does not seem to mess with our DNA, as large doses of chromium picolinate may do. After all, your goal is to help your body, not hurt it."

"So where do I get the good chromium from?"

"From real food like meats, apples, spinach, green peppers, wheat germ, even bananas, but if you are going to supplement with chromium, look for the ChromeMate trademark on the ingredient list or for the words chromium polynicotinate. You never want to take too much of any mineral, and chromium is no different. I tell clients never to exceed 200 mcg per day. Please note that no one should take most minerals every day, as they are capable of accumulating in your system, especially if your liver function is impaired at all. So you see, David, you could be taking a cinnamon extract that if taken in too large of a dose could inhibit your liver function at the same time you are taking a mineral that can accumulate. Sorry, David, it takes hard work to get the right supplements. I've had to order Ceylon cinnamon on the internet. My wife and I use it on oatmeal, in coffee, and on baked apples. We buy it on eBay, of all places. We still use the cheap form of cinnamon if we are in a coffee shop, but only in moderation. We know it can help blood sugar levels, and acts as an antioxidant, but we are worried it may be too much of an irritant for our livers to use too much of it. We do use the good form of chromium ChromeMate but not every day. Just like we do with the mineral selenium, we only take chromium on the weekends and not every day. You don't want to be deficient with your minerals, but you don't want to overdose on them either."

GLYCATION

"Got it, Doc, I will investigate further. It makes me appreciate why so many doctors tell their patients not to take so many supplements. Because there are so many side effects known and unknown. I know common cassia, or Chinese cinnamon, can't be as bad for you as *excess* nutmeg turned out to be, causing mental disorientation, but it deserves to be looked it. You have given me a real wake up call. Stating that, how do you explain to your patients the dangers of sugar overload and the cross-linking damage it causes?"

"Good point, David. I actually give them a little history lesson so they can get a reference point and understand how this whole sugar overload process began in our society."

"Interesting, Doc. I mean, you've got me hooked. So explain it that way to me."

"Great, David. First off we all know that humans have a sweet tooth, and right-fully so. As hunter-gatherers, we foraged for hundreds of thousands of years. Our taste buds developed the feel for sweeter plants, grasses, fruit, berries and tubers. The sweetness was usually an indicator that these foods were safe to eat, unlike many bitter plants that were too high in alkaloids. So it is only natural for us to find these foods satisfying. Note, primitive people did not have modern farming techniques that stripped down food products where the husks, fiber, protein, minerals, and vitamins had been removed. The result today is many foods are overly processed. Most processed grains are high in sugar content and produce a huge glycemic response within our bodies."

"That makes sense, Doctor, simple carbs turn into simple sugars."

GLYCEMIC INDEX

"Doctor, so by your words, I take it that you believe in the Glycemic Index and its impact on our diets. Do you cover that index with clients?"

"Absolutely, David, as you may know David Jenkins came out with this nutritional index back in 1981; he measured carbohydrates and how quick they get assimilated within our bodies. Too quickly and we get a high glucose level in our blood. He found some carbs give us a quick rise in blood sugar, which is damaging, while other carbs gave a slower response. Before the Glycemic Index became well known we all were making false assumptions about most of the carbs we ate."

"How's that, Doc?"

"Well David, some carbs that we assumed were good for us turned out to be quick releasing carbs instead. These quickly increase our blood glucose levels, possibly causing health concerns down the road, especially if we consumed these types of foods all the time."

"So stay aware of the index, right, Doc?"

"Right, David. It's easy enough to explain, so all nutritionists and doctors should. Foods with a Glycemic Index of 55 are considered low, while those between 56 and 69 are medium, with anything over 70 being high."

"Sounds simple enough, Doc. Do you give your clients a chart of this or a list of foods and their Glycemic Index?"

"We show them this but urge them to get their own reference booklet. It's an eye opener. I mean, we expect white bread to be high on the index but most of us are surprised to see whole wheat bread high on the list as well. Likewise, many, quote, healthy cereals are high on the Glycemic Index list as well."

"I know, Doc. Since my wife and I believe in the Glycemic Index and its usefulness, we have dramatically lowered our intake of many of these bad carbs.

We no longer load up on lots of high glycemic carbs like corn, potatoes, beets, and sweet potatoes. Instead we focus on low glycemic vegetables like cabbage, lettuce, broccoli, green beans, and such. And of course, Doctor, it goes without saying that my family gave up on a lot of those, quote, health snacks like baked potato chips, corn chips or supposedly healthy crackers, which are really high on the Glycemic Index without offering much in any real nutritional value."

"Good to hear, David, most Americans are doing the opposite. It's hard to have an anti-aging lifestyle if you are consuming too many high glycemic carbs. Especially aging is high fructose corn syrup, which in my opinion causes a lot of glycation within the body."

"Right you are, Doc."

The doctor continued, "While in nature we might encounter a patch of honey in the wild, our bodies were never meant to burn these types of calories day-in and day-out. Hence we lack any real defenses against the damage this high carb diet does to our system. It messes with our insulin, our livers, our immune system, and on and on. It's very destructive to our health. I then tell them about a food chemist named Louis Camille Maillard."

"Let me guess, was this in the 1920s?"

"Almost, David. It was around 1912, and Maillard discovered that sugars such as glucose react with proteins in a process called glycation, which is a binding of sugars and proteins or sugars and fats. This whole process produces an end result of impaired molecules. It may dramatically impact their very function. Later, a researcher by the name of Johan Bjorksten who was well aware of this glycation process, noted it was similar to what we consider normal skin aging as we move up in years. He noticed a resemblance of damage occurring on film processes similar to what occurs to human skin. He proposed a theory that this occurs in our cells, tissues, and organs. This glycation process, or cross-linking, makes our bodies much less efficient. So he proposed that what we consider normal aging may, in reality, be excessive glycation and cross-linking damage. High blood sugar levels in diabetics, and the damage and rapid aging it causes, seem to corroborate his theory."

212

"I do recall his name, Doc. He really hit the nail on the head with that theory, but don't we have this glycation process going on no matter what our diets are?"

"Of course, David, but I look at it like swimming in a pool of water or a pool of water mixed with gasoline. One is a lot safer for you than the other."

"I understand, Doc; some glycation is normal, but don't push it."

"Right, David. I then wake up patients to the fact that food companies want to sell product and don't care what steps they take to do it. They push a highly refined product that is void of nutrition and full of glycated products or AGEs. They rationalize that everybody deserves a sugary treat like candy, Pop-Tarts, doughnuts, soda, fruit drinks, and so forth. Most Americans assume their breakfast cereals are safe, but most products are hidden sugar traps and full of toasted AGE products. So we have to be on the defensive. We crave natural sugars to an extent, but have to realize we are being offered false foods. With a little training, it becomes easier to just say no to garbage foods like this. These food companies know this, so they get our children hooked while they are still young by adding sugar to baby foods, advertising junk breakfast meals, and selling fruit drinks like they have some nutritional value."

"People understand all this, Doctor?"

"Yes, David, if you explain it over 5-10 minutes, they do indeed get it. Often, they start giving me their own, real life examples. Once they get it and are put on the defensive, they see what the 'health nuts' have been saying for years. We are being offered too many poor quality food products which are illness promoting, not nourishing or health promoting."

"So, you tell them too much sugar can be a bad thing."

"Right, excess sugar can be very mischievous within the body. Since glucose can react with proteins, you have excess sugar gunking up the works. We expect a certain amount of sugar damage, or glycation as we call it, because it is a normal part of metabolism. However, an excess leads to an increase in cross-linking damage and advanced glycosylation end-products. This gunks up our body."

"Doc, when you say gunked up, what do you mean?"

"David, we discussed that high sugar can cause cells, tissues, and organs to become stiffer from cross-linking damage, but it also affects the heart of our cells, the DNA. Remember, our bodies are amazing; we can survive on junk diets for years and years. I've heard of people living on simple rice, bread or noodles for years. But no one is saying that is healthy. We now know that too much in simple carbs is the same as too much sugar – very health destroying. Health is a path; you are either moving toward good health or away from it."

"Is there a test we can do?"

TESTING

"Everybody needs to have their blood tested for long-term sugar levels. This test is called the A1C test. Most people have heard by now that high sugar levels are harmful and aging. What they don't know is this test can show how good you've been at keeping your sugar levels in line. The hemoglobin A1C test checks out how much glycated hemoglobin is in circulation. That biomarker is representative of your average sugar load over the last three months. You want your A1C levels to be 5% or less. Many Americans, especially diabetics, are testing at 7% or higher."

"But, Doctor, what do you do if your test results are too high?"

"David, to get your A1C levels under control, you need to do several things. One, don't consume so much sugar. It's hard because it is added to so many foods. It goes by many names, such as dextrose, sucrose, fructose and lactose. Two, especially toxic to our bodies and what causes our A1C levels to soar, are foods with AGEs. There are foods that have been overcooked. So stop consuming fried foods, barbequed, charred, overly baked, etc. This food is not only high in overly glycated products, but has had its antioxidants destroyed as well. A very aging combination within our bodies."

"So, Doc, that might explain why some of the low carb diets give people better blood results, less carbs equals less sugar in the system."

"That's right, David. Eat less sugar, less over-cooked food, and fewer simple carbs. Also exercise often, take your antioxidants, and supplement with your anti-glycating agents like carnosine, DMAE, lipoic acid, and benfotiamine."

"So, Doc, will taking digestive enzymes help with a diet of too much sugar and too many simple carbs?"

"I don't think so, David. This high blood sugar condition that causes glucose to attach to our proteins and that is causing damage doesn't need enzymes. So taking enzymes won't help. While I like and use digestive enzymes, the only time I would not use them is when you are eating excess sugar. In fact, you may cause the sugars to digest too fast, causing more damage."

"OK, avoid foods with a high glycemic index."

"Absolutely, David. Low sugar foods and smaller meals are the way to go. To further help reduce glucose levels, take a brisk 20 minute walk after meals."

OTHER BAD STUFF

"So, Doc, I get what you are saying about fried food and food that is overcooked, it produces this toxic stuff, which is hard for the body to process. Anything else we should know about these overcooked foods?"

"Yes, David, I am glad you mentioned that. First off, I always tell people not to fry anything, as that type of food is never found in nature. It seems that any cold-pressed oil that is normally healthy for you if consumed in moderation can become a toxic time bomb, even in moderation, if overcooked. Aldehydes are produced when you fry oils and these can cause cancer and brain degeneration. We worry about those types of oils increasing conditions like Parkinson's disease and Alzheimer's. Surprisingly, healthy oils like flaxseed and sunflower oils handle the excess heat really poorly. Other oils like peanut, macadamia, olive, and coconut oil seem to fair better when heated. But to be safe, avoid all fried foods. Many people are surprised when a family member or themselves come down with these degenerative disorders and often say they don't understand where these disorders come from. However, once you understand how

215

they can be created by a bad diet, you will want to pass on that fried appetizer platter at your local restaurant."

"Wow, Doctor, I knew fried food was bad but I had not heard of that finding."

"Dave, it has been known for a long time and often studies will come out re-affirming what I just told you. I recently saw an article from the journal Food Chemistry where a study was done at the University of the Basque Country in Spain, and they reported on the toxicity of such oils. But for those of us in the nutrition field, we are not surprised in the least."

"Doc, if this is so commonly known amongst nutritionists, what else might be common knowledge that I should report on?"

CANCER CAUSING

"David, something that everybody should have a firm understanding of is the cumulative damage overcooked food can have on our bodies. I have seen several prominent vegetarians develop stomach cancer. Now, we are not surprised when a heavy meat eater develops this type of cancer. After all, many of them burn their meat or consume processed lunch meats full of nitrates. But we are surprised when a vegetarian contracts this type of cancer. Why?"

"OK, Doctor, you have my attention, why indeed?"

"It's speculation, but plant foods have been found to be mostly protective, so what is it in a vegetarian diet that might be causing an increase in stomach cancer? There could be several reasons. One is, overly salted food or pickled food can cause stomach cancer. But number two, in my opinion, is something that is deemed more innocent yet could really be the culprit in many cases. That something is known as acrylamides."

"Yes, I've heard of them. They are produced from toasting of a product, correct?"

"Right, David, they are created anytime you overheat a food product. So frying, baking, or broiling will create them. When you boil or steam your food we don't see many acrylamides forming."

"So, Doc, how does this finding lead you to a theory of why some vegetarians develop stomach cancer?"

ACRYLAMIDES

"Well, David, when people are consuming no animal products they are filling up their diets with something. Often, you will observe a non-meat eater consuming much more grains. Many times, those grains are overly processed. They may consume more baked goods, more toast, more roasted nuts, more grain cereals that have been baked at a high temperature. Doctors report that many vegetarians fall in to the trap of eating too many simple carbs or too much sugar. Unfortunately, they may consume the same type of food over and over, exposing themselves to a possible cancer-causing set of agents called acrylamides."

"So what specific foods contain the most acrylamides?

"I can't tell you for sure, David, but I was surprised to see how many were found in common breakfast cereals. No one wants to report on that story as cereal companies spend a tremendous amount on advertising. One that ranks high in acrylamides was one of my favorite cereals over the years, called Wheatena toasted cereal. They ranked four times higher than another favorite of mine over the years, Cheerios. But, David, we can mitigate a lot of the potential damage, possibly, by consuming antioxidants with our cereals like a lot of Americans are doing. Blueberries and strawberries would be a wonderful compliment to your breakfast cereals."

"OK, you have me concerned. How does Rice Krispies and Corn Flakes rank, as I note they are heavily toasted?"

"They rank much lower in acrylamides than the two cereals I mentioned to you, David. My point is that you can still consume these products but realize that you do not want to consume them everyday as many Americans do, all the while thinking they are doing something totally healthy. Everything in moderation."

"So, Doctor, you mention this to people. How do they handle it?"

"Quite well, actually. I just tell them never to consume fried food or potato chips. Some are worse than others. Chips that have the life baked out of them like baked chips that are low in fat, kettle chips, and stuff like Pringles chips would score real high in acrylamides. Then I warn them not to consume overly baked goods day in and day out. Sorry, but you will never see this stuff in the news. The food companies behind these products are powerhouses when it comes to advertising budgets. It is as it always has been, 'buyer beware.'"

David said with a grin, "OK, I got that. So was all this discovered years ago like in the 1920s?"

Smiling back, the doctor replied, "Actually, no, David, I first heard about it back in 2002 when a Swedish study found these harmful acrylamides in starchy foods like French fries and potato chips. While mostly found in overly baked goods, scientists have also now found these acrylamides in other foods deemed healthier like olives, prunes and even coffee."

"So are you concerned about those other foods as well, Doc?"

"Not really, David. Remember what I said, consume foods with their own antioxidants since that probably protects you. At least olives, prunes, and coffee contain some powerful antioxidants. But it does reinforce what I said earlier, everything in moderation."

KEY POINTS
GLYCOGEN CROSS LINKING THEORY

- Follow all the steps mentioned previously to reduce damage on the cellular level.

- Avoid all added sugar food and drink products, especially high fructose corn syrup.

- Avoid refined food products and hydrogenated oils and hydrogenated fat.

• Never consume fried foods of any type.

• Avoid consuming overcooked food of all types, especially fried eggs, barbecued meats, charred food, and processed baked products.

• Watch your oxidative load and don't overdue oxidative damage by consuming a processed food diet or by over exposing yourself to too much sun, excess radiation from medical body scans and airport check-in body scanner machines, too many medical X-rays, radon gas, or by using oxidative agents like excess alcohol or any tobacco product in any amount.

• Avoid all pesticides, solvents or other toxic chemicals.

• Consider supplements like carnosine, DMAE, cinnamon, chromium polynicotinate (nicotinate, chromium bound to niacin), and benfotiamine (B1), all in moderation.

• A dosage of carnosine, 500 mg per day, should work well with 200 mg of DMAE per day. Many people double those amounts a few days a week.

• Avoid excessive doses of common cinnamon (*Cinnamomum cassia*). A small amount each day is helpful for blood sugar, but an excessive amount may inflame the liver.

• Avoid cheap chromium picolinate. It has been shown to be destructive to DNA when tested in test tubes. Get chromium from food sources or use chromium polynicotinate or the brand ChromeMate.

• Take a brisk 20 minute walk after meals to reduce glucose levels.

15
DNA Telomeres Theory/ Planned Termination
Theory VII

"IN THE HISTORICAL words of John Donne, 'Perchance he for whom this bell tolls may be so ill, as that he knows not it tolls for him...' So it is with life. The body has a clock that ticks down slowly. When that clock called your telomeres stops ticking then many types of cells are told to stop reproducing themselves. The end result is your life slowly starts to end."

"So enjoy it while you can, huh, Doc?"

"That's right, but we will see this generation and many future generations enjoying a lifespan that our ancestors could only dream of."

"What do you see ahead?"

"Well, there is much research currently going on with telomeres and an enzyme called telomerase, and for good reason. Telomeres may be the ultimate currency of life. If your cells' DNA have adequate telomere length, then they may continue to reproduce. If they do not, or if the telomere shortens too much, cell replication will come to a sudden stop. It's like feeding coins into a music machine. When you have coins you hear music, you live. When you don't have any coins left, the music goes silent, your cells die off."

"You almost make it sound poetic, Doctor. I am fond of my music. I don't want it to stop. Are you saying we can really do something about it?"

"Absolutely. What have you heard so far about DNA telomeres, so I don't bore you by repeating too much information?"

"I've heard bits and pieces over the years. Telomeres are at the end of DNA strands and protect the DNA from falling apart. They get shorter each time a cell's DNA replicates itself. Finally, getting to the point, Dr. Leonard Hayflick spoke of what is now known as the Hayflick Limit, usually about 50 replications for most cells, though more or less replications for various other cells before these cells ultimately quit reproducing and die off."

"Good description, David. These telomeres protect the end of DNA strands. Were you aware that our bodies can use an enzyme to replenish these telomeres?"

"Not really, Doctor, but I suppose the body must be able to do this with some cells, like our germline cells and stem cells, right? I mean these types of cells don't seem to age, do they?"

"Great questions, ones we should ask a microbiologist or geneticist. From what I know, stem cells do retain their full telomere length, but are not protected from the onslaught of everyday oxidative stress and damage to the cell's structure and its DNA. Now, in regards to germ cells, this may be the greatest story ever told."

"How's that, Doc?"

"Well, for starters, they are deemed immortal. These cells are what allow for human reproduction. Evolutionary biologists theorize that our germline cells are handed down generation after generation from one common germline ancestor, reaching back through time over a million years, if not a lot longer.

Each of us is created when the germ cell from a man passed via a sperm cell, fertilizes a woman's germ cell, contained in her egg. This joining creates a new life, and I observe that we are all born young then we slowly start to age."

"So, you are saying that these cells are immortal and that we all are part of an endless chain, started millions of years ago?"

"Apparently so. I do note that the germ cell, along with the stem cell, can be damaged as we age. This would explain why older couples may have some developmental problems with their offspring. These germ cells are referred to as your germline. They include various cells in your reproductive tract, like gonocyte cells, that are responsible for sperm and egg production. These germline cells are part of an endless chain going back over time. Somehow, they are able to transfer their data, their information, and their life force from generation to new generation. Truly the most amazing feat I can imagine. But also, something in our bodies allow these cells to retain their youth. Could it be the enzyme telomerase?"

"Sounds very interesting, Doctor. What does research show?"

"Quite a bit, David, we know germ cells have protection mechanisms within them. According to Professor Gregory Hannon, of Cold Spring Harbor Laboratory, they have their own molecular immune system. In addition, we know that germ cells seem better able to repair genetic damage, but perhaps in addition, they have longer telomeres and access to the enzyme telomerase. Some speculate that many of our cells lose their ability to import the enzyme telomerase into their cells, causing the same effect as if they didn't have enough in the first place."

WHY TELOMERES STOP

The doctor paused just a little before continuing. "We know telomeres are essential for protecting the ends of our chromosomes. They keep the chromosomes from fusing to other chromosomes and allow for smooth replication of our genetic material. After replication, the cell that just replicated has less of these protective telomeres caps. As they reproduce more, they continue to have less telomeres caps to the point that they stop replicating. Even as the telomeres are getting shorter each time the cell reproduces, the body does have a substance it produces, which could directly influence the telomeres. This enzyme telomerase can preserve the caps or even lengthen the caps on the end of our chromosomes. However, the body does not generously direct it towards all of our cells, only specific cells like the germline cells.

"Alexey Olovnikov, a Russian scientist, during the early 1970s stated his theory that the loss of these telomeres caps on our chromosomes pushed us to what Professor Hayflick called our cell's life limit or the Hayflick Limit. The further research of three Nobel winners, Elizabeth Blackburn, Carol Greider, and Jack Szostak illustrated how the enzyme telomerase protects our telomeres. You can look at Elizabeth Blackburn's lectures on YouTube to gain fascinating insight of this whole process. We know germ cells, stem cells, and some white blood cells have access to this telomerase enzyme. So does it reside in these cells or are the cells just more receptive to this enzyme? I can't say."

David replied, "But, Doc, wouldn't using telomerase enzymes cause more cancer? I mean that is the problem with cancer cells, they won't stop reproducing, right?"

"We don't know the answers yet. We can just speculate about what you just said. I would note that cancer appears more often in older cells that have shorter telomeres. But is it the aging of the cell or the shorter telomeres responsible for the greater incidents of cancer or something else? So yes, telomeres may be involved in cancerous cells being able to reproduce constantly, but may also be the key to preventing a cell from going cancerous in the first place. But, David, to answer your question, inhibiting telomerase in cancer cells would be a huge step in controlliner cancer. Researchers are studying this as we speak."

"So, Doctor, is this a catch-22 situation? Too little telomerase and your cells get old, leading to an increase in cancer and too much telomerase and you might find cancer cells on their path to immortality and endless replication?"

"Don't know, David, but I feel that the enzyme may be the key to anti-aging, so I would side with every step you could take to preserve telomeres or, if possible, lengthen them."

"Incredible, Doc. Do we know how to do that already?"

"That is what scientists are working on now. They are close to finding solutions for extending our telomeres safely. However, for the time being, we should all strive to slow down the rate of telomere decline. I work with clients all the time in trying to preserve what telomeres they have left. We did not know exactly why certain health steps were helping people, but now knowing about this telomere research, it all makes sense. So back to telomeres, I also point out to people that preserving telomere length will reduce cancer risk, not increase it. Keep in mind, the body if kept healthy, fed correctly with no hydrogenated oils or processed food, and nourished with what it needs, will be very resistant to cancer at any age. Of course, toxic chemicals, radiation, irritants, or excess estrogen from excess dairy foods or pesticides, can cause cancer at any age."

DOLLY'S STORY

"David, let me tell you about Dolly. She was a beautiful baby, at least on the outside. She looked exactly like her mother because she was cloned from her mother."

"Right, Doctor, I heard about Dolly, the cloned sheep, that was awhile ago. Wasn't she the first cloned mammal?"

"Right you are, David. She's gone now but she gave us a lot of knowledge about the cloning process and, perhaps, what we can expect from it and not expect. Great research and great lab work led to the creation and birth of Dolly, these scientists changed our perception of what was possible in the world of biology. It also told us something important about telomeres."

"OK, you have my interest, what did it tell us?"

"Sad to say, Dolly did not start life completely as a newborn. While she looked young on the outside, her telomeres, which she received directly from her 6 year old mother via a nuclear transfer cloning process, were already the same age as her mother since they took one of her mother's cells in the first place to do the cloning process. These cells were already aging."

"Hmm, I think I know where you are going with this...the relentless ticking of the telomeres."

"Good, then you see that the telomeres that Dolly started with were the same age as her mother's telomeres."

"So, Doctor, based on what you said about telomeres, her cells were already aging ahead of schedule. The telomeres in her cells were aging like they were in her mother's cells."

"Right, David, the best way I can describe it is to say, Dolly was like an old gift in a new box."

"So how did this impact her?"

"Dolly lived less than 7 years. She was put down due to health problems. Most sheep live 11 to 12 years. So, in effect, looking at her telomeres, they showed her to be 12 years old, a full life indeed."

"Interesting, Doctor, what this means is in order to address successful cloning in humans some day, we need to address the biological time clock of our telomeres and if we can improve on that, we may be able to reset our own telomeres. That research could add years to our lives."

"I think so, David, but keep in mind, while it is no guarantee of extending our lives, it should indeed, do exactly that. Also, it may dramatically improve our quality of life as we age, as short telomeres seem to negatively impact our health. So it may give us two main advantages: extending our life and adding life to our years."

PRESERVING TELOMERES

"Tell me more, Doc. What can the average person do to preserve their telomeres?"

"Thought you would never ask, David." They both laughed. "David, number one on my list is to reduce stress. Do what you have to do to reduce the feeling of being overtaxed, overworked, and overly concerned about outcomes and such."

"OK, Doc, reduce stress. That sounds simple enough, doesn't it?"

"Depends. Reducing stress means reduced cortisol levels. Doing this keeps your body's hormone levels healthier. High cortisol can make you feel helpless or overwhelmed. To reduce your cortisol levels, you need to focus on reducing all negative emotions as they enter your thinking. For instance, change your thinking to more positive thoughts or reactions when you start feeling thoughts like fear, regret, self-criticism, or chronic worry talk that naturally goes on in our brains when we are not careful in monitoring self-talk. For instance, many people tame negative emotions like fear and jealousy but fail to negate thoughts of self-loathing."

SELF-LOATHING

"Hold on, Doc. What do you mean by self-loathing?"

"Well, David, humans are brought up to have critical thinking skills. They are necessary for our own survival. Too often, however, we fall into the routine of constantly criticizing others because they fail to live up to our expectations. Many times these expectations are unrealistic or created so quickly that no one could live up to them, as we were often unaware of them ourselves just prior to thinking that others should react a certain way. The perfectionist attitude, which dooms anyone from being perfect or meeting our needs. Now here's the thing about criticism. It's very toxic. Subconsciously, we turn that negative judging view inwards on ourselves. We aren't good enough, we fester on mistakes we have made, we self-judge our actions, we doubt ourselves, etc. This is where the term self-loathing comes in. It is a negative emotion and one must take care to eliminate it whenever you become aware of it. So as I say, eliminating stress means changing how you look at the world and how you look at yourself."

"Sounds good, any other steps for reducing stress then?"

"Yes, David, stop the physical factors leading to stress as well."

"Such as?"

"Reduce your caffeine intake as that drives up cortisol levels. Exercise often as that reduces stress, allow more time for getting things done, eliminate many tedious tasks altogether, delegate stuff, get a good night's sleep, take a warm bath, eat healthy, and a real important step we all can take..."

"Which is?"

"Commune with nature every day for at least 20 minutes. Something about being around natural surroundings calms our animal spirits."

"Right, Doctor, I agree. I mean a nice walk outdoors always seems to put things in perspective. I had no clue that high stress levels reduced your telomere length. Any other suggestions?"

HOMOCYSTEINE

"Yes, David, it's important to keep your homocysteine levels down."

"Why's that, Doc?"

"High homocysteine levels are a bad thing for our bodies. As we discussed before, it is definitely a biomarker you want to have under control."

"Explain."

"As you know, high homocysteine levels can damage the lining of our arteries, increasing our risk of heart disease and stroke. But almost all people are unaware that high homocysteine levels are hard on your telomeres, as well."

"I never heard about that part of it. So what does it do exactly?"

"It shortens our telomeres. Why? I couldn't say for sure, but shortens them it does. I suppose it negatively affects methylation and that negatively affects our DNA. As you know, David, many of us get high homocysteine levels from not having enough folate in our diet, others get high levels from consuming too much protein, especially from animal products producing high levels of methionine which can lead to high levels of homocysteine, and some of us are just naturally prone to having high homocysteine levels."

"Well, it sounds like we are back to folic acid again, aren't we?"

Laughing, the doctor added, "I didn't think about that fact, David, but you are right, using real folate along with vitamins B-6 and B-12 may help lower your homocysteine levels. But as we discussed, always use natural folate when possible."

"Gotcha. Any other steps?"

"Check your thyroid function, as that could be causing higher homocysteine levels. While you're at it, have your doctor check your kidney function and review any medications you might be on for its effects on homocysteine levels. Also, I should note that many people have had good luck with a supplement called trimethylglycine."

"Right, Doc, I've heard of this supplement, but most people call it TMG for short. It's a methyl donor compound, correct?"

"Correct. It is a widely held theory that TMG may assist in the process of being a methyl donor, which helps DNA from expressing harmful genes. It is thought that our ability to produce or utilize methyl donors decreases with age, hence, one of the reasons we get ill more often as we age."

"Is that it then, Doctor, for homocysteine?"

"Note quite. An interesting tidbit, David: Women tend to have 10% to 15% lower levels of homocysteine than men, but only during their reproductive years. Also, I use a large amount of vitamin C for treating high homocysteine levels. It seems to help the homocysteine convert to a less harmful substance and allows the blood to flow better. At least that's how I think it's working on patients. But I also would note that high vitamin C levels by itself, helps preserve your telomeres as well."

CYSTEINE

"A lot to remember, Doc. I've heard of bodybuilders using the supplement cysteine. Why would people take that type of supplement?"

"Great question, David, I have to tell you that when dealing with antioxidants, when possible, it is always better to have your body produce its own antioxidants instead of just loading up on handfuls of supplements. Now, when you mentioned taking N-acetyl-L-cysteine, or NAC as we call it, or L-cysteine, studies have found that those two supplements can increase one of the of the bodies most powerful natural antioxidants called glutathione. That is one of the preferred antioxidants our cells like to use. If you can naturally increase the glutathione levels in your body, then your body can decide when to use it and what it will use it for. Much better. Hence, you get people using cysteine supplements to increase their bodies' own natural glutathione levels especially when doing heavy or prolonged training."

"Ok, Doc, that makes sense, but I also heard that anyone taking the supplement L-cysteine should also be taking vitamin C with it. Is that correct?"

"That's right. I have heard the same advice, use vitamin C, especially when taking the form of cysteine called L-cysteine. Others don't feel it is necessary to take vitamin C with N-acetyl-L-cysteine, but let me make it clear, while these supplements, L-cysteine and N-acetyl-L-cysteine, are both potent antioxidants, they don't typically have a lot to do with high homocysteine levels. That type of homocysteine we have been talking about concerns how the body processes the amino acid methionine, or to put it correctly, our body's inability to process it correctly. We have two pathways to process it, remethylation and transsulfuration. Don't ever take large quantities of any supplement unless being directed by a medical practitioner for some specific health crises."

"Give me an example, Doc."

"I would use high quantities of N-acetyl-L-cysteine for someone who's over-consumed Tylenol. In fact, hospitals will often use an intravenous drip of this supplement to help protect the liver from the serious side effects of too much

Tylenol. Both forms, however, might be suitable for mushroom poisoning as well. While I use N-acetyl-L-cysteine often, I only use small amounts of L-cysteine when needed, and when I do, I add vitamin C."

"Why do you recommend vitamin C when taking L-cysteine?"

"The answer is twofold. One is that L-cysteine can lead to rapid detoxification within the liver and vitamin C would greatly aid in this endeavor. The second reason is that too much L-cysteine can lead to the conversion of cysteine to cystine, which is a crystal-type form. That is obviously not good for the arteries or kidneys. Doctors have seen these crystal type formations in people's eyes and internal organs. That is why mega doses of any supplement seldom makes sense. Some bodybuilders use high amounts of L-cysteine but like many things in bodybuilding, it doesn't always make sense nor is it really safe. We see less bodybuilders using these supplements now, as studies have shown that lipoic acid can increase your natural glutathione levels quicker. That is why we often recommend a small amount of a supplement called lipoic acid."

LIPOIC ACID

"Lipoic acid, Doctor? You recommended that for protecting our cell membranes, didn't you?"

"Yes, lipoic acid was brought to my attention by the research and writings of Lester Packer, the director of the Packer Lab. He brought to the public loads of research on antioxidants and their real value. He mentioned in one of his books the value of lipoic acid. Since then, I have seen these lipoic acid supplements evolve."

"Evolve how?"

"Well, David, after studies showed lipoic acid increasing our bodies' natural master antioxidant glutathione, researchers also found that lipoic acid helped lower blood sugar levels, reduced oxidative stress, and helped other antioxidants like vitamin C and E, and even Co-Q10, recycle so they could be used again by the body, researchers found ways of producing an even better form of lipoic acid. We are using lipoic acid in many anti-aging regimens."

"A better form of lipoic acid? How?"

"At first we only had alpha-lipoic acid to work with, but then they found they could commercially produce a better form called R-Lipoic acid, much more bang for your buck as the saying goes."

"So Doc, you heard about this through the Packard lab? Just so I can research it further. What year was that, do you recall?"

"David, Lester Packer published a book on antioxidants just before the year 2000. But, I have to tell you that alpha lipoic acid was discovered a lot earlier then that. Scientists found out about it back in the late 1930s, and Dr. Irwin Gunsalus was credited with synthesis of a supplement in the 1950s, which proved helpful in treating various liver disorders."

"To summarize, Doc, you recommend lipoic acid, N-acetyl-L-cysteine, or cysteine with vitamin C. What about vitamin C, do you ever use that just by itself?"

"Absolutely. I take 2000 mg per day. 1000 mg with my afternoon meal and 1000 mg an hour after my evening meal. But remember, while I like to use synergistic formulas, most any vitamin C will do. Just try to find one that has something else with it to make it better for you, like bioflavonoids."

"What form of vitamin C do you use?"

"My wife and I take an ascorbic acid formula that includes some mixed bioflavonoids, quercetin, and magnesium at our first meal and a non-acidic form later after our last meal."

"Oh, you take magnesium each day?"

"Most days, David. It is a master antioxidant for the body, helping prevent a lot of disorders."

"Such as?"

"Well, I feel it helps your heart valves from becoming calcified by allowing calcium to be properly absorbed. Also, it helps in preventing high homocysteine levels."

"I am surprised to hear that, Doc. So minerals can be really good for you?"

"In moderation, David. Remember what I said about iron?"

"Yes, I do. Excess iron is very oxidative. OK, Doc, I get it, stress and pollution decrease our stores of vitamin C. So that is why we should supplement."

"Very good, David. I think you came to the right conclusion. Bad air, like bad habits, quickly destroy anybody's good health."

"Any more suggestions on telomere health?"

TA-65

"Yes, remember the first things we mention about prevention, antioxidants, and caloric restriction? All of them apply towards your telomeres. You can be tested to see the chronological age of your telomeres. Stress and a bad lifestyle can quickly diminish their length. A few companies are working on, and even currently selling, a proprietary supplement that may actually extend your current telomeres. One of the most promising is called TA-65."

"OK, Doc, what's TA-65 about?"

"Well, TA-65 is supposed to produce the enzyme telomerase within your body. It is derived from astragalus. Taking regular supplements of astragalus is a thought, as it helps immunity and may also act as an adaptogen, allowing you to handle stress better. However, saying this, it would not be possible to get enough of it into your system to equate to what TA-65 does."

"So TA-65 is derived from astragalus, Doctor, but astragalus alone doesn't do what TA-65 does?"

"That's right, David, just like the supplement resveratrol. In which a pill gives you the equivalent amount of resveratrol contained in a hundred bottles of wine. You would need bushels of the astragalus plant to equal what is contained in the one capsule of TA-65."

David laughed. "What a picture that would be, a person eating bushels of astragalus."

"Really, David, they would die from mineral poisoning or a fiber blockage first before getting enough of the ingredients needed."

"Any other tips on preserving telomeres?"

"If you don't feel the TA-65 route is for you, and that is a big if, since we don't know enough about how it may behave in your body long term, I would consider a more natural protocol offered by Gary Null."

"OK, Doc, I've read several of his books. I don't recall anything about telomeres."

"I don't either, David, but his anti-aging protocol would flood the body with micronutrients, chlorophyll, vitamins, and bioavailable minerals in their proper form and portions. So his protocol is acting in a natural way to rejuvenate the body from the inside of the cell out, protecting the cell's RNA and DNA, allowing for proper gene expression, and allowing the body to naturally repair mistakes. All in all, a great way to go."

"What does it involve?"

"A lot of items like stress reduction, juicing, consuming organic foods, avoiding toxins, and such. I would do him a disservice by trying to break his protocol into a sound bite. His books should be read by anyone who is serious about extending their lives or adding quality years."

David and the Doctor continued discussing the topic of telomeres and David was aware that not all cells replicate themselves as we age. The brain and many heart muscle cells stay just the way they are, which makes them fallible in the long run. The doctor stressed that even with telomere therapy, we may all sooner or later just wear out, which he said was another theory of aging to be discussed later.

KEY POINTS
TELOMERE THEORY

- Follow all the steps to anti-aging such as prevention, caloric restriction, antioxidants for free radical damage, protecting your cells' membranes, preserving your mitochondria, and preventing excess cellular, tissue, and organ cross linking damage via the glycogen cross-linking theory.

- Tame inflammation.

- Keep stress in your life to a minimum. Use tools like exercise, long walks, yoga, meditation, communing with nature. Establish a network of friends, be realistic about issues, and in dealing with people don't be a perfectionist. Practice forgiving others and yourself for mistakes that will always be made.

- Monitor your homocysteine levels and reduce them if necessary. Consider using the supplement TMG (trimethylglycine) to help.

- Telomeres affect cells' ability to replicate so it may go a long way in preserving and extending your life. Various supplements may help such as TA-65 offered by a company named Geron. As of yet, no real studies have been published on the effects or safety of TA-65.

- Take vitamin C each day. At least 1000 mg twice a day.

- Consider a quality magnesium supplement and take daily.

- Strive to consume natural, non-synthetic versions of vitamins B, C, and E.

- **Exercise on a regular basis.**

- **Everyday consume some fresh vegetable juice that contains green plants.**

16
The Inflammation Theory
Theory VIII

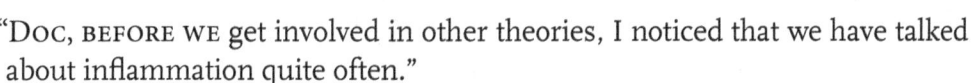

"Doc, BEFORE WE get involved in other theories, I noticed that we have talked about inflammation quite often."

"That's right, David. It wasn't well known 20 years ago, but people are waking up to the fact that we have a huge problem in our midst – excess inflammation."

"Right, Doctor, many people talk about it, but how do you define it?"

"Good point. Yes, many people do talk about it and, like a lot of things, you can have different reasons for inflammation in the body...so, lots of causes but one major effect, a shift of the body towards an inflammatory response and its resulting damage. The type of inflammation that is so damaging is chronic inflammation. That is our bodies' response to harmful things that we expose our bodies to."

"Interesting point, Doctor, so actually there are many causes of inflammation. What, in your view, is the most common?"

"Hard to say, David, excess sugar consumption along with an overload of simple carbs would definitely be inflammatory, but so would eating a diet of processed oils. I mean a diet of trans fats or hydrogenated oils, as they call them, can quickly compromise anybody's health. Especially when you add an abundance of processed omega-6 oils. The body uses up a lot of its own natural antioxidants dealing with this onslaught."

"Are you saying omega-6 fats are bad?"

"No, not at all, if you are consuming a moderate amount in a natural state, you will do well, especially if you are also consuming a moderate amount or equal amount of natural omega-3 fats with them."

"OK, Doc, so are we back to the concept that inflammation is tied to your diet?"

"Not always, David. I mean infection, injuries, diseases, parasites, bacteria, viruses, stress and pollution can all be causes of inflammation. Lots of chronic inflammation, however, manifests itself in people today causing autoimmune disorders on a huge scale. I mean, once our bodies find themselves compromised or confused, then disease patterns are allowed to take hold."

"Like what diseases?"

Slowly releasing his breath, the doctor responded, "David, you're asking the golden question, which is seldom addressed let alone discussed. It's hard to quantify, but let me try. You should note that 70% of all chronic medical conditions are related to inflammation as are many autoimmune disorders. Why? Bad diets lead to chronic inflammation, just as long-term stress leads to chronic inflammation, and on and on it goes."

"OK, Doc, I'm detecting a long list of maladies that are about to flow out of you, am I right?"

Smiling, the doctor nodded. "David, almost all of the major diseases as we know them or that we think as normal parts of aging are, in truth, consequences of inflammation. Things like diabetes, cancer and most heart disease."

"What else?"

"It's possible that most autoimmune disorders are also related to chronic inflammation. The list of those disorders are almost too numerous to mention, but I will give a handful, like asthma, arthritis, chronic fatigue, irritable bowel syndrome and lupus."

"So, Doctor, is it fair to say that you think many diseases and disorders are caused by inflammation, and inflammation is caused by a bad diet of sugar, simple carbs, and bad fats and oils?"

"Right, David, but let's not leave out excess salt and salt substitutes like MSG."

"Any other tips to further reduce inflammation?"

"Yes, get a good night's sleep, drink pure water that is free of fluoride and chlorine, and get outside with nature each day, like we were meant to do. Make sure you are not too high in minerals like copper and especially iron. Follow all the health steps we discussed so far and inflammation will not be a problem."

Looking at his notes, David smiled before saying, "Wow, Doctor, I get it. Use the steps you mentioned like prevention, caloric restriction, antioxidants from mostly natural sources to protect from free radical damage, avoid excess sugar consumption and its glycogen cross-linking damage, protect your cell membranes inside and out, along with protecting your mitochondria, take steps to preserve your telomeres, and you will naturally avoid most inflammation. Is there anything I left out?"

Laughing, the doctor added, "David, I really love a good listener."

They both laughed. They exchanged notes over the next several hours. The doctor explained that all the steps he mentioned previously prevented most chronic inflammation. A healthy diet containing fish, berries, salads, vegetables, fruits, and anti-inflammatory powerhouses like cherries, ginger and turmeric. David noted that the doctor repeated over and over again that heat-treated oils, hydrogenated fats, or too much of omega-6 oils could push someone into an inflammatory state. Of course, David already knew that basic bad habits like drinking excessive alcohol, smoking, and a stressful lifestyle could keep someone in a pro-inflammatory state.

The doctor explained that natural inflammation processes were referred to as acute inflammation, a natural and usually very quick response to some type of injury, while chronic inflammation usually produced by a faulty diet and lifestyle was the risk factor that must be avoided long term to gain a healthy and long life.

David knew that inflammation was natural in the body when the body encountered a cut, wound or insult, but also relieved when the doctor informed him that moderate exercise could reduce chronic inflammation.

The doctor told David in his opinion that the three main causes of chronic inflammation were processed food, hydrogenated oil, and the lack of magnesium in our food and water.

INFLAMMATION CULPRITS

The doctor explained to David that the average and unaware American has no chance in maintaining a healthy body long term, unless, they are aware of the five main causes of inflammation. He called these five factors H.E.A.P.S. He explained them as:

<u>H</u>ydrogenated Oil & Fats
<u>E</u>xcess Omega-6 Oils
<u>A</u>rachidonic Acid
<u>P</u>rocessed Food
<u>S</u>ugar Excess

When David inquired on how arachidonic acid factored in, he was surprised to find that excess arachidonic acid can be extremely inflammatory to humans. It is found in animal products, especially eggs and poultry. It may help explain why those that regularly overconsume these animal products have higher rates of cancer and heart disease. The doctor explained that current livestock practices in the United States found factory farms feeding excess omega-6 rich grains, such as corn and soy, to their cattle, pigs and poultry to fatten them up. This increased the levels of omega-6 in their tissue and also increased their arachidonic acid levels. Normally, these animals naturally ate a more balanced diet consisting of a lot of omega-3 fats in addition to the omega-6-fats. So now Americans found some of their favorite foods becoming increasingly more inflammatory.

Most grocery stores and restaurants also loaded their shelves with omega-6 rich cooking oils like corn, soybean, safflower, sunflower, peanut, and the worst oil possible: cottonseed. What makes cottonssed oil so bad? It is highly contaminated with pesticides. Also, many salad dressings are loaded with the same oils. Avoid using too many omega-6 based oils, as they will be inflammatory when consumed in excess. Baked goods found in most grocery stores, restaurants and doughnut shops are hidden havens for these oils as well, and worse: highly inflammatory partially or fully hydrogenated oils.

The doctor explained that certain carnivores, like tigers and lions, require arachidonic acid as an essential fat, but humans did not. We can create our own arachidonic acid within our bodies from food consumed. Of course, the doctor explained that there are other causes of inflammation like not getting enough magnesium in our food or water. This also could lead to a pro-inflammatory state.

LEAKY GUT SYNDROME

Doctor Tessler explained that eating a high sugar diet along with processed foods—void of their enzyme potential as most processed foods are—makes it highly inflammatory. Much of today's foods have had their enzymes destroyed and their natural phytochemicals compromised to such a large extent that they offer only a fraction of their true nutrient potential. This occurs when food is processed to insure a long shelf life. Often these products are precooked, baked, dehydrated, powered, canned or frozen. This often leads directly to poor or incomplete digestion causing the compromised food product to impact the permeability of our intestines, called leaky gut syndrome, which then causes a strong immune reaction leading to inflammation. This is not the only cause of this condition but this along with alcohol abuse and allergic reactions are listed causes. This may lead someone directly to life draining maladies like myofascitis, inflammatory bowel disorders, fatty liver, fibromyalgia, or other inflammatory disorders.

B.E.

The doctor spent time discussing an acronym he called B.E., an abbreviation for balance and excess. He stated that you can balance your oil and fat intake to a certain extent. Make sure you are consuming enough omega-3 oils to offset the amount of omega 6-oils. Our bodies require both of these essential fatty acids in moderation. Important to note, you can balance these two oils only to a certain extent. An excess of omega-6 could lead to a pro-inflammatory state regardless of how much corresponding omega-3 oils you are consuming. If more oil consumption is desired, consider the more neutral mono-saturated oil like olive oil. It is mostly an omega-9 oil with a smaller amount of omega-6, followed by an even smaller amount of omega-3. Most oils do in fact contain some omega-3 and omega-6. Some nutritionists state we can consume a higher ratio of omega-6 versus omega-3, but lately others are stating that it should be more in balanced to tame inflammation. People should be wary of all oils as they were not naturally part of our diet. They are, for the most part, a highly processed, concentrated fat product. Also, consider fresh avocados (mono-saturated) for a healthy fat source along with a small amount of cold processed coconut oil (saturated fat).

KEY POINTS
INFLAMMATION THEORY

- It's crucial to follow all the previous steps outlined to tame inflammation.

- Avoid processed food.

- Avoid too much sugar.

- Avoid all trans fats, partially hydrogenated fats, or rancid fats. All of these processed fats are toxic. Heat-treated fats are unnatural to the body and will quickly make any body inflammatory.

• The start for reducing inflammation within your body starts with diet. Reduce all simple carbs, such as sugar, processed food, packaged foods, fried foods, fast foods, junk food, white flour, soda pops of all types including diet, canned or bottled fruit juice, which are usually just sugary fruit imitations, excess alcohol, etc. Ditch these simple carbs, as they cause inflammation.

• Balance the good fats you consume by making sure you are consuming, in moderation, the best omega-6 fats, such as nuts, flax seed, cereals, avocado, borage oil, sunflower and pumpkin seeds. It's crucial to include an adequate amount of omega-3 fats as well such as flax seed, chia seed, quinoa grain, and walnuts and cold water fish. Many oil and fats, such as olive oil, are neutral; these are called monosaturated. Consider fresh avocados and cold processed coconut oil as additions to your diet.

• Monitor your inner terrain. Bad diets, stress, and lack of exercise can make your body inflammatory. A bad lifestyle will allow various bacteria and fungus to take over too much of your biological territory or your inner terrain as it is also called. This can result in a host of problems such as H. pylori bacteria giving you ulcers, yeast infections, fungus disorders, leaky gut syndrome, autoimmune disorders, and a host of other afflictions. You need to consume a minimally processed diet of real foods in their natural state and consume a diet that is mostly alkaline.

• Never smoke and limit your exposure to polluted air, water or food.

• Take steps to distress such as long walks, quiet times, meditation, gardening, hobbies and sports. Prolonged exercise, if not taken to excess, will reduce inflammation within the body.

• Avoid toxic people. These are people who are negative, gossip constantly, complain too much, or belittle others. People that constantly doubt or demand that you prove something can be energy draining. These people lower your immune system while also driving up your cortisol levels, a major stress indicator.

- Exercise on a consistent basis, walking at least 30 minutes minimum each day.

- Use supplements like turmeric, ginger, vitamin C, green tea, and a good source of omega-3 oils from cold water fish or krill capsules.

- Consume raw food with any cooked food to garner some natural enzyme potential. Supplement with digestive enzymes with meals and between meals to tame inflammation.

- Use a magnesium supplement most days to tame excess chronic inflammation. Best forms are magnesium citrate, magnesium orotate, magnesium glycinate, and magnesium chloride.

17
The Thymic-Stimulating Theory
Theory IX

"So far, Doctor, we have covered theories that we can do something about. What theory of aging, however, do you feel we have less control over?"

"That is an interesting and deep question, David. I have often wondered about society's expectations regarding one's aging. Quite frankly, it stinks."

"How's that?"

"Well, society, in general, gives a very negative view on growing old. Here in this country, two gerontologists, Elaine Cumming and William E. Henry, proposed a theory on aging people called disengagement. It states older people naturally refrain from many social activities and that is normal with aging. I don't fully agree; I feel it's more about society pushing our elderly into tight corners, than elderly people wanting to be left alone. Our society and its businesses market to the youth market and make life all about the young consumers. Yes, older people do withdraw some because they can't be as active in some things or perhaps they feel they have done it already. But I sense the reality is that many older people have lost touch with much of their social network.

Why is that? It's just natural for them to lose contact with multiple friends and family members they had while growing up and during their formative years. People spread out, friends pass on, times change, so this is a real factor for losing their support base. Consequently, elderly people often feel cut off from and out of sync with society. They feel they don't belong yet the reality is, they belong as well as any other segment. So many elderly people go along with this misguided thought process of feeling left out and quit living full lives."

"Really, Doc? What do you mean?"

THE SHOULDS

"Look around you. I call it the shoulds. People have the expectation that older people should move slower, should play less sports, and should not do young people things like roller skate, ride mountain bikes, climb mountains, scuba dive, etc. The list goes on and on."

"That's right, I never thought about it that way. I mean, I take martial arts classes and, you're right, I never see anyone over the age of 65 working out there."

"That's a shame, David. Some of the world's most knowledgeable martial arts experts are in their 70s. Your class is missing something."

"I know, Doc, but even with my father, I notice him withdrawing from life. In fact, I think he is fighting depression."

"I wouldn't doubt that, David. Society has turned a blind eye towards our elderly and downplays their significance on almost every level. I suggest you look at television to see what I am saying. The only elderly role model I recall is Matlock, and God bless Andy Griffith for his charm, wit, and problem solving abilities, but he was not in the best shape for a senior. We need more types like Jack LaLanne to wake up people to how vibrant your senior years could be. He lived vibrantly to his mid 90s."

"So how do we address that issue, Doctor? It seems so complicated, almost like it's written in stone already."

"It's a mindset, David. I guess everyone needs to focus on themselves in this area. Stay fit, stay active, stay involved, stay independent, stay educated, and seek out friends of all ages. Build up your own safety network of people who see you for who you are, a very alive and vibrant person!"

"Great points, Doc, but I can see why someone would think that many elderly are secluding themselves from people."

"You're half right, David. That is sad, but not all cultures are like this. Look at the Japanese. They respect age a lot more than we do here, and, you guessed it, people there live a lot longer. They are intentionally included, not excluded, and the only withdrawal you see of older people there is when they go off to take a nap in the afternoon. The same goes for many cultures in the world."

WHY WE FAIL

"So what really happens as we age, Doctor? What have you seen that takes people out of the game called life?"

"Everything we've talked about, and more, of course. I see many elderly people having a health crisis, like falling and breaking a hip, a heart attack, a stroke, or a bout of pneumonia. That one event can start a chain reaction or a negative cascade towards failing health and often this precedes their untimely demise."

David asked, "So how is that a theory of aging?"

"Think about it, David, once your immune system goes, or if it is compromised, death can follow quite quickly."

"Oh, right, Doctor, I see where you're going with this line of thought."

"So, David, one must keep up their immune system to help survive these crises as they come up. I have many elderly patients that had a heart attack, or a bout of cancer in their 70s, and go on to survive to their late 90s. So having a strong immune system and a will to continue can make a huge difference in longevity. Also, remember, David, I mentioned caloric restriction can rev up the immune system. Something about it helps preserve our T-cell function. We are better able to fight off colds and infections."

"I have heard things, Doc, like fast when you have a cold to greatly diminish its duration."

"That's right, David, but getting back to your question, how is the immune system a theory of aging, let me relate that as we grow older our immune system tends to grow less vigilant. Why is that? A real possibility is that our thymus gland starts to shrink, as it does, so we have less immune cells patrolling our bodies."

"Doc, describe why this would cause aging?"

"Well, I can think of several ways. One is that we need a strong immune system to fight off disease, sickness and cancer. However, another way a weak immune system causes aging goes back to what we discussed before regarding the reasons we age. I mentioned cell senescence."

"Yes, Doc, that's our cells knowing when to terminate, right?"

"Right, David, but that's my point. If too many cells don't die off when they should, you get too many cells in the body that are old and ineffective. Worse, some of them start producing toxic byproducts. So having a strong immune system would allow your body to clear out these defective cells, thereby promoting youthfulness."

HOW TO PRESERVE YOUR IMMUNE SYSTEM

"Doc, what can you tell me about the thymus gland?"

"Quite a bit, but not everything. You see, in medical school we were taught that the thymus gland wasn't important. Of course, that was many years ago and we now know better. In fact, the thymus is control central for certain lymphocytes. These lymphocytes are known as T-lymphocytes, a type of white blood cell. The thymus doesn't produce them but shelters and nourishes them until they fully develop then releases them into our system to protect against infections. All mammals have a thymus, but they can be located in different areas of the body. Ours is under the breast bone of our upper chest area. They are quite large in humans while we are young, but reduce dramatically in size as we head towards adulthood. It gets smaller as we age; leading many to speculate that this is the reason our immune system faces a reduction in its vital force. I should note some researchers' state the thymus does not shrink in all mammals. One of many theories circulating is that when we consume processed, cooked, or denatured food, it causes the thymus gland to shrink as we age. I have not looked into these studies but if correct it should serve as a wake up call concerning eating a processed diet. When you hear of people referring to an animals body part as sweetmeat, they are usually talking about the thymus gland. And many hunters will tell you that the sweetmeat on a wild animal is plentiful."

"OK, I can research those studies, Doctor, and I agree, if true it could be very meaningful, but regarding the spleen, doesn't the spleen produce lymphocytes, too?"

"Well, David, most are produced within our bone marrow, but it just goes to show how connected our organs are. People that have had their spleens removed are much more prone to infections, especially sepsis. So the spleen must be producing some type of lymphocytes as well. Scientists say it's the white pulp within our spleens that produce some of these lymphocytes. So it is a duel purpose organ, producing lymphocytes and getting rid of old red blood cells. Now the thymus gland, which many thought of as separate from the rest of the endocrine system, is indeed a part of this system. And like other glands, it does indeed send chemical messages, so it is indeed part of the endocrine system. This thymus acts as a reservoir for T-lymphocytes to mature some before doing their job in protecting the body against infections. Often ignored by science and the medical world, the thymus may be a major key in living an extra long life."

"How's that, Doc?"

"Well, if your thymus is not functioning up to speed, you could see yourself catching infections much easier, or worse you could perish from pneumonia, infections or even cancer. And, as it goes, many elderly people pass away from pneumonia and cancer."

"Cancer?" asked David.

"Sure, David, remember T-cells refer to cells that pass through the thymus. If they are not on the job then the potential for cancer increases dramatically. In addition, to attacking viruses and bacteria, our immune system goes after our own cells if they are malformed, dysfunctional, or cancerous."

ARE THERE ANY SURPRISES?

"Doctor, one of my favorite questions, as you may know by now, is 'Are there any surprises?' I mean regarding the lymphatic system."

"Right, David, you do like to ask that surprise question, and it's a great question. It makes me think. Usually, I come up with something unique about what we are discussing. Let me ponder a moment here, as you know the thymus doesn't get much respect, but yes, I do have some surprising information on the thymus."

"Great, let me have it."

"Many years ago doctors thought an enlarged thymus was a sign of disease. They were not aware that very young people have a large thymus gland, as it was incubating and training newer T-cells. Now the doctors had done autopsies quite often, years ago, as it was a common practice. They did autopsies on babies that died of sudden infant death syndrome and found they had very large thymus glands. They made the assumption that these large thymus glands had suffocated the babies. This was because of the location of the thymus gland to a human's trachea, or windpipe as most people call it."

"Excuse me, Doctor, you mean autopsies if people died in unpredictable ways, right? Not from natural causes?"

"Actually no, they used to do autopsies in most cases. This was a great way to find out what really killed people. Often, the doctor thought one thing had killed a person but upon autopsy, found out an entirely different cause of death. These investigations led to a large advancement of what actually was killing people. What was really going on? It gave us doctors a lot more understanding of the body's weak points or vulnerabilities. It gave us a better view on disease pathology and, more importantly, it also kept a doctor honest with themselves."

"Honest, Doc?"

"Well, the autopsy report often showed the doctor that what he thought killed the patient was, in fact, not correct. It made doctors less cocky, in my opinion. I mean, if you lost a patient, you also saw a report on that. Someone else looking at what occurred. A huge benefit for the medical sciences."

"How would performing more autopsies help us now?"

"I can't say for sure, but many patients die from their treatments, medical mishaps, or toxic drugs. Autopsies might help put an end to some of this nonsense."

"OK, back to children having larger thymus glands. How did this pose a problem?"

YOU WANT TO DO WHAT?

"Well, David, well-intentioned doctors would get a sick infant and observe a large thymus gland. They thought that this large thymus gland was a problem, so they would radiate it, greatly reducing its size."

"Really, Doc? What did that do?"

"As you know David, radiating an organ is not usually a good thing. It did shrink the thymus gland, and for a long time most children still did well in spite of this misguided treatment. That was until years later when many of them developed thyroid cancer. That was because the radiation used on the thymus also radiated the thyroid at the same time. Thousands of thyroid cancer cases were caused by these treatments. Remember those autopsies I mentioned? Well, when they did autopsies of healthy children that died in accidents, they started noticing that infants' and children's thymus glands were naturally bigger at those ages. Nothing was wrong with the thymus gland's size."

"Wouldn't they have noticed that with the autopsies on sick children as well?"

"Not really. Many times when a person is sick, their thymus will shrink in size as it fights an infection."

"So that was the surprise, Doctor? Our thymus gland starts big and gets smaller as we age, nothing to worry about, right?"

"Right, David. In the early 1960s a research scientist by the name of Jacques Miller researched the thymus gland in depth. He found that if you removed the thymus gland of an animal at birth, then that animal loses much of its immune system. So hence, he proved the value of the thymus gland. The gland used to be thought of as a waste processing plant for T-cells. We now know better. We need more researchers like Jacques Miller."

"Wow that was a great insight. Any more surprises?"

"Well, yes. Amazingly, if you remove the thymus gland long after birth, the effects are not anywhere as severe. So strange, to say the least."

"Any more surprises, Doc?"

THYMUS EXTRACT

Smiling, the doctor replied, "There's that surprise question again, David. Let me think. OK, yes, recently a story was written about a very sick patient suffering from pneumonia. The patient wasn't going to make it. A doctor gave a series of thymus injections, allowing for a recovery that was deemed nearly impossible. So the door may be open to using thymus extract in the future for elderly folks who are not responding to antibiotics, etc."

"Thymus extract? Is that safe?"

"Right, David, I certainly would not use an animal's gland product unless I was desperate. I mean, you would have to make sure it was from an uncontaminated animal like a cow from New Zealand or Argentina, where no cases of mad cow disease have ever been reported."

"OK, that makes sense in a lot of respects, but how do we keep our thymus gland active so we don't need injections?"

"Number one in my book is exercise. Using a mini-trampoline daily will get the lymph fluid moving within your body as well as possibly stimulating your thymus gland. Along with that, David, I would add a yoga pose called the cobra, which forces you to stretch your chest cavity as you reach upward during this stretch."

"Any other tips, Doc? I mean, if this gland is so important, why aren't we all trying to protect it?"

"Good point, David. Science needs to study the thymus a whole lot more. We can speculate that a healthy diet and lifestyle will help protect your thymus gland, but how much it helps, we do not know. So following all the previous anti-aging steps we covered already should help. Also, make sure you consume a good diet of mostly fresh food, not overly processed, including lots of uncooked fruits and vegetables and that should go a long way."

"Interesting viewpoint, Doctor. You're saying we have our own antibiotics within our body which, everyday, helps fight off infections."

"Good analogy, David. Our immune system originates from several different points within our body, such as our bone marrow, which produces our white blood cells or leukocytes, as they are called. But keep in mind that our immunity is linked throughout the body like white blood cells in our blood and lymphocytes in our lymphatic system."

"The lymphatic system? What does that have to do with our thymus gland?"

THE LYMPHATIC SYSTEM

"Quite a bit, David, as you know, the body is divided up into operating systems like the cardiovascular system, nervous system, endocrine system, but often ignored is the lymphatic system. A series of tubular tissue that runs throughout the body allowing germ fighting lymphocytes to do their job. They are defenders against bacteria and wipe out viruses and malformed human cells. If they did not, you would soon perish."

"So it is like another circulation system, similar to our blood supply?"

"Yes, but instead of the heart pumping this fluid, the body uses several other methods for circulating this lymph fluid. In fact, this lymph fluid comes initially from our blood circulatory system. The lymph fluid is created from our blood supply's plasma as it makes its way through our capillary system. Our blood contains about 60% plasma, and this plasma migrates out from the blood system into the lymph system. This protective lymph fluid bathes our tissues and dramatically protects the body from viruses, bacteria, malformed cells, and other pathogens. It escorts this bad stuff to the lymph nodes where they are destroyed. It also allows fats and fat soluble vitamins from our digestive tract to be passed on to the cells in our body. Then the lymph fluid cleans our tissue as it makes its way via a one-way path that moves its fluid up the body. Once the lymph fluid has completed its journey of feeding our body's cells and tissues, killing invaders, and cleaning our body's tissues, the majority of this fluid gets added back to our blood supply at the top area of our necks, called the thoracic ducts. So, just so you know, our lymph system is connected to our spleen, tonsils, adenoids, and, of course, our thymus gland. An amazing system and nature's way to circulate some of our white blood cells where the tissues get bathed in this protective fluid."

"I see, Doctor, so everything really is connected."

"Right, David. So stimulating your lymph fluid circulation may aid your thymus gland as well. The thymus gland produces thymic hormones, which help control our body's immune system. All of our glands work together in various feedback loops. If you lose your thymus function, it just may signal the rest of your endocrine system to shut down your remaining life force. So the Thymus Theory of Aging may be directly related to the Neuro-Endocrine Theory of Aging."

"Any other tips to restore our thymus gland, Doctor?"

"It is a field that is wide open to speculation, but I have heard of alternative practitioners using low doses of melatonin with their patients, a small amount of zinc may help restore thymic activity, DHEA may help, human growth hormone may cause an increase in T-cells, a supplement called indole-3-carbinol, which can block testosterone in men from being converted into excess estrogen, DIM for excess estrogen should do the same in women, and last but not least, coconut oil."

IMMUNITY AND CANCER

"A Dr. Ray Peat felt that simple cold processed coconut oil could help the thymus gland. I haven't heard how that's been working out for people, but I do note that coconut oil doesn't taste bad on a piece of lightly toasted whole grain bread, especially if you add a little honey to it."

David laughed, "Really, Doctor, it's hard to know what really works or doesn't work, isn't it?"

"I know, David, but I remember these strange stories, and I think Dr. Ray Peat may be on to something. Our diets really matter. Perhaps bad fats suppress our immune system as well as being so oxidative. According to an article by Dr. Peat, he saw a report that said Albert Schweitzer, who operated a medical clinic in tropical Africa, said it was many years before he saw any cases of cancer. He believed that the appearance of cancer was caused by the change to the European type of diet, especially the types of fat they introduced. In the 1920s, German researchers showed that mice on a fat-free diet were practically free of cancer. Since then, many studies have demonstrated a very close association between consumption of unsaturated oils and the incidence of cancer. So does coconut oil, a naturally saturated form of fat, help the thymus gland directly? I don't know, but eating healthy fat most certainly will keep ill health at bay.

I would mention that studies show antioxidants help the thymus as well as some folks stating that a little bit of real licorice along with ginseng can help the thymus gland and immune system. They say to use ginseng often, but not every day unless you are older than fifty. The same would go for Echinacea, which should only be used for several weeks at a time by anybody, as using it all the time lowers its effectiveness quite a bit."

MELATONIN

The doctor continued, "It appears melatonin, a supplement that can induce deeper sleeping, can increase your immune system, especially as we age. Studies have shown that melatonin helps restore thymus function. Therefore, anyone over the age of 50 may benefit from taking 1 mg of melatonin before sleeping. I use a time release tablet. As people grow older, they may want to increase that dosage. At age 60, you may want to start taking 2 mg before bedtime, at age 70, start with 3 mg. Experiment with different brands, as some are much more effective than others. Always sleep in a dark room as it will help your body produce more melatonin."

"What studies were those?"

"Too numerous to recall. I've seen research papers from China, Turkey, Italy and others showing melatonin helping the thymus gland and improving immunity function. It appears also to be a strong deterrent for cancer."

"Cancer, Doctor, really? I have not heard too much about that."

"Whatever works, David. I feel it's a strong preventive measure. It not only stimulates the immune system but appears to help the cancer cells destroy themselves."

"You mean apoptosis?"

"That's right, David. It tells the cancer cells that it's OK to self destruct. Our pineal gland slows down in its production of melatonin as we age and, interestingly, cancer rises as we age. I also note a Swedish study and Finnish study that showed totally blind people having lower cancer rates, presumably because their bodies were producing more melatonin."

"That makes sense, Doctor; after all, bright light or daylight diminishes our melatonin levels."

"That's right, David. However, if your pineal gland is healthy and you are getting a good night's sleep, you should have a healthy melatonin level. Unfortunately, people seldom have either as they age."

"Your advice?"

"Sleep in a dark room and, as you get older, take melatonin."

David added, "Finally some simple advice anyone can follow."

"Right you are David, and by the way, I should mention that once you are properly taking care of your thymus, make sure to take care of your thyroid gland too."

"How's that?"

"An improper thyroid gland will also dramatically influence your immune system and general health."

"How so?"

"A proper performing thyroid will allow your body to remove waste from your cells and allow for better hormone balance."

"Your advice then would be what?"

"Avoid fluoride, bromide, and use supplements like iodine."

FOUR SUPPLEMENTS FOR IMMUNITY

"Can you suggest any other supplements for boosting your immunity?"

"Several, David, but you should only use them periodically, not every day."

"How so, Doc?"

"Well, I recommend using four various supplement protocols on a cycle basis. For instance, you would use that supplement for a month only then take a week or two off, before resuming them. I use four various supplements that way: astragalus, ginseng, and mushroom extracts containing three commonly used types: maitake, reishi, and shiitake. One other supplement can be taken more often, especially if suffering from something like cancer. That supplement is IP-6. Of course, it's crucial to let your doctor know that you are using any of these supplements, especially if being treated for any medical condition."

"Tell me more, Doc."

"Use ginseng for increased immune strength. It also is known to protect against cancer and is used for males as a sexual aid. You can cycle on and off with this herb a little longer, this simply means to use ginseng for a month or two and then take a month off. If you are 55 or older then you can usually continually take ginseng on an even more consistent basis, as you will usually derive more benefit than possible side effects. However, to be safe it is always wise to cycle on and off of any herb as this will lessen the possibility of having too much build up in your system and also will allow your body to keep getting a response from the herb. People with high blood pressure must monitor themselves well while taking ginseng, as it can raise blood pressure in many people. Panax ginseng, also called Korean ginseng, may work best but many people use American ginseng as well. I use both together in small amounts on a consistent basis."

"What about astragalus?"

"Many people use this herb around the world as it seems to increase the response of our immune system. I use it periodically but not every day. I take it if I feel I am coming down with something. Often, then, that malady never manifests itself."

"Doctor, I heard many Japanese use mushroom extracts. Is that the type you are talking about?"

"Right, David, shiitake mushrooms are used quite often there to treat cancer and to boost the immune system. They also use the maitake mushroom and the reishi mushroom. All three may help fight cancer and all three appear to boost our immune system. Make sure you buy them from a reputable source."

"Doctor, I know mushrooms are fungus, and I also heard of people dying from eating certain mushrooms, so my question is how safe are mushrooms to consume?"

"If purchased at your supermarket, they are very safe. But, David, you make an excellent point. Some mushrooms will kill you. The death cap mushroom, when eaten by people, gives a slow death by destroying your liver. These mushrooms are usually identified as having white gills underneath that create white spores, but why take a chance. Don't go picking your own mushrooms unless you really know what you are doing and when buying mushrooms at open markets and such keep aware of the old saying, 'buyer beware.' Speaking of mushrooms and their ability to impact your body, reishi mushrooms have been shown to help your liver. So there you go, two different mushrooms and two very different impacts on your body. Use only mushrooms from a trusted source and do your research. Also, David, as you may know, cooking makes most mushrooms safer to eat as it destroys much of any harmful substances. With death cap mushrooms, no amount of cooking will help. Hence they are deadly indeed. Also, some people have picked deadly webcap mushrooms, which destroy the kidneys."

"You are scaring me, Doctor, So don't pick your own mushrooms unless you really know what you are doing, right?"

Laughing, the doctor replied, "Great advice, David, more than you know. Millions of mushrooms are consumed in this country without incident but every years several folks will consume some wild found mushrooms thinking they know what they are doing or, ironically, several cases are related to people trying to harvest mushrooms which may contain psilocybin which have mind altering properties. I think of many mushrooms more as medicine than food: to be used cautiously. So like other powerful agents some can cure and others can kill. Some famous people are assumed to have died from mushroom poisoning."

"Such as?"

"Well, we can't know for sure, but it is mentioned that Charles VI, the Holy Roman Emperor, died from eating mushrooms and many speculate that even Buddha died from poisonous mushrooms, as they may have been in the last meal he ate. When they describe his death it certainly parallels mushroom poisoning. I also will note that I do not eat a lot of mushrooms myself, since in the United States we are sold mostly white button mushrooms or portobello. Many people believe that these two mushroom varieties may help your body fight off cancer but I am not so sure. It is essential that you cook these mushrooms first as they contain a small amount of cancer-causing hydrazine. So heating negates its harmful effects. I see many people adding raw white button mushrooms to their salads like that is OK. I would not add them unless they are cooked. It's my view, but mushrooms are something that should only be eaten in moderation. While I eat them, I do not eat them every day."

"Whys that?"

"Both the white button mushroom and the portabello may contain some natural carcinogens, which should be greatly negated by cooking. So while they offer good nutrients, it may come at a price. Just like pickled food, they should be used in moderation. I am sorry to say, David, nobody in the food business will tell you this. It is bad for business."

KEY POINTS
THYMUS THEORY

- Follow all the previous steps as outlined as they will all benefit your immune system.

- Consume a natural diet heavy in uncooked food consisting mostly of vegetables, fruit and berries.

- Consume lean sources of protein never over cooked.

- Consume fat in its natural state, never hydrogenated. Avocado, olive and coconut oils that have not been hydrogenated or heat-treated are good for the body in moderation.

- Sprout grains and nuts before consuming by soaking in water overnight. This biologically activates the enzymes and makes the food more bio-available and nutritious. It also keeps your body from using its own enzymes purely for the digestive process.

- Exercise often, jogging, fast walking, doing jumping jacks, or using a mini trampoline. These stimulate the lymph system.

- Reduce stress in your life. High cortisol levels greatly diminish your immune system.

- Periodically take micronutrients like zinc. Safely use up to 50 mg per day. If taking everyday, however, add 2 mg copper since too much zinc will deplete copper.

- Consider thymus extract if your immune system remains weak for a prolonged period. Make sure you select extracts made from cows from Argentina or New Zealand, two countries free of any mad cow disease-causing prions.

- Do supplement with probiotics in capsule form or, if consuming dairy, have yogurt and kefir several times a week. Much of our immune system lies in our digestive tract.

- Supplement with vitamin C and other antioxidants.

- Sleep in a dark room and, as you age, consider a melatonin supplement.

- The herb astragalus helps wake up the immune system, especially the thymus gland. Use in moderation and cycle on-and-off. Never take a herbal preparation on a neverending basis.

- Various mushroom supplements may aid in boosting your immune system. One such supplement includes three types: maitake, reishi, and shiitake.

- Use the supplement IP-6 periodically.

- Use ginseng for increased immune strength. It also is known to protect against cancer and is used for males as a sexual aid. Cycle on and off with this herb; this simply means to use ginseng for a month or two and then take a month off. If you are 55 or older then you can usually continually take ginseng on an even more consistent basis, as you will usually derive more benefit than possible side effects. However, to be safe it is always wise to cycle on and off of any herb, as this will lessen the possibility of having too much build up in your system and also will allow your body to keep getting a response from the herb. People with high blood pressure must monitor themselves well while taking ginseng, as it can raise blood pressure in many people. Panax ginseng also called Korean ginseng may work best, but many people use American ginseng as well, especially since they know where it is grown and harvested.

18
The Acidification Theory
Theory X

THE DOCTOR WENT on to explain about another theory of anti-aging called the Acidification Theory. He felt it held a lot of merit and went a long way in explaining many of the ailments in modern society. He discussed this in depth with David.

"So, Doctor, what's the next theory of aging we should cover?"

"A very important one, David."

"Aren't they all?"

"Yes, I suppose so, but this one is easy to do, or as they say about ailments, easy to fix."

"What is that?"

"Have you heard about the Acidification Theory of Aging, David?"

"Not really. Tell me more."

"Our body needs to maintain a certain pH level or death with result. During an operation, an anesthesiologist will track the acid buildup in the blood and body to ensure that a patient doesn't die. However, on our own, we often neglect the fact that our body's acid levels can be harmful. The pH level varies depending on what part of the body we are dealing with. Obviously, the stomach will be more acidic than the rest of the body, as it digests our food. Overall, the body likes to maintain a pH of around 7. It's crucial to understand that too much of either an acidic condition or too much of an alkaline condition can kill us."

"So how does this scale work?"

"The pH scale reflects parts of hydrogen and ranges from 0-14. Anything over 7 is more alkaline. As you move lower on this scale from 7 towards 0, things are more acidic. The body's blood likes to be slightly alkaline with a pH level of 7.3 to 7.4."

"OK, so the blood is more sensitive to pH levels?"

"Yes, very much so. It is interesting to note that moving up the scale of pH, let's say from 7 to 8, may seem like a small increase, however, like the Richter scale used to measure earthquakes, 8 is ten times more than 7. Not simply one digit more. Why is this important? Our bodies might do OK at 7, but our blood needs to be around 7.4. The energy portion of our cells, the mitochondria, needs to be at a 7.5 pH level."

"How sensitive is the body to this pH range?"

"Simply put, too high of an acid level will cause enzymes to lose their ability to function. It will also destroy our proteins, which the body needs to maintain life."

"This is all news to me, Doc, is this a reason we get ill?"

TWO FORMS OF SICKNESS

"David, many people feel that an acidic body is much more vulnerable to diseases and ailments. Sickness can be divided into two broad categories: sickness from outside and disease from the inside. Sickness from the outside would include contagious viruses, bacteria, food poisoning pathogens and such. Disease from the inside includes high blood pressure, heart disease, Alzheimer's, diabetes and cancer. Other afflictions also may be included like autoimmune disorders, fatty liver, colon problems, arthritis and asthma. Being acidic allows for an increase of all these afflictions."

"So what causes it?"

"The culprit for a high acid level is usually our diet. Either what we are eating or what we are drinking. The culprits? Processed foods, trans fats, sugars, high glycemic food choices, and too much meat and dairy. Liquids that are acidic to our bodies are items like soda pop, coffee, wine, tea, milk and overly processed sugary drinks."

"So don't consume too much of these acidic foods?"

"That's right, David, but note, many people assume that it is the pH of the food or liquid that makes it acid or alkaline. While this can be the case, it is not always so. Scientists will burn off the food or liquid being tested in a container and measure the ash remains. A pH test determines whether that ash is acidic or alkaline. Therefore, fresh orange juice may be acidic but actually might register as alkaline if tested using the pH ash test."

"OK, tell me more."

"If the body remains acidic for too long, it sets up our inner terrain for infections and diseases. Of course, you don't want to the body to be over alkaline either, as that condition can be harmful as well. Either extreme in pH can be deadly."

"What else?"

"Chemicals in our environment and stress can also produce an acidic tendency within our system. The Acidification Theory of Aging notes that when we are younger, our bodies are more alkaline. As we age, the body gets more acidic. Therefore there must be a connection between these two states. A more alkaline body also utilizes oxygen better, hence we have more energy."

"So, the body wants to maintain a slightly more alkaline state?"

"Yes, David, the body needs to maintain its homeostasis, its equilibrium, its perfect environment for operating. It does this by regulating its temperature to ward off pathogens and also creates the correct pH level. This allows numerous chemical reactions to occur. These enzymes need the right environment to act as catalysts allowing life to operate. This is part and parcel of homeostasis, the biological necessity of all living things to remain in balance or to maintain their equilibrium within to allow life to continue."

"OK, Doc, I have heard that our body has a harder time maintaining homeostasis as we grow older. So that is a theory of aging right there, that failure to maintain our systems is why we may die. Is that correct?"

"Yes, a crucial part of homeostasis is the acid-alkaline balance. Why is this so crucial? The Acidification Theory of Aging states that if acid levels get too high, the body takes immediate action to alleviate this problem. It buffers the acid and/or moves it to a less vulnerable area other than our blood supply. Our blood supply needs to be slightly more alkaline than the rest of our body; therefore, the body will take excess acid and store it in other body parts, hopefully to be dealt with later. So in effect, we get acid deposits amongst our organs and tissues. After a set amount of time, our bodies become acidic overall and a perfect terrain for sickness and disease. This acid effect is cumulative and thus mimics what we assume is normal aging. Young people when tested are more alkaline, older people more acidic, and sick people, especially those with advanced cancer, can test very acidic."

"This all really makes sense to me, Doctor. How do we deal with it?"

"There are many ways for the body to deal with excess acid. Three of the primary buffer systems are the protein buffer system, phosphate buffer system, and the bicarbonate buffer system. So if the blood supply becomes too acidic, it will use various buffer systems to take up excess hydrogen ions to decrease acidity. The main thing we have to do, to live a disease-free life and longer life, is to make sure that we are making our bodies more alkaline and not too acidic. We need to consume a mostly alkaline diet."

"Which is?"

"I feel like a broken record, David, but eat a natural plant based diet and that will almost always be an alkaline diet. Aim for about 80% plant-based food and only a little acid forming foods like eggs, meat, and dairy. Also, avoid acid forming drinks like sugary drinks and alcohol."

"It makes sense to me, Doctor, I can see why you say all these theories are related and I can appreciate how they are connected. As I said before, once you know the logic behind it, it really does make sense. I also, feel this will be an easy practice to put into place."

"Indeed it is, David, but I do believe people need to be informed on why it is so important, otherwise they will constantly reach for acid forming comfort food thinking that it isn't really that bad for them. Now they will know how harmful it can really be pushing your body into an acid state, causing fatigue, compromising your immune system, and creating pockets of acid waste in your body if you eat poorly."

"It's kind of like running up a load of credit card debt, right, Doctor? I mean when you eat poorly, that acid is being deposited into your body somewhere and creating mischief either now or later."

"I guess so, David, I never looked at that way but as we both know, if you accumulate too much debt, you will go bankrupt someday. So I guess if you are not careful, you will bankrupt your health by being too acidic."

KEY POINTS
ACIDIFICATION THEORY

- Follow all the other previous steps mentioned.

- Our bodies have a multiple buffering system. One uses our body's minerals to neutralize this acid. This can lead to mineral depletion with the negative effects of our system being too acidic and also our bodies then have fewer minerals within our systems for other needs.

- Food consumption needs to be mostly alkaline versus acidic. Most people should consume about 80% alkaline and 20% acidic foods. Liquids are included in this, too.

- All the previous steps to anti-aging covered lead to a naturally alkaline body.

- In the words of a famous biologist and scientist Henry G. Bieler, "Germs seek their natural habitat—diseased tissue—rather than being the cause of diseased tissue." This may be at odds with modern germ theory but explains a lot of sickness and disease.

- Arm your body with the tools it needs. Consume mineral-rich food such as vegetables and fruits. Organic food usually contains more of these minerals.

19
The Enzyme Theory
Theory XI

"Doc, as we discuss each theory of aging, I sense how important that theory may really be. But almost all the time, as I feel that theory may be the answer we are looking for, you give me another theory that sounds like it may offer more promise."

"I understand what you are saying, David. It's amazing to think of some of these theories and what the impact could be by understanding them and using them to improve our lives."

"Do you feel a few of them might be more important than others?"

"Not really, David. I mean, if you violate the laws of nature there will be consequences. It's not like driving where you can break a few rules of the road now and then and get away with it. With nature, if you overeat, ignore prevention, eat the wrong fats, run your body into an inflammatory state, or remain acidic, you will pay the price."

"So, what are the last two theories of aging that you want to address?"

Laughing, the doctor replied, "Slow down, David. We will take them one at a time. I need to stress that the dozen theories of aging we are covering are the theories of aging I feel we can easily address. Some of the other theories may be more difficult. So one theory I want to share with you now is about enzymes and how crucial they are to our health and our existence."

"Great!" replied David, "I studied a little about enzymes in school. I agree that our existence is predicated on them. I mean, I learned that without enzymes we would not be able to take advantage of food, produce energy, or even function. Right, Doc?"

"Right, David. Enzymes are the molecules that act as catalysts allowing for an increase of various chemical reactions. Without them, our bodies would cease to function. What else have you been taught about enzymes?"

"Only that various reactions may still occur without them, but at such a slow rate that it is almost not worth mentioning, as we would be long gone."

"Good point, David. Enzymes can accelerate a reaction a million-fold, so they are essential for life as we know it. Also, you may know that many poisons inhibit normal enzyme reactions, hence that is what makes them so poisonous."

"No, I didn't know that. So you want your enzymes to perform optimally. Does that make sense, Doc?"

JUST RIGHT

"Yes, our bodies require the right temperature, the proper pH levels, and chemical environments for enzymes to perform their functions for our optimal health. This is crucial and, yet, often ignored."

"So how does this present itself as a theory of aging or anti-aging?"

"That is what I want to discuss. Enzymes are so crucial to life and health, but in my view, they don't get enough respect. Outside of manufacturers of alcohol and yogurt, they are ignored. We, as a modern society, have acted ignorantly on such matters. Sure, we talk about macronutrients such as proteins, fats and carbohydrates, and even vitamins and minerals, but enzymes? They are barely discussed."

Smiling now, David said, "So here I am, Doc – discuss them."

With a grin, the doctor said, "Here's the point and the theory. Without proper enzymes and proper enzyme activation and utilization, we cannot achieve optimal health. Without proper use of enzymes, we will age much faster."

"OK, Doc. You have my attention. What are we doing wrong, or what should we be doing different?"

"As you know, enzymes are catalysts, they accelerate various biological and chemical reactions, but that is not the whole story. We need enzymes to break down our food and to repair our bodies. When we consume food with its enzyme potential compromised or destroyed, we are hurting ourselves and impacting our life potential."

"You mentioned destroyed and compromised. How do we do that to these enzymes, Doc?"

"We know about 5,000 enzymes and counting. Enzymes, when heated, can become denatured or destroyed. So by consuming a diet of cooked and processed food, we are robbing our body of some of the food's best attributes. Food in its natural state offers its enzymes."

"OK, Doc, that makes sense."

"David, remember when I told you that younger people have a higher pH level than older people?"

"Yes, you said younger people were more alkaline and older people are much less so. How does that relate, Doctor?"

"Well, younger people also have more enzymes in their body. When their saliva is tested, there is more of the enzyme amylase. This is the enzyme used for digesting carbohydrates. So a healthy level of enzymes within the body could be seen as a healthy biomarker and a lack of enzyme function a sign of failing health. Dr. Howell mentions in his book *Enzyme Nutrition*, a 1937 study done by Meyer, Golden, Steiner, and Necheles, where not only was the enzyme amylase higher in young people, but so was the enzyme pepsin and the pancreatic enzyme trypsin was dramatically higher."

David smiled. "Meyer, Golden, and who...Jeez, I didn't know law firms did medical research."

The doctor laughed. "They do sound like a law firm, don't they? But remember, David, I told you there was a lot of good research done in the 1920s and 1930s. In fact, every decade adds to our knowledge, but there is so much information out there and special interest groups keep putting their own spin on things."

WHAT CAN WE DO?

"Then what can we do about it?"

"We all need to focus on consuming food in its natural state. Things like fresh fruits, raw vegetables, some raw fish, fermented food, unprocessed nuts. If consuming grains, it's best to soak them so the sprouting process activates and increases the enzyme activity dramatically. The last thing you want to do is overcook your food."

"What do you mean by overcook?"

"Anything over 116 degrees Fahrenheit is believed to destroy the natural enzyme potential of food."

"Doc, you're not saying that we shouldn't cook our meat, are you?"

"No, David, since factory farming has reached every sector of agriculture and food production, I would not go raw with meat. However, saying this, it's crucial to make sure that you are consuming as much food in its raw state as you can. This will keep you from getting too enzyme depleted. Remember,

David, that man in his natural state ate raw meat for thousands of years. Even cavemen didn't always cook their meat. In our lifetime, we still had Eskimos around Greenland consuming a good portion of their meat raw. Researchers in years past found Eskimos in extremely good health and in high spirits. In fact, scientists could not find any heart disease amongst them and very low cancer rates. The only real negative to their high-meat diet was higher incidences of osteoporosis. Of course, things have changed with the use of modern food in their diets."

"So the enzyme theory states that we should get our enzymes from food itself instead of relying on our body's enzymes to digest and process food?"

"Well said. Actually, Dr. Edward Howell felt very strongly that our bodies only had so much enzyme potential within itself. If we used up those enzymes to digest dead food, we'd have less enzymes for our body to carry on needed processes such as repair. He felt that this was a major reason we age too fast. So, in a sense, we become enzyme depleted."

"Fascinating, Doctor. I've never heard this before. It sounds similar to a theory I heard that we only have so many heartbeats and such."

"David, I've heard that theory on heartbeats before, but I don't put much weight into it. However, regarding Dr. Howell's theories on enzymes, I do indeed give it a lot of weight."

"How's that?"

"Dr. Howell speaks from experience. I feel he has laid out his positions well, and I find them very compelling. Unfortunately, too many people dismiss them. I feel America's health would be a lot better if we listen to him. Really listen. Dr. Howell gives us a historical perspective on how food used to be consumed, more in its natural state with its enzymes intact. The result? Far less sickness and illness, at least in regards to modern maladies like heart disease, diabetes and cancer."

"Tell me more about his theory."

273

"In short, food in its natural state contains its own enzymes, which if you eat this food raw, it will help the digestion process greatly as it is bringing active enzymes into the body along with its macronutrients like fat, protein, and carbohydrates and its micronutrients such as vitamins and minerals. Also, if you do consume cooked food, then your body must use its own enzymes, leaving less for the body to use for other purposes such as body repair. Furthermore, Dr. Howell felt this could lead to overall enzyme depletion."

"So is this why I've heard people refer to food's vital force?"

"It certainly would make sense, David."

"So what are your thoughts on this theory?"

"Well, it can be argued that we only need a small amount of enzymes, as they can be used over and over again. I will also add that modern science doesn't seem to accept Dr. Howell's theory. Saying that, I note that people that follow Dr. Howell's principles appear to be much healthier and more vibrant than the population as a whole. We may not know why his principles seem to work but I would not dismiss him so easily. His book, called *Enzyme Nutrition*, lays out the case for raw food and gives compelling examples. I like his thought processes. I would incorporate much of his thoughts and principles into an anti-aging lifestyle. I would presoak my beans and grains the night before cooking them, as I feel it would make nutrients more available. I would not overheat them to over 200 degrees either. It will make for slow cooking, but I feel it would be more nutritious. There are some things, however, that need to be cooked or else they are hard to absorb."

"Such as?"

"Beans, grains and some vegetables need to be cooked to reduce their natural plant defenses that can bind up nutrients or cause negative reactions to people. Many nuts, seeds and spinach are high in something called oxalates. Sprouting nuts and seeds by soaking them overnight then rinsing them usually takes care of the problem. With spinach, just don't consume it every day, but even then it's not a problem for most people unless you have a problem with calcium metabolism. Many nutritionists will warn of phytates, but these are not a problem if you get into the habit of soaking phytate-containing food such as seeds and nuts. Be aware they are also found in oatmeal, wheat and rye. Considering how often these foods are consumed you seldom hear of any concerns. Seldom is calcium totally locked up by these phytate-rich foods. To be safe, use sprouts from alfalfa and other grains in moderation. By the way, that is why foods like potatoes and green beans are best cooked."

"Any more on the theory, Doc?"

"Yes, David, critics may argue about enzymes in raw food compared to cooked or processed food. They state our bodies can handle the lack of enzymes by producing our own but they miss two important points."

"Like?"

"One, being why should we use up our own enzymes when the food is willing to allow us to have its enzymes for free? Two, people who consume a mostly raw diet are some of the healthiest people I've seen. It's hard to argue that cooked food is better. I mean, cooking destroys the structure of food, diminishes its vitamin content, and produces toxic byproducts in meat if cooked too much."

"Doctor, speaking on enzymes, I was taught that our stomach acid is so strong that it will destroy all the enzymes that enter the digestive system."

"I am not surprised to hear that, David. Doctors are taught in med school that the hydrochloric acid our stomach produces neutralizes the enzymes found in food. So any good student would conclude that it doesn't matter if you eat live fresh food or processed dead food. Too bad these medical students don't do their homework."

"How's that, Doc? What are they not learning?"

"David, people like to simplify things. Teachers often tell their students that digestion begins and ends in the stomach. They explain that our stomach acid is so strong that carbs, fats and proteins are broken down in the stomach and absorbed later as they make their way through the lower intestine."

"Well, Doctor, I am blushing a little here, because that is what I was taught."

"I know, David, many people are. Let me say a few things. One is that digestion starts in the mouth. If you don't think so, try a little experiment. Take a bite of bread or a bagel. Chew it for a minute and you will find its been converted into a liquid. Try the same with a bite of fruit or even a piece of meat. Pre-digestion starts in the mouth, especially for carbs. That's crucial. The more work your salvia does or your teeth do, the easier it is for your food to be digested correctly. Two, the stomach acid is not just for digesting, but it's also there to kill bacteria, viruses, parasites and such. It is also important for helping digest proteins mostly and fats a little. Third, it is not just the high acid content that digests proteins but the low pH created by the acid that allows the stomach's own enzyme pepsin to be activated. This is the primary enzyme used by the body to digest protein. So in reality, it is not just our bodies' stomach acid that digests proteins like meat but it's the enzyme pepsin as well. Fats are partially broken up here also, but the real job for digesting fats occurs later, as it is emulsified with bile that is produced by our livers. So a major portion of real digestion occurs after food leaves our stomach and enters our small intestine, which may be small but it sure is long, measuring over 20 feet."

"So chew your food! Right, Doc?"

"Right David, and then some. Growing up I had the privilege to be exposed to the teachings of Horace Fletcher. He taught people that we all need to chew our food much more than we think. He recommended to chew your food 50 to 100 times before you even think of swallowing it. People used to say 'Fletcherize your food,' instead of just saying, 'chew your food well.' He also proposed that we chew our liquids a little before swallowing to allow our salvia to start the digestion process. Famous people like John D. Rockefeller followed his advice and lived to an old age."

"Well, was he right, Doc, or was he a nut job?"

"Funny David. I think he was mostly right. They said Mr. Fletcher had incredible strength and endurance, which he said resulted from proper chewing of his food. He also stressed concepts such as not eating large meals when angry, sad or if overly hungry. Things that now pass for common sense may have started with Fletcher's observations."

"Ok, Doc, I see, but like I said, I was taught that the stomach did most of the work and after hearing what you just said, it just doesn't seem that way."

"Right David, I have several clients that had most of their stomach removed due to medical problems. They have survived for many years and have actually done quite well."

"Really, Doc? How can that be?"

"David, years ago they would have died but with our understanding of what nutrients our bodies need to survive, like folate and vitamin B-12, these folks can actually survive now. They also use supplements like digestive enzymes, take vitamin B-12, folic acid and a good multiple vitamin. As long as they eat correctly they thrive, no stomach or stomach acid needed."

"So Doc, you are saying enzymes from live or fresh food can pass through the stomach and be used by the body?"

"That is my belief. I think many enzymes cannot function if the pH level is not right or if the temperature is not correct. However, once getting through the stomach a small portion may again become active once the environment is correct. Also, to a much lesser degree, many enzymes provide some benefit at the beginning stage of digestion, like in the chewing process, allowing those foods to be utilized more efficiently, especially when chewing completely."

"Makes sense to me, Doctor, but you are in agreement that enzymes are affected by the stomach acid?"

"Oh, absolutely, David, especially animal enzymes like those that dissolve protein. After all, the stomach is where these types of enzymes are activated and used the most. Having said this, even the stomach's strong acid doesn't completely digest proteins. Enzymes produced by our own pancreas finish that job in our small intestine. So in life there are few absolutes. Next time someone tells you that your stomach does all the digesting, you will know better."

"Are there some other absolutes open to debate, Doctor?"

"Of course there are, David. Take food fanatics that say we should eat everything raw. While I think we need at least half of our diet to be raw, I would not go crazy with this notion. For instance, some foods are best eaten after they are cooked, especially various starches like beans and tuber plants like potatoes. Even though millions of people in the world today consume cassava root as an excellent carbohydrate source, it can be deadly unless cooked properly. And I note that seeds, nuts and grains seem to harbor anti-vitamins like phytates, which bind up minerals in many foods. Therefore these foods are better sprouted or cooked before consuming. I note these phytates can bind up calcium, iron, magnesium and zinc. Some cooking can also improve bioavailability of certain foods, so once again I am not saying to eat everything raw. But also, I would say it is a very bad thought to eat all of your food cooked. I am not sure if it is the destruction of enzymes that cooking food causes or if it's cooking's by-products that cause harm. Like I just said, there are few absolutes in nutrition but I will give you one of mine, 'eat at least half of your food raw.'"

OTHER ADVANTAGES

"Any other advantages to real food?"

"Yes, you will avoid a lot of chemicals, preservatives, hidden allergens, food coloring, sugar, and salt. Just look at fats as an example, once we started heat-treating and hydrogenating fats they became inflammatory and health destroying."

"So, Doctor, eating a mostly raw natural diet, with its nutrients intact, is what you said earlier about eating close to the earth."

"That's right, David. I feel you will see rapid improvement with your immune system, higher energy levels, significant weight loss, and many people will see a much nicer complexion within eight weeks. Just add raw instead of cooked food to your diet. Give it time."

Smiling, David asked, "Any other insights?"

"Yes, several. While critics argue over enzymes and critics mock Dr. Howell for stating that food has some vital force within it, they can't argue over the results someone gets following a mostly raw diet."

OTHER INSIGHTS

The doctor grabbed an edition of Dr. Edward Howell's book *Enzyme Nutrition* off the bookshelf. He opened the book to various pages. He pointed out the doctor's work on food and gland size. He quoted several findings concerning rats that were fed a high sugar diet and on dogs given a heavy dextrose intravenous infusion. The surprising results were damage to the pituitary gland and the pancreas gland. Dr. Howell stated his view on "The Adverse Effects of Dextrose on Pituitary and Pancreas" with the following quote, "Heat-treated, enzyme-free, refined items of food caused the most drastic deviations in pituitary gland size and appearance.

"Furthermore on the defense of eating food in its natural state, Dr. Howell noted 'raw fat is not fattening.' He stated, 'A pound of raw beefsteak may add only protein to the tissues and not put on any fat. On the other hand, the same amount of cooked beefsteak may give the eater a little unwanted fat.'"

He explained to David that Dr. Howell's work seemed to illustrate that processed food, especially sugars, negatively impact our glands and that eating real fat in its natural state did not cause obesity. However, the real astounding insight from Dr. Howell's writing was the final passage he quoted to David: "It can be accepted, as a working rule, that the enzyme potential is limited and withers as time marches on. The more lavishly a young body gives up its enzymes, the sooner the state of enzyme poverty, or old age, is reached."

Dr. Howell pointed to numerous studies in his book illustrating the gravity of this finding yet is ignored by the majority of the American public. Ignorance is truly life shortening in this respect. Once an individual understands Dr. Howell's message, they can take steps to truly feed their body with real food. This alone should spare them of most modern diseases and common ailments. Best of all, real food boasts energy and extends life.

Dr. Tessler explained to David that Americans need to get back to reality on what real food is supposed to be. He explained that our eggs are no longer as healthy, as the hens are fed a dead food diet. Our milk, butter and cheese is overly pasteurized, and our beef is grain-fed instead of being allowed to feed on grasses on the open range. Adding to this insult is that we are overcooking any real food we have to the point that we are negating so much of its real life energy properties.

People who turn to eating an all-out raw diet need to know that many raw foods are off limits. Soybeans have a high amount of inhibitors called trypsin. That is why several cultures ferment soybeans to disarm this inhibitor. Many seeds, nuts and grains have various enzyme inhibitors. If they did not, these live foods would sprout, grow or turn into plants and trees. That is why raw food activists recommend soaking or partially sprouting most of these items. It makes these foods more bioavailable and, in several cases, far less toxic. Unfortunately, the large calorie choices such as meat, fish, and dairy are either overcooked or pasteurized. This destroys their enzyme giving ability, pushing our bodies into a negative enzyme balance. The pancreas enlarges on such a diet as it must secrete its own enzymes to allow for digestion and assimilation. Surprisingly, the pancreas will enlarge if eating cooked or processed food or if you try to consume raw food that has too many inhibitors in them. Many people have turned to digestive enzyme supplements for this reason.

ENZYME SUPPLEMENTS

"So, Doc, what about enzyme supplements, do you recommend them?"

"Yes, I do, David, usually the two main common types of enzymes supplements people are using."

"Which are?"

"Digestive enzymes while consuming food and systemic enzymes between meals."

"What's the difference?"

"Digestive enzymes are taken before or during a meal and are mostly used by people who feel these enzymes help digest their food. People who have that bloated feeling after eating, or complain of excess gas often state that these digestive enzymes help them. In addition to digestive enzymes, we also see individuals using additional digestive aids such as betaine hydrochloride and pepsin to increase stomach acid production as they grow older, since our digestive processes often diminishes as we age. If you recall, I mentioned that one of the main purposes of our stomach acid is to activate the enzyme pepsin, a powerful digestive force within our stomachs. Many people also believe that using digestive enzymes with their meals, especially with cooked foods, leads to better food assimilation. They reason it's not just what you eat but what your body can assimilate that makes a real difference. Also, others use digestive enzymes under the belief that by doing so they spare their own body from having to use a lot of its own digestive enzymes. Many of these types of enzymes are derived from plant sources.

"The other main kind of enzymes used are systemic enzymes. These enzymes are usually enteric coated, which is important, otherwise they will not fully survive the journey through the stomachs acid environment. They are designed to be taken on an empty stomach so they can then release their enzyme potential in the body's lower intestines, just like natural enzymes from the pancreas would do. These types of enzymes are often used to fight inflammation and to potentially ward off cancer. Many of these enzymes are derived from animals such as pigs under the theory that those enzymes would more closely match what our own body produce."

"Interesting, tell me more."

"Well, Dr. Howell pioneered the use of digestive enzymes. These were plant and/or animal based enzymes that were taken with food to aid in that foods assimilation. He felt these digestive enzymes would be helpful since most people were eating cooked or processed food that had its enzyme potential destroyed. He reasoned this was important in order to spare our bodies from having to use too many of its own enzymes. These enzyme supplements usually contain at least three main types of enzymes: protease, amylase, and lipase. Some contain many more types of enzymes."

"Hmm," replied David, "I know the protease enzyme helps digest protein, amylase helps digest carbohydrates and lipase helps with fat digestion. So, all of this seems somewhat logical to me, Doctor, if that's the way the body really works. What do you think?"

"Can't say with certainty ,David, but as you said, it does seem somewhat logical, but as far as I know, I have not heard of any detailed studies for this theory or against. Yet, I've met many people that swear their digestive problems have gotten better while using enzymes. However, as you know, this is known as anecdotal evidence, which means it is only based on their experience, not very scientific to say the least. Having said this, I do use them quite often."

"Why's that, Doctor?"

"I feel it can't hurt me and may, in fact, be helping me to preserve some of my own body's enzymes. As you may know, our pancreas is a busy organ not only secreting trace amounts of insulin, but also producing over a pint or two a day of other liquids including a lot of enzymes like trypsin, chymotrypsin, lipase, and more."

WHY RECOMMEND ENZYMES?

"OK. Doctor, but since you are talking about enzyme therapy, I do remember you telling a person in the coffee shop that you might have recommended enzymes for his wife. Why was that?"

"Right, David, that person was telling me about his wife, who had suffered through pancreatic cancer. I told him about a fascinating concept using enzymes to fight cancer. It's used by some alternative health practitioners."

"So is there something to it?"

"I think there might be, David. When I tell you of some of the history behind it, you will see why it's recommended for some people. I told you about the two types of enzyme therapies, digestive enzymes being used with food and systemic enzymes being used on an empty stomach. The treatment for cancer involves using mostly systemic enzymes. It's about quantity and timing of the enzymes into the body and there is a history behind it. For instance, while Dr. Howell explored and wrote about enzyme therapy, he was not the first."

"History? Such as?"

DR. BEARD

"The tale of three doctors: Dr. Beard, Dr. Kelley, and Dr. Gonzalez."

"Go ahead."

"John Beard, a doctor of science and a professor at the University of Edinburgh, brought forth the hypothesis that the body's pancreas secreted various enzymes like trypsin, which helped digestion and, maybe more importantly, may keep cancer at bay."

"Wow, that's amazing, I mean I never heard of this before."

"Nor have most people, David. You're not alone and the reason I am not surprised is that Professor John Beard died in 1924 and his research was written around 1902, over a hundred years ago."

"A long time ago, Doctor, so was he a quack?"

"No, David, he was no quack and he spent years researching this stuff. He was nominated for a Nobel Prize on embryology."

"OK, Doctor, I see, he studied embryology, the study of cells at its most basic stage, right when it starts developing into life. So I would imagine his theory and work have been explored extensively, right?"

"Not really, David. Various doctors claim to have had good results with enzyme therapy, but I know of no double blind studies or any other in-depth research being done on his enzyme work either to prove it or disprove it."

"So what was his thinking about these enzymes?"

TROPHOBLAST CELLS

"A fertilized egg quickly starts to grow with some of it becoming the placenta, which will contain the embryo, and the rest becoming the embryo itself. That growth rate is extraordinary in its speed and scope. It may be one of nature's greatest processes. That fertilized egg develops into an embryo, which then continues its journey into a newborn, providing that journey is not interrupted. Note, that all of this growth of the embryo transpires in a sac called the placenta. This placenta is initially comprised of interesting cells called trophoblast cells which are created just before the newly formed embryo. These trophoblast cells have the ability to implant themselves in a woman's uterine lining and develop a blood supply directly to them and the surrounding placenta, all the while growing quite quickly without facing any immune attack from the mother's body."

"So how does this matter to us?"

"Hold on, David, it will all make sense. Think about it, an embryo is a foreign growth in a woman's body. The placenta is the vessel that shelters that entity, the baby, nourishes it with nutrients, and provides the baby's blood supply, yet is not attacked by the mother's immune system. How is it that the body does not attack the placenta and the baby it contains? Something generated by the placenta, probably the trophoblast cells, tells the body it's OK to let it stay, to grow, to thrive within the woman's uterus, at least for awhile. Keep in mind that the woman's uterus is very hormone sensitive."

"And then?"

"Professor Beard observed that after the placenta finds a way to attach itself to a woman's uterus and it grows enough to accommodate the new embryo being developed in the womb, that some time later, chemical signals generated by the woman and more so by the newly formed embryo itself slows the growth of the placenta and normalizes the tissue within the placenta, and keeps it in check from growing continually."

"What was that chemical signal for stopping the growth of the placenta, Doctor?"

TROPHOBLAST CELLS & ENZYMES

"Great question, David. He observed that just before two months had lapsed since inception of the fertilized egg and the growth of the placenta tissue, right before the embryo starts being called a fetus, the embryo's pancreas starts generating enzymes. It was at that point in time when the placenta stopped its aggressive growth. The trophoblast cells that initially formed the beginning of the placenta started as aggressive, undifferentiated cells that invaded the uterine tissue and later transformed to a much more stable form of cells which are more differentiated and noninvasive. Professor Beard went on to observe this in all the animals he tested. The timing was different for each species, but in each case a signal was generated via the embryos pancreas. Once the embryos pancreas becomes active, the growth protocol for the surrounding placenta slowed. The professor was intrigued because the newly formed embryo was not using these pancreatic enzymes to digest food since the embryo was not consuming nourishment through its digestive tract yet. So the professor proposed the theory that it was pancreatic enzymes that stop the growth of the placenta."

"Interesting, Doctor, tell me more."

GERM CELLS, VAGRANTS, TROPHOBLAST HYPOTHESIS & CANCER

"You see, initially the placenta attaches to the mother's uterus and is not rejected, even though it is an aggressive growth. Professor Beard reasoned that the embryo's enzymes are crucial to triggering the stop to the growth process of the placenta. He reasoned that soon after an egg is fertilized and it grows only slightly, then being called a blastocyst, special cells start growing extensively, possibly directly from our germ cells. These cells are called trophoblast cells.

285

They can grow quickly and become the placenta, but most certainly retain the ability, at that stage, to become various body parts and organs of a new human being as well. Soon after, a large portion of primordial germ cells find their way into the embryos sexual organs called the gametes and reside there waiting to create a new life when yet another future egg and sperm combine to complete fertilization.

"The doctor observed that when we are born we retain many germ cells throughout our bodies from those germ cells that did not make their way into our sexual organs. Dr. Beard called these vagrant germ cells.

"Dr. Beard hypothesized that if our pancreatic enzyme function diminishes too much, these vagrant germ cells may act on that as a formative growth wake up call. When they do wake, they may try to form trophoblast cells as that would be needed first in order to create a container for a newly created embryo. His thought was straightforward. Since it was originally our bodies' pancreatic enzymes that told the trophoblast cells to stop their aggressive growth in the uterus when we were embryos, then it stands to reason that the lack of this signal from the pancreas within our own bodies as we grow older could cause cells to start growing again. It may be one of the main regulators of cancer within all of us."

David was quick to respond, "Right, now I get it. You were suggesting these types of enzymes to the person in the coffee shop, so that by including these enzymes in his wife's system they may have helped to fight off the cancer, or perhaps turn off the cancers growth signals."

GERM CELLS GONE WRONG

"Correct, David, perhaps these enzymes would turn off the growth of certain germ line cells or, as Dr. Beard said, germ cells that turned on and became similar to trophoblast cells. By the way, just to be clear, the germ line cells I am referring to have nothing to do with germs that cause disease but are the germ cells that carry the seed of life with it from one generation to another."

"Of course, Doctor, I understand that."

"Well, then, Dr. Beard thought that perhaps stray germ cells in our bodies retain the ability to grow, leading to interesting but negative consequences. So by using enzyme therapy, he might be able to prevent those outcomes."

"Such as?"

"Actually David, it is more like 'what if?' What would happen if a germ line cell activated itself even without being fertilized? Your body would discover it had within it a tumor with some interesting properties. If the cell tried to develop into an embryo, a tumor could develop called a teratoma. This tumor usually is composed of various body tissues, such as a combination of mixed body tissue containing brain, teeth, hair, and bone. Other, more virulent tumors have been noted within our sexual areas like a man's testicular area. Apparently, according to Dr. Beard, the germ cells there may try to turn on inadvertently and create growth tissue. However, what Professor Beard thought might be much more common is when the germ cell turns on thinking its first job is to create a placenta, thereby creating trophoblast cells, which are highly invasive, similar to cancer, if not cancer itself. Since Dr. Beard observed that the placenta was created slightly before the embryo and the placenta developed with aggressive trophoblast cells, he concluded that cancer would indeed be a much more expected outcome than the usually less dangerous teratoma that could be possibly produced if a germ cell tried to develop into an embryo."

"Gotcha, Doctor, continue."

GERM CELLS, GAMETES & MISCHIEF

"Well, David, with the creation of a new life, the fertilized egg within the placenta tissue carries with it the eternal seed of life, the primordial germ cells. These germ cells eventually get incorporated within the newly formed embryo. It is believed that these germ line cells are not only immortal but lead directly to the creation of stem cells within the embryo. These germ cells go on to exist within the embryo, which after just eight weeks is then referred to as a fetus. For males these germ cells migrate to the area of the body that will someday produce sperm. These are known as our gamete cells. For the female, these cells migrate towards the ovaries. Dr. Beard observed that many of these germ cells never make it to these locations and are sitting throughout our body possibly ready to do mischief at a future date. These are the cells Dr. Beard referenced as vagrant germ cells. After all, these cells can continue to grow without restriction under the right circumstances."

"So Dr. Beard had some original thoughts on this process, what else did he think differently about?"

WHAT CELLS CAUSE CANCER

"Several items, David, with most of them being mind expanding, to say the least. But what I found very interesting was that Dr. Beard thought that other scientists may have it incorrect when they state that cancer originates from normal, healthy cells that have gone wrong. These cells would supposedly suffer damage then convert from a highly specialized cell to a poorly formed cell and miraculously develop the ability to keep producing more bad copies of themselves. He felt it made more sense to assume that a cell that had the ability to start off primitive and replicate indefinitely as a more simple answer. That primitive cell possibly being a germ cell, what we may now identify as a stem cell. For some reason, it gets activated by some type of hormone, or cellular insult, and begins producing more bad copies of itself, or according to Dr. Beard, a lack of pancreatic enzymes might allow this switch to turn on. A germ cell would have that ability if activated to start."

"Any updated news on this?"

"Sad to say, David, but most scientists remain ignorant of Dr. Beard's work, so they may not be asking the right questions."

"Such as?"

"Is cancer simply germ cells wanting to grow outside of the fertilization cycle? Also, if this is the case, what might trigger this reaction?"

"Your thoughts, Doctor?"

"David, I know cancer is complicated. There are many forms of cancer and I believe that there is not one cause nor one cure. But I do believe that some cancers may be related to these vagrant germ cells as Dr. Beard called them. In fact, he believed that if these germ cells become activated they would cause the majority of all cancers. Perhaps these cells really do exist in our body and researchers should look into it. Dr. Beard had no doubt that they did, as he observed them in all the species of animals he studied over a twenty year time period. I also feel there are many triggers to initiating cells into a misguided growth mode such as irritation, radiation, inflammation, hormones, chemicals, acidic conditions and low oxygen levels. And if Dr. Beard was correct, low pancreatic enzyme levels may be a cause as well."

"Low oxygen levels, why do you think that Doctor?"

"Several reasons, David. When the trophoblast cells first start implementing themselves into the cervix of a woman, and for a few months afterwards, it does so in a very low-oxygen environment. Researchers have commented about this low-oxygen environment. They felt it was necessary to protect the newly formed embryo from free radical damage but that just doesn't seem right to me. Also, at a later date after Dr. Beard passed away, a Nobel winning scientist Otto Heinrich Warburg, held a hypothesis that low oxygen levels could lead to cancer. Keep in mind that when the pancreas functions fully it also produces an alkaline solution which would increase oxygen levels. So were the low oxygen levels along with a lack of the embryo's pancreatic enzyme function a reason for these trophoblast cells to grow so quickly and rapidly establish a blood supply and thereby acting the same as cancer?"

"Go ahead, Doctor, I think I'm following this line of thought."

A BOX

"Regardless, these germ line cells may be the start of life longing to beget more life. It's about life's journey and its process of change, evolution, advancement, and continuation. Dr. Beard also proposed that life is about the immortal cell lines creating a physical body to contain it. A human being is nothing more than a container to carry the immortal seed of life called our germ line cells."

"Doctor, are you saying that our bodies are simply an elaborate container that is used to convey the seed of life from one generation to another?

"Yes, David, you see Dr. Beard observed that while two germ cells joined together to form a fertilized egg, and that entity quickly grew into a placenta and embryo, he also observed that newly formed germ cells would wait on the outside of the newly created embryo in its yolk sac until it was time to move in. Then they would make their way to the gamete area of the embryo which holds the reproduction cells of our bodies, almost like they were waiting for a new box to hold them. But as I mentioned before, he also observed that not all of these germ cells found their way to the right area."

David quickly replied, "OK, I see, those misplaced germ cells are what Dr. Beard referred to as vagrant germ cells. But, Doctor, I don't want to get distracted, can you explain his cancer theory in a way my readers could understand?"

BEARD'S HYPOTHESIS

"Well, David, saying it was a theory may be too strong, but for sure Dr. Beard stated a hypothesis that these vagrant germ cells may develop into cancer at a later date. Keep in mind that he based this on years of observation while studying embryos and their development. He observed that a new born baby is essentially a foreigner within its mother's body, yet the reproduction process allows the baby and its surrounding placenta the protection it requires. How? Chemical signals to not attack the placenta or fetus are sent, while a blood supply is established and nourishment is directed from the mother's body. Meanwhile, the baby's body starts the rapid building process of formatting a new human-being, free from any real immune attack by its mother's system. Once the placenta is established and the baby's own pancreas starts generating enzymes, the growth of the placenta is moderated and it does not continually grow. Dr. Beard thought that the baby's own pancreatic enzymes stopped the growth of the placenta tissue. This may not only be the answer for stopping fast growing placenta tissue growth but a possible remedy for cancer as well. Dr. Beard observed that life forms that do not utilize a placenta have dramatically lower cancer rates."

"Doctor, when you say it that way, it does sound similar to cancer, I mean the rapid growth, the blood supply, the nourishment given and that the baby is not really a part of its mother's body, yet is not attacked by the immune system."

"Right, David, you see now why it got my attention, the similar characteristics exhibited by cancer are similar to that contained in the creation of a new life. The doctor being an embryologist would indeed be more open to this observation."

"Could you sum that up, Doctor?"

"Well, we all start off as an embryo within a placenta. The doctor believed that some of the cells from our early conception that formed the placenta, which he called trophoblast cells, remain in our body possibly as germ line cells, trophoblast cells, or even stem cells. Of course, Dr. Beard did not know about stem cells at that time but by his description he may have been the first person to really describe them. These vagrant germ cells lay dormant, perhaps never to be a problem. However, for many, these cells start up causing uncontrolled growth, first in one of our organs and, if left unchecked, our entire body. The doctor noted while these cells were needed early in our development they can cause cancer later in our lives. Now the real big question is what kept these cells in check while we were still an embryo? Dr. Beard concluded it was enzymes."

"I see, Doctor, but that also begs the question why would germ line cells turn on and try to change into an embryo or those placenta cells called trophoblasts if they are not fertilized? Also, it begs the question that perhaps those vagrant germ cells are supposed to be in other body parts since we need stem cells to produce our red and white blood cells non-stop."

"Good point, David, Dr. Beard did not have an answer for that but only stated he thought it a real possibility that vagrant germ cells, which did not make it all the way to the gamete areas of the baby, would be sitting in that body possibly waiting to do what germ cells are made to do, grow. But you are correct on one point, David, stem cells are definitely found in other areas of a newborn, such as the baby's umbilical cord as well as their bones where they produce white and red blood cells constantly. Its up to researchers to determine how these cells originate as this could answer this question."

"Gotcha, Doctor, but back to Dr. Beard's hypothesis, why would enzymes keep trophoblast cells in check?"

WHY ENZYMES?

"David, something was stopping the rapid growth of the trophoblast cells. Dr. Beard thought these cells are held in check when the embryo's pancreas is more fully developed and starts producing enzymes at a sufficient level, just before it reaches eight weeks of age. He saw this occurring in all the animals he studied. When the embryo started generating enzymes, the growth of the trophoblast cells in the placenta slowed. In fact, if the embryo died or was aborted, often the growth of the placenta tissue kept accelerating causing an invasive cancer. Of course, Dr. Beard believed it was the embryo's pancreatic enzymes slowing the growth of the placenta, but I do not know if the doctor was aware that our pancreases also produce an alkaline mixture as well, which is used later to negate the effects of the strong acid produced by our stomachs during digestion. So I wonder if it was the alkaline environment or the enzymes halting this growth. But either way, it certainly appeared that something in the pancreas was slowing the growth of the trophoblast cells and tissue."

PANCREATIC ENZYMES

"Now I'm seeing this hypothesis more clearly, Doctor. Dr. Beard was saying pancreatic enzymes may be the controlling agent for keeping aggressive cell growth in check during our lives?"

"That's correct, David. Now do you see why a person should keep their pancreas in good shape?"

"Wow, Doctor, this is a lot to take in. First, you tell me that the placenta is acting as a growth within a woman's body, similar to how cancer acts, and then you tell me that the embryo's newly-formed pancreas is control central for controlling this growth."

"I suppose I'm saying that, David, or to be more correct, Professor Beard is stating a possible hypothesis."

"What does the American Cancer Society say about Beard's hypothesis?"

"Not much, David. On their website they gloss over it fairly quickly, stating that no real research has been done on it and they see no real value in it."

"But, Doctor, isn't that why we donate money to them, to make sure the research gets done?"

"Right you are, David, but it sure seems like the American Cancer Society has no problem with any form of damaging radiation or harsh chemotherapy, but God forbid if you want to give some enzymes to someone."

"Someone must be working with the science of enzyme therapy, right?"

"Not any major research sources that I know of, David. A few doctors are working with enzyme therapy but I know of no universities or drug companies working on it. Many professional researchers are seeking grants for trophoblast research but most are underfunded, if funded at all. Also, any research being done on trophoblast cells is focusing on a lack of a strong trophoblast presence within the uterus causing miscarriages and a medical condition for the woman called preeclampsia or, more commonly, pregnancy induced hypertension. I would like to see studies on the ability of germ cells, or trophoblast cells as Dr. Beard stated, to start growing on their own, years after being implanted into a new human body by the creation process early on. Placenta cells contain the genetic mixture of both parents, but I wonder if the initial trophoblast cells do as well or are they similar to the mitochondrial genetic code, which is entirely donated by the woman's side. Why do I want to know this? Because, I still can't fathom why the woman's body does not attack the trophoblast tissue when it first starts taking hold."

"Many questions, Doctor, and lots of research to be done someday. So tell me about the other two doctors you mentioned?"

DR. KELLEY

"Right, David, this brings me to some of the other doctors that are noteworthy for working on enzyme therapies. I first must mention a past dentist by the name of Dr. William Donald Kelley. He stated that he himself had pancreatic cancer and was told to go home and get his affairs in order. Instead he did his own research and rediscovered, by accident, the power of enzymes. I say by accident because initially he was unaware of the enzyme work of Professor Beard. Dr. Kelley said he got better from simply consuming raw food and raw juicing, similar to the advice given by Dr. Howell, and also by taking copious amounts of digestive enzymes orally several times a day to relive his indigestion. Not knowing about Dr. Beard's theory that enzymes may be the cure for many cancers. From that point on he reestablished his health and went on to help many others in their struggle to do likewise."

"Tell me more, Doc?"

"Dr. William Kelley saw the relationship between enzymes, protein, and cancer. He also was an avid reader and researcher. He theorized that our bodies' inability to process excess protein as a major reason that may cause cancer to grow within us. He felt that we must increase our pancreatic enzyme production in order to fight off cancerous growth. He felt that not only did pancreatic enzymes help to digest food in our intestines but also circulated freely in our blood system destroying cancer cells. Along the lines of Dr. Howell, Dr. Kelley recommended plenty of raw food and fresh raw juices so these enzymes would be available for our own digestion along with giving our pancreas some enzyme relief. He felt that raw food, raw juice, supplements, and additional enzymes were so powerful and useful that he would have his patients slow down the program periodically so the body could remove any destroyed tumor. His therapy included much more than enzymes. He wrote a book titled *One Answer to Cancer*. In this book, after he had researched the works of Dr. Beard and successfully treated many cancer patients himself, he summed up nicely the major points Dr. Beard was making."

"Which were?"

"He summed it up by stating that when human eggs are fertilized, three cell types are initially developed: primitive germ cells, normal body cells, and trophoblast cells. His explanation is simple for why a woman's body develops trophoblast cells leading to the full development of the placenta. If this did not occur, then the newly fertilized embryo would not have anything to attach it to the cervix nor could it obtain nourishment. He also felt that as we develop we have thousands of displaced germ cells remaining in our body, so is it any wonder that we have the potential to develop cancer in so many places?"

"Sounds just like what you were saying about Dr. Beard."

"Yes, David, but Dr. Kelley had a way of saying it much quicker. Dr. Kelley also summed up the reason for cancer. Instead of just stating it was a lack of pancreatic enzymes, Dr. Kelley also felt it was helped along by the presence of the female sex hormones, which might drive the development of a vagrant germ cell. When you think about it, many women and most men do start to have too many estrogenic hormones within their bodies as they grow older. Women with high estrogen and estradiol develop breast cancer and men with high estradiol develop prostate cancer. The inability to break down hormones properly increases with age and especially with a bad diet or lack of exercise. Cancer appears much more often as we age. I could go on and on about Dr. Kelley's track record but it speaks favorably for itself, that's if someone is willing to really look at it. His book, *One Answer to Cancer*, was a cutting edge book that was way ahead of itself and its contents full of hard to find information. I sense that many in the alternative health field have gained valuable insights from Dr. Kelley's writings."

DR. GONZALEZ

"Thanks, Doctor, I will check that out. Now, what about Dr. Gonzalez? "

"David, in recent years, Dr. Nicholas Gonzalez saw first hand the impact of Dr. Kelley's treatment protocol by observing many of Dr. Kelley's patients and by going over Dr. Kelley's records. He was convinced enough by Dr. Kelley's protocols that he developed his own treatment program for cancer patients based on much of Dr. Kelley's work. Dr. Gonzales had kept detailed records on his own patients and has had much success, especially with cancers that are usually considered terminal. So that leads me to believe he is on to something. He's written several books on cancer and recommended treatments to guide people by. One book I recall is titled *One Man Alone: An Investigation of Nutrition, Cancer, and William Donald Kelley*, and also another great book, *The Trophoblast and the Origins of Cancer*, that was written by him and another medical doctor by the name of Dr. Linda L. Isaacs. They both dig into the science behind it and review Dr. Beard's ideas in detail. Simply put, it may be one of the most fascinating books I have ever read."

Laughing, David replied, "Don't worry, Doctor, you're not the only person who likes these types of books. I will review them in detail as you definitely have got my curiosity aroused."

"That's all I could hope for David."

KEY POINTS
ENZYME THEORY

- Follow all the previous steps mentioned.

- Investigate what foods can be eaten raw.

- Learn to sprout grains, nuts and seeds before consuming. According to Dr. Howell, squirrels bury nuts not to hide them but to germinate them, thereby releasing the maximum food value.

- Consider quality digestive enzymes. They can be taken with meals and in between meals.

- If you eat like everyone else, you can expect the same results. Eat close to the earth by saying no to processed food.

- Pasteurization is a heat treatment therefore modern milk and cheese products are sold without their true enzyme potential.

- Eat less, as that uses less of your enzymes and also allows your enzymes to repair your body.

- If eating cooked food, incorporate raw food with them.

- Chew your food thoroughly.

20
Mineral Overload Theory
Theory XII

THE DOCTOR AND David met in the doctor's study and the doctor brought up the subject of minerals.

He explained that we were all taught that various minerals are needed for the body. We are told to get our calcium, sodium, magnesium, potassium, phosphorites, iodine, zinc, copper and especially don't forget the iron.

Often not known by most people is that we require other minerals in trace amounts such as manganese, selenium, sulfur, silicon, cobalt, bromine, boron, chlorine, chromium and molybdenum. Less known trace minerals that are utilized by the body in very small, micro amounts include aluminum, arsenic, fluorine, nickel, tin and vanadium.

The doctor explained that minerals came in various forms and that depending on which form the mineral was in would impact the body's ability to utilize each mineral properly. The difference in various forms of minerals could be dramatic. The doctor also informed David that he paid attention to veterinarians for a lot of his mineral advice. He explained that vets knew important aspects about minerals and their impact on animals' health, well-being, and even their reproduction ability. These doctors, many times, knew more about minerals and health than most medical doctors.

Often scientists felt that trace minerals were trace minerals, were trace minerals. It did not matter if they came from inorganic salts, sulfates, oxides or chlorides. However, the livestock industry discovered that organic trace minerals gave a much better outcome. When money is involved, truth often comes out. The livestock people also found out that minerals should be balanced instead of just one mineral given at a time. For instance, it has long been known that too much zinc reduces copper levels and vice versa.

THE DOSE MAKES THE POISON

Another important point on minerals was that too little can be harmful to an animal, just as too much can be harmful, the Doctor explained. In fact, too little or too much of various minerals will lead to certain death. It is like the story of Goldilocks and the three bears. When tasting the bears' porridge, Goldilocks replied, "This is too hot. This is too cold," and to the last bowl, where she said, "This is just right." So goes it for the proper mineral intake.

Thereby sits the crux and premise for a theory of aging that is often ignored, yet may hold a real key to longevity. The Mineral Overload Theory of Aging.

In the doctor's study, he and David resumed their discussion.

"Doc, I know you talked about minerals before, but how do minerals make it to a theory of anti-aging?"

"As we discussed, David, too little or too much can dramatically impact your body."

"Some examples?"

"Sure, David, too much potassium in your body, especially your blood, will result in hyperkalemia."

"What does that do?"

"Well, hyperkalemia can give you an irregular heartbeat or lead to cardiac arrest."

"Ouch, Doc. What else can mineral overdoses do?"

"The list goes on. Excess calcium will cause damage to your kidneys and even your bones. Taking too much zinc will deplete copper, iron, and magnesium levels. Too much copper can be even worse, causing liver failure, mental problems, and a host of other potential problems."

"Wow, Doc, so as you said, minerals in moderation."

THE CAUSE, THE CURE

"Right. In many countries, the lack of various minerals like selenium in the soil, leads to high cancer rates, while too much selenium leads to convulsions or even death. Also, some minerals, like cadmium and arsenic, can cause cancer."

TOO MUCH OF THE WRONG KIND

The doctor went on to say, "Various minerals and metals are crucial to our health, some we require in moderation, others not at all. Consider our modern industrial economy; it finds unnatural substances being produced and entering our food chain. Just one example: the need for batteries has allowed two very bad substances, cadmium and lead, to be added to most people's diet through manufacturers' and other companies' waste disposal practices. The cadmium, in some ways, may be worse than lead. Scores of manufacturers pour their waste products into our environment where it soon wreaks havoc. Accumulation of cadmium takes place as waste products accumulate in crayfish, shellfish and shrimp. Humans consume these toxic by-products gradually and cadmium is one of those toxic metals that accumulate over time in your body like a ticking time bomb. Out of the blue, a person may develop pancreatic cancer, never connecting their consumption of contaminated aquatic seafood products to their disease."

"So, Doctor, how do we protect ourselves?"

"Well, since many people are trying to increase their consumption of seafood and omega-3 fatty acids, you really just need to be aware of where your seafood is coming from. If your seafood is farm-raised or coming from polluted watersheds like the Chesapeake Bay area or the Gulf of Mexico, you are best off limiting yourself to just two servings of this seafood a week."

"I understand that viewpoint on seafood from polluted areas, but why did you say to limit your farm-raised seafood?"

"As you may know, David, farm-raised seafood is often lacking in real omega-3 potential, as these fish and shrimp are fed low cost commercial diets in a contained area and not fed their natural diet of other rich omega-3 sources."

"So what can we do if we already have been exposed?"

"I will sound like a broken record, David, but follow all the other steps to good health we have been talking about and, especially important, do not smoke, as cigarette smoke contains cadmium. Also make sure you are getting adequate levels of zinc in your diet. Zinc and cadmium like to occupy the same position in our bodies. So adequate levels of zinc may help displace high levels of cadmium. Of course, don't overdo any mineral, even the good ones. Remember, however, high levels of zinc can also displace copper, therefore, I would recommend a mineral supplement that contains 100% of the required daily amount of zinc but also includes up to 50% of our daily requirement of copper."

"Now, Doctor, I've heard it said that pancreatic cancer is often inheritable. Also, people who are overweight or suffer from type 2 diabetes have a much higher rate of this cancer. But, truthfully, I have never heard that this cancer was tied to contaminated seafood consumption."

"Mostly true, David, what you say may be correct, but you left off the list people who smoke, drink excessively, or eat too much processed lunch meats that are high in nitrates and, sad to say, a real possibility for people who consume too much shellfish found in the coastal waters of the United States, especially the Gulf of Mexico and spots on our east coast."

"OK, Doc, are you saying that slow accumulation of toxic metals is taking place through contaminated seafood found in industrial waters could be our undoing?"

"Right, David, consistently, people get more cancer as they get older because, perhaps, their bodies have had time to accumulate more toxic metals. And, speaking on batteries, lead is a major poison problem, it accumulates in our systems just like arsenic."

"So, Doctor, death by metal poisoning, done slowly so we don't even see its real destructive effect."

"Right, David, and we all need to be diligent. Our great-grandparents could get away with eating lots of shellfish, but we need to keep our intake to a minimum. The same can be said for some other common items that most people assume to be safe no matter what."

"OK, Doc, I'm going to bite on that one. What are you referring to?"

"Rice, David. Plain, simple rice."

"Good grief, Doctor, is nothing sacred?"

"I know, David, but here in the United States a lot of our rice is being grown in contaminated water. Rice sits in water as it grows, so it stands to reason that any contaminated substance in the water would impact the crop being grown. Arsenic levels are often too high. Rice grown in California is usually much better, but rice grown in cotton producing states like Louisiana, Arkansas, Missouri and Texas may have too high of arsenic levels since arsenic containing insecticides were used for years and years in these states for cotton crops. Too many people consume rice thinking it is a health food without giving it a second thought. And, David, too high of arsenic levels have been found to be a strong cancer inducer, especially concerning skin cancer."

"Whew, Doc, it can get exhausting staying on top of this stuff?"

"Right, David. But ignorance kills. Most Asians know to rinse their rice thoroughly before cooking and many even add extra water up front and then they drain the excess after the cooking process, which would naturally lower the arsenic levels. In Japan, over prior years much of their rice was contaminated by cadmium, causing a disease known as 'Itai-Itai,' which, translated to English means, 'It hurts-It hurts.' Cadmium poisoning often affects the bones, kidneys and the pancreas."

"Amazing, Doc, two different areas of the world, two different poisons, cadmium and arsenic, impacting rice eaters. What else is happening out there that we are not aware of?"

"Right, David, that's why we all need to educate ourselves. We should reduce as many known health threats as we can. It takes work, but your health is worth it."

"But, Doctor, it takes time, money and energy, doesn't it?"

"Yes, but I made an important observation years ago..."

"Which was?"

"Too many people use up their health in the pursuit of making money, only to find then, they must then spend all their money trying to regain their health. In short, your health is your greatest asset. Yes, it may take a little work to protect it but it is well worth the investment."

"OK, Doctor, so all minerals can be harmful if consumed in too large of an amount. How does that give us a theory of aging?"

"David, it has long been known that calcium builds up in the arteries of many heart disease patients years before they have a heart attack or stroke. We call that calcification process hardening of the arteries. If that is not enough to scare you, radiologists find it very common to see intracranial calcification when they perform CT scans."

"What else?"

THEORY OF AGING

"David, too little in the way of mineral consumption may induce aging just as too much can. However, concerning excess levels, the concern to a few researchers is iron excess."

"Well, Doc, it must not be too big of a problem if only a few researchers seem concerned."

"That was my opinion at first as well. However, the more I looked at their contemplative theory, the more I realized that they may be on to something."

"Such as?"

"A logical viewpoint on why most animals age in the manner that they do. I mean, when you understand their theory, it makes a lot of sense. David, science has known for a long time about the dangers of iron overload in the human body. The body has very sophisticated ways of dealing with iron excess, however, soon its defenses are overwhelmed."

"Really, Doc? Tell me a little about it. You see, all everybody hears is how good iron is for you."

"I know, David, and a lack of iron is bad for people, as you will feel tired, have trouble concentrating, perhaps get headaches, and feel out of sorts. Many people notice they are short of breath or their skin appears pale or they have an irregular heartbeat. Often these people are diagnosed with iron deficiency anemia, the most common cause for anemia. We all need adequate iron levels to function, to thrive, to live. No doubt about it. But, of course, David, there are numerous forms of anemia, too many to mention. However, the most common forms I've seen are due to either a lack of iron, vitamin B-12 or B-6, or a lack of folate."

"I hear you, Doc, but can't loss of blood due to internal bleeding lead to anemia as well?"

"You are right, David. We always need to make sure that you are not bleeding internally as that can be a cause. I've seen ulcers and even hemorrhoids cause this condition. We also need to rule out cancer as a cause."

"So 'See your doctor as soon as possible,' right?"

"Absolutely, David. Many disorders, if addressed early, can be taken care of. It's important to note that many people, and even physicians, assume the cause of most anemia is from iron deficiency. That is why we do medical tests. Saying this, too many people start taking iron supplements and they can overload their systems to the point of causing heart disease, diabetes, cardiomyopathy, cancer or liver failure."

"Really? So how do we get tested properly?"

"Doctors perform various tests, such as a hemoglobin test, serum iron test, total iron-binding capacity test, and serum ferritin. It's crucial that you get more than just a hemoglobin test. That test may show you as normal when you could have iron overload or PCT – or porphyria cutanea tarda – an enzyme disorder. It's crucial not to overload your system with iron, as that is very aging."

"Interesting, Doc. If high iron levels may pose a problem, why don't we hear more about it?"

"David, the world is well aware of iron deficiency, but not iron overload. One researcher E.D. Weinberg, wrote a book specifically for the medical community called *Exposing the Hidden Dangers of Iron*. In this book he reports on the 'iron hypothesis.' He stated, 'In 1981, Dr. Jerome L. Sullivan proposed that the lower incidence of heart disease in premenopausal women as compared with men and postmenopausal women is due to the lower amount of body iron in the former group. In the Framingham heart study investigators found that "men had significantly higher serum ferritin concentrations than females." This finding tends to support the hypothesis that females who are still menstruating and therefore losing iron are somewhat protected by this process against heart attack.'"

HIGH IRON LEVELS

"E.D. Weinberg goes on to point out that not only was monthly blood loss, due to menstruation, helpful in protecting against a heart attack, since losing blood reduces iron levels, he pointed out that actions that are deemed health promoting, such as exercising, taking aspirin, and drinking tea also reduce iron levels. He points out that reducing iron levels by using iron chelators could be helpful in protecting against heart attacks. He notes that inhalation of any iron particles increases the chance of cancer as well as any injections of iron may cause an increase of infections and death."

"So, Doctor, where does that leave us?"

"Don't hide from truth. Face what real problems confront us and do something about it."

"Such as?"

"David, everybody should get their blood tested for iron levels. If anywhere near high levels are detected, you should take immediate steps to reduce your iron levels."

"Doc, I know chelation therapy helps, but what else would you recommend?"

"You are right, chelation, which actually means 'to claw,' will remove excess iron, lead and other minerals and metals. Doctors mainly use a chemical called EDTA, which when infused into your blood system will bind with metals and escort them our of your system. While this will help many people, there are simpler ways to accomplish this. For instance, simply not consuming too much red meat which contains heme iron, will go a long way. Adding tea to a meal or two each day will keep iron from being absorbed too much from your food, and a real big aid would be to donate blood often. Giving blood is a great way to reduce excess iron levels."

"Great advice. Any other suggestions?"

"Another simple step is to not consume orange juice with your meals, as that causes iron to assimilate within the body. So will consuming vitamin C with your meals. And, of course, don't take iron supplements. Many times iron is lurking in our multiple vitamins and in our breakfast cereals."

"Could you explain in a few sentences how that gives us a theory of aging?"

EXCESS IRON

"Our bodies need iron to survive and low iron levels are an epidemic on our planet. A lot of that is due to malnutrition and parasites. Iron-poor blood or low iron induced anemia is rampant. Our bodies need adequate levels of iron to function. After all, our bodies and blood systems are designed to use iron to carry oxygen to our cells. We need optimal iron levels to prevent damage to our DNA, mitochondria, and to function. But too much iron can be deadly. Our body has no physiological way to get rid of high levels of excess iron. Excess iron is oxidative and toxic to the body. Doctors find excess iron in the brains of those with Alzheimer's and severe overdoses of iron will ruin the liver, cause heart attack or strokes. So excess iron in our bodies may be what ultimately leads to premature aging and an early death."

"So when you say excess iron kills, are you referring to the medical disorder hemochromatosis?"

"Yes and no, David. Yes, certainly hemochromatosis, which is the inability to handle iron correctly, is deadly. Thankfully, we now know how to treat this disorder. And no, the iron overload I am referring to is similar but much more subtle."

"How's that?"

"Well first off, let's address patients with hemochromatosis. They need to lose some of their iron. Actually, they need to let go of some of their blood quite often, as this reduces their iron overload. They should not drink alcohol since that causes iron levels to rise and excess iron can cause liver cancer, so that is another reason not to drink. Often, patients are told not to consume vitamin C with their meals since this causes more iron to be absorbed. However, saying this, everybody needs to be aware of their iron levels. Why? Untreated excess iron levels will kill you after causing great mischief with your organs. Hemochromatosis can kill quickly, while slightly elevated iron levels may kill slowly."

"So what happened to people suffering from hemochromatosis in the past?"

"They usually died, often from heart attacks, strokes, organ failures, or liver cancer, a horrible way to go. David, I told you I use a resveratrol supplement called Longevinex. Do you recall?"

"Yes, I do, Doctor. After you told me, I looked into their product and, I agree, it appears to be one of the better resveratrol products on the market. I mean a lot of companies are just throwing some resveratrol in a pill or capsule without regard to quality or content."

"I agree, David. You have to buy from a trusted source. It was while looking at Longevinex's website that I came upon the work of Bill Sardi. He covers the theory of over-mineralization quite clearly. He states 'that the rate of over-mineralization within our bodies parallels the rate of aging.' Furthermore, he states 'the gradual overload of minerals, particularly calcium and iron, which are the predominant minerals in bone and blood, explain a great deal of aging, and partially if not totally explain the free radical, the mitochondrial, the hormonal and the calorie-restriction theories of aging.' I have to tell you, David, that when I read that, I felt like finally someone has explained a major reason we are aging so quickly."

"I hear what you are saying, Doctor. I mean, with what you told me about high levels of iron in our systems and the mischief it causes, I can see why you feel this theory has merit."

"David, not only does this theory seem probable to me, but Sardi goes on to offer further explanations that drive the point home. Since Sardi laid out the theory so well, I feel it would be a disservice to try and articulate it, as he did such a fine job."

The doctor looked through a stack of papers neatly arranged on the shelf behind his desk. Quickly looking over these papers, he said, "Here we go, David, let me quote Bill Sardi correctly. 'During growth years, all the iron that is ingested is directed toward the production of new blood cells (millions must be produced every second) and calcium is shuttled to develop bones. So it is very difficult to develop iron or calcium overload during youth. In fact, this may explain why the first two decades of life are largely free of disease.'"

"Very good, Doctor. I can see why his reasoning appeals to you."

"David, it is scary how well Sardi's theory fits the picture of aging. Sardi talks not only about the effects of too much iron but about the increasing rate of calcium and calcification within our bodies. I mean, look at all the atherosclerosis that occurs in people later on in life, after they have had time to accumulate minerals. Furthermore, women who have consistently lost blood each month due to menstruation lag men in having hardening of the arteries and/or hardening of the aorta or calcification, as they may call it. However, once women quit losing monthly blood flow after menopause, the rates for both sexes and atherosclerosis starts equalizing."

"I see, Doctor, it all makes sense."

"It sure does, especially when Sardi points out that our arteries and heart are not the only body parts that harden. Something just as important, something our body needs to regulate itself also calcifies."

"What's that, Doc?"

"Our pineal gland, located at the base of our brain, begins to calcify in almost all people as they age due to calcification and, also, excess fluoride will cause sever pineal gland disfunction."

"Really? Is that why older people sleep less? Because their pineal gland is not producing enough melatonin?"

"That's the thought, David. So I place a great deal of importance on this theory and its implications."

"Let me guess, most scientists dismiss this theory, don't they?"

OCCAM'S RAZOR

"I think so, David. I mean, it is too easy of an answer for such a complicated dilemma like aging. But remember Occam's razor, a philosophy principle, *pluralitas non est ponenda sine necessitate.*"

"Yes, Occam's razor. I never learned to say that quotation in Latin, but basically doesn't it state, 'When you have two competing theories that make exactly the same predictions, the simpler one is better?'"

"Right you are, David. That is a simple way of putting it. I would say it even simpler. What appears obvious, may just be the truth. Now, thanks to Bill Sardi's way of explaining things, I feel it could be an obvious reason we age prematurely."

"What can we do about it?"

"Lots, David. We need to get our iron levels tested. It wouldn't hurt to test copper levels, lead levels, mercury levels and iodine levels, or your thyroid function. Remember everything in moderation. Studies show often people do not get enough magnesium or take megadoses of vitamin D. This may cause some folks to develop calcification of the soft tissues or calcification of the aorta, heart, and other vessels. That is why I never tell people that more is better. While we need adequate amounts of vitamin D, too much may hurt people. Taking vitamin K-2 along with vitamin D may help. According to Dr. Weston Price, who spent years researching health and diets around the world, natural sources of vitamins A and D were vital to health because they acted as catalysts to allow minerals to be absorbed. Vitamins A and D may compete, so don't take too much vitamin A, as you may not then absorb enough vitamin D. Vitamin A deficiency is rare in the U.S., but borderline vitamin D deficiency is not. Without them our bodies simply will not absorb or assimilate the minerals properly. Dr. Price felt an additional fat soluble nutrient, which he called

X, was present in healthy, natural animal foods and researchers speculate that what Dr. Price called X is in reality vitamin K-2."

"So, Doc, how common are vitamin A, D, and K deficiencies?"

"Here in the U.S., vitamin A deficiency isn't a huge problem, but lack of sufficient vitamin K is. Around the world, especially Africa, lack of sufficient vitamin A is impacting millions of infants and children, often leading to blindness and death. Vitamin D is another deficiency for most people. But, David, remember, our bodies need enough of these vitamins to prevent a deficiency but don't overdose on them either. Too much of proform vitamin A can be harmful."

"Interesting, Doctor, I would agree that everything in moderation makes sense. I am curious when was this Dr. Price researching this stuff? Let me guess...the 1920s?" David smiled waiting for the doctor's response, knowing he probably was not far off the mark.

Laughing now, the doctor replied, "David, I do know that Dr. Price was born around 1870 and passed away in the late 1940s, but to answer your question I don't know when he first proposed his theory about factor X, but David, I can't help it if the research from the past stands the test of time!" They both shared a laugh.

The doctor and David sat for hours discussing what could be done and what could not be done to thwart aging in all of its forms. David felt a lot more confident after this talk than he had before. He realized that all of us that are currently living and in fair health have a world of possibilities ahead of us. It is in our best interests to follow the steps we know that are proven to help delay aging, so that when new anti-aging compounds, strategies, insights and discoveries are made, we can take advantage of them. David also walked away sensing that many people were already implementing anti-aging strategies and such protocols into their life. While the majority of humans remain ignorant, there are many informed and dedicated people doing something about aging now. The future did indeed look much brighter and healthier at that.

KEY POINTS
MINERAL OVERLOAD THEORY

- Follow all the previous steps mentioned.

- Avoid fluoride, as it can cause severe pineal gland disfunction.

- Consume some vitamin D-3 and K-2 together, several days a week.

- Don't over use calcium supplements. If using, make sure they contain equal amounts of magnesium.

- Obtain most of your vitamin A through food, not supplements.

- Do not consume rice grown in the southern U.S.A. daily, due to a possibly high arsenic contamination.

- Do not overconsume shellfish and shrimp from the Gulf of Mexico, as it may contain cadmium and other toxins. Limit these items to twice a week.

- Get your iron levels checked first. *If above normal*, use the following steps:

  - Consume less red meat.

  - Donate blood at least four to six times a year.

  - Don't take vitamin C with your meals but instead take it in between meals.

  - Drink tea with main meals as it may reduce iron availability.

  - Drink alcohol in moderation, if at all.

  - Consider taking a baby aspirin daily.

- Exercise since sweat contains iron.

- Don't use cookware that exposes your food to direct contact with iron, aluminum, copper or non-stick coatings. Do not use glazed containers, especially with acid foods.

- Don't use iron supplements or use multiple vitamins that contain iron, or consume iron-rich food like fortified cereal product.

21
Any Other Surprises?

DAVID KNEW THAT himself and the doctor would not be talking for a while, so he used that time to ask the doctor his favorite question, "Doc, are there any other surprises you want to tell me about?"

"Several, David, but we will need much more time to discuss them."

"Well, can you give me a hint so I can be better prepared to ask some intelligent questions the next time we meet?"

Smiling, the doctor responded, "David, you honor me; I mean what I have to tell you is that some things that have occurred historically are already being forgotten. And, sad to say, some things that were really important."

"Such as?"

"Well, the forms of medicine that used to be practiced in this country and around the world are being crowded out to the point that they seem irrelevant, but having lived around those types of medical practices, I can tell you that it will be our loss."

"Why's that?"

"Many of the past remedies really worked and were a lot less toxic to the people receiving those treatments. For instance, homeopathic doctors had much better success with flu cases during the Great Flu Pandemic of 1918, which wiped out millions of people. Also, various theories over the years, which make a lot of sense, are ignored or smeared so people don't follow up on them. It is a sad loss for all of us."

"There you go, Doctor! You can't tell me something like that and expect me to wait to hear what you are talking about, can you?"

Laughing at David's words and expression, he responded, "I suppose not, but we will need at least a full week so we can discuss all of those items."

"Well, besides discussing the other theories of healing and medical practices, what else were you going to discuss with me?"

"Yes, all of that we just spoke of, David, plus other theories on aging, theories that are ignored yet still make a lot of sense, and different views and philosophies."

"Not to sound like a broken record, but I will say it again: Such as?"

"Well, as a quick example I will ask that you look up a theory called hormesis and also that you review the history of another branch of medicine that has almost gone extinct in this country: homeopathic medicine."

"Well, OK, Doc, but first tell me what hormesis deals with."

"It deals with our body's real response to different toxic substances in our environment, and that may include several types of antioxidants."

"So, does this theory state antioxidants are good or bad for us?"

"Great question, it actually does deal with antioxidants and a lot of other topics, but let me say that according to this theory, we need some harmful stuff in our lives as it helps the body produce the needed response to those substances and in doing so helps our bodies in the long run. Some researchers point out that certain antioxidants may work by eliciting a certain response from our body and not by their actual antioxidant status. So maybe just taking lots of antioxidants could be harmful."

David replied, "Hmm, that might help explain something I noticed. I note you often say that you don't take antioxidants every day. Why is that? I mean if they are so good for us why shouldn't we load up on them?"

The doctor responded, "Good point. It is commonly believed that more is better. I don't feel nature works like this. In fact, more may be a problem. I feel the body has evolved to go without many things often and for long time periods. So the body devises ways of dealing with these shortages or weaknesses. In fact, there is a theory out there that states our bodies require some stress to perform optimally and to prolong life. It causes our body to become adaptable. If you think about our history, there must have been long time spans when we had to go without various foods, suffer extreme conditions, and yet still we survived."

"OK, Doctor, it sounds like that German philosopher that said, 'What does not kill us makes us stronger,' right?"

"Nietzsche is the philosopher you speak of, David, and the funny part is that another German came up with a theory that directly relates to that saying. In fact, they both lived in the same time period and in the same country, so maybe Nietzsche got the idea from him."

"Really? How's that?" replied David.

"Have you heard of a scientist by the name of Hugo Schulz?"

"No, who was he?" asked David.

HORMESIS

The doctor continued, "He was a German pharmacologist that noted in the late

317

1880s that the growth of yeast could be stimulated by small doses of poisons. Further work was done by another German named Rudolph Arndt, who came up with some interesting work using animals during the 1920s and 1930s, but many people tried to discredit his work because he spoke about this theory in conjunction with homeopathic medicine, and many in the medical community hate anything to do with homeopathic medicine. This did, however, give rise to a theory formulated by the work of both Schulz and Arndt that stated, 'For every substance, small doses stimulate, moderate doses inhibit, large doses kill.' It was a provocative concept. This led to a theory years later developed by scientists C.M. Southam and J. Ehrlich called hormesis. It was first published and covered in a journal called *Phytopathology* back in 1943."

"Why was that such a provocative theory, Doctor?"

"It mimics what seems to happen in real life. We endure a little hardship and are better for it. It's like a tree that grows tall in a strong wind area. Its roots seem to go deeper and its branches are more flexible. Yet scientists feel it can't be proven. It seems to work in limited situations when tested, especially when tested in various life forms. They can give a small amount of alcohol, and it seems to make the animal live longer, but too much makes it live a shorter life. Some poison seems to infer a life-promoting adaptive response. They have experimented with several other life forms with different results. In some experiments, it works and in others it doesn't. The real issue is that there is something to this and it is not being explored enough. It may really be a key to this mystery we call life. We should, as a society, study this phenomena closely to see where it may be helpful to us. So that is why I do not simply load up on antioxidants. Many quote antioxidants don't really work the way people think. Some are not really providing antioxidants but allowing the body to produce an adaptive response to the supplement, therefore, conferring the health benefit. If you want to really study this aspect of anti-aging, I suggest looking up the writings of Vince Giuliano. He has written extensively about this topic and seems to be on the leading edge of seeing how all this fits together."

"Really, Doctor, I can see why people would be confused. I will look it up and maybe do an article on it. I mean I can see the title page already, "How I punished my body and became better from it." They both laughed.

Hesitating for a brief moment, the doctor quit laughing and said with a lower voice, "All kidding aside, you know, David, you may have touched on just what we have been talking about."

"How's that?" asked David.

"Well, you know that hard exercise helps the body create its growth hormone. So by doing a few heavy lifting exercises before bedtime you could really rev up your human growth hormone production. It's like what we have been talking about, a little pain equals a lot of gain."

"Really, Doctor? By heavy lifting, what exercises do you mean?"

"By doing some heavy squats, bench presses, or dead lifts, you could really be turbo-charging your body into a growth phase. So grow while you sleep!"

"Good news, Doctor, obviously I don't want to do aerobics before going to bed but some heavy weightlifting will be no problem." They both chuckled again before David added, "Before I forget, why do people hate homeopathic medicine?"

HOMEOPATHIC MEDICINE

"I can't say for sure, but I feel it is because most people don't understand homeopathic medicine or they simply cannot comprehend it."

"Come again, how could it be so difficult?" queried David.

"Well, David, do you understand how homeopathic medicine is supposed to work?"

"Not really, Doctor, I mean I have heard of it. I also know that many famous people believe in it."

"Right you are David, Queen Elizabeth, the Queen Mother, used it and lived a very long life. My understanding is that many in the royal family still use it. John

D. Rockefeller used homeopathic medicine and lived to age 99. Several past presidents of the United States used this health practice, as did the late Pope John Paul II. Homeopathic medicine is hard to explain, but I will try; it is a lot like finding isolated natives living on a part of some secluded island around, let's say, Borneo. If you showed them a television set, they would have a hard time understanding how that television got a picture on it, especially if you explained that picture is being broadcast from thousands of miles away. They simply would refuse to believe it because, of course, they cannot really conceive it."

"OK, so explain it to me." said David.

"Well, once you understand the Theory of Hormesis, it might start making sense. This theory covers how the body may create a favorable response to a small amount of poison. Biologically, our systems know how to handle poisons, toxins and stress in small amounts, and it may develop a healthy response to that stimuli. For instance, if a person is facing starvation, the body may develop some protection mechanisms for allowing the person to live longer with less than living with a bountiful food supply. Later observations by other scientists gave credence to this, David. Some scientists believe that stress, if not overwhelming to an animal, may actually prove beneficial. Hence, they argue, caloric restriction may work because it produces a stress response within our bodies. Likewise, strenuous exercise may do the same."

"Really, Doctor, how is this theory accepted?"

"Not too well amongst most people. That is why I said it is similar to homeopathic medicine. Both are hotly debated yet both seem to have something to them. Homeopathic remedies are said to have none of the active ingredient within them because they are diluted mixtures. Homeopathic uses a concept called the law of similar. That is where a substance that produces a stuffy nose can be used to treat a stuffy nose. How? By using that substance in such a small amount that the body produces a small response to it but keeps it from producing a large response. That is what you are trying to create, a similar but much smaller reaction. In the case of homeopathic remedies, this small response keeps the body from producing a huge response and, therefore, keeps the person from getting sicker. In fact, it may even solve the original problem that person was having. So a person suffering from an ailment is given a very small dose of medicine that will produce that same symptom they are suffering from. This is just one problem medical people have with homeopathy. How can this work? And how can such a small diluted substance effect such major changes. That leads to the second problem they have, they simply believe that the dose is too small to have any real effect. They feel it must be the placebo effect. This is amazing because they should know that one small drop of various poisons, undetectable to the human eye, can instantly kill a person. You may not be able to see it, smell it, or taste it. But something is there. With homeopathic medicine the substance that remains is virtually undetectable but something of its chemical, biology or energy structure remains. So the major question remains: Can such a small dose really have an effect on a person's anatomy?"

"So most people don't use this type of medicine here anymore?"

"David, around the world, homeopathic medicine is doing well, but here in the United States, many of these doctors were assimilated into the American Medical Association years ago. Then powerful powers, that probably had ties to the drug industry since they were commissioned by a very wealthy industrialist Andrew Carnegie, made reports on schools' training and used those reports to attack the homeopathic schools and naturopathic schools in this country. This forced many of them to close or convert to traditional medical schools. I know because this occurred at the University of Michigan in Ann Arbor, Michigan, my original home state. Now, you cannot find a trace that there once was such a school and adjoining hospital. You see, homeopathic medicines were so cheap that their doctors did not have to charge much for them. Not profitable for the drug companies either, who were fond of patented medicines, since they made so much profit. These drug companies may have had direct ties to the agency doing the reporting on the schools' academic programs. So, like they tried to do with Native Americans, most American homeopathic physicians and herbal healers known as the Eclectics were assimilated, and their culture and teachings were downplayed."

ECLECTICS

"Eclectics? Tell me more about them," asked David.

"You've made my point, David. From your expression I feel you never heard about them before, have you?"

"No, Doctor, I feel a little embarrassed, I never heard that term before, who were they and what did they do?"

"David, I am not surprised by you not knowing, most people have never heard of them. It is like a lot of things, new places replace old places, new styles replace old styles, and so it goes... The Eclectic movement lasted over a hundred years and was essential to many Americans' well-being. They really served their purpose. They were also known as healers for everyday people. A cross between a doctor and a herbal healer. They created a good niche for themselves because they first would do no harm to a patient. That meant they did not bleed their patient like most medical doctors were doing back in that time, nor did Eclectic physicians use overdoses of mercury, as was the norm for regular doctors. In fact, their hundred-plus years on the scene curing and helping people finally helped lead to most doctors abandoning their liking for bleeding and using such excess doses of toxic things as mercury, lead and arsenic. This and with many medical doctors using herbal medicine in addition to their regular drugs caused the difference between the two types of physicians to diminish. At about that same time, traditional doctors were handed some powerful weapons such as vaccines for several different afflictions, anesthesia, much improved surgical outcomes, more stringent education requirements for their newer doctors, better and more organized hospitals, and a trade group that promoted their interests and suppressed the competition. Finally, with the advent of sulfur drugs and antibiotics, most people just preferred to see a regular traditional doctor. All of this together leading to the eventual demise of the Eclectic branch of medicine."

David asked, "What years was this type of medicine popular?"

The doctor responded, "It lasted from 1825 until 1939. The remnants still remain as the art and advice given by many herbalists and naturopathic physicians. However, their schools, libraries and students cannot be found. All that remains are some of their medical textbooks like *The American Eclectic*

Practice published in 1857, or better yet, their main textbook published around 1907 by Dr. Rolla Thomas, called *The Eclectic Practice of Medicine*. Eclectic means searching. So for over 125 years they advocated three main principals. First was reforming traditional medicine so it was not so harmful to the patients, second, was advocating for any treatment as long as it was proven to work and third, which is very important, placing the patient's long-term health first and foremost in importance. To a large extent, modern doctors and scientists have created successful treatments to treat many disorders and have created weapons against many diseases, but the truth is, today, too many patients are hurt by their treatments. Their long-term health is not valued as much as a quick response to treatment is valued, thus often overlooking the real underlying problem."

"Doc, the description you give makes me think that you feel there is a place for Eclectics today."

"Yes," said the doctor. "Perhaps there is a real place for Eclectic medicine to be brought back via modern medical schools and taught as being as important as any other area of medicine. Taking care of the needs of the patient should be the primary concern and the reason people go into medicine. This should be paramount in importance. Many years ago doctors were guilty of something we now call heroic medicine. The treatment was so strong that it killed the patient, yet they continued their ways for hundreds of years. Things like bloodletting and the giving of mercury compounds. The Eclectics helped steer traditional doctors away from these treatments. Now we need to lead the medical community away from excessive use of radiation, chemotherapy, invasive testing methods, and way too many questionable surgical procedures. Perhaps the latest development and reemergence of naturopathic medicine can influence modern medicine the same way the Eclectic healers influenced past medicine. That is my hope at least, after all; you do recall what I said at the beginning when we first sat down together, the primary mission of any good doctor should be, 'first, do no harm.'"

"So Doctor, I can see you have some strong views on medicine today in this country. I feel you think we can make it less deadly to people, but can we do this as well as keep the costs in check?"

KEEPING MEDICAL CARE AFFORDABLE

"Great point, David. We do have some incredible things going on in modern medicine, and we can do a lot. But that doesn't mean we should be doing many of the things we do. As an example, we are fighting the war on cancer the wrong way. Many medical people and scientists want to win it their way or not at all."

"How's that?"

"Well, we know prevention really works. What is so wrong with heading down that road big time and stopping much of the cancer from forming in the first place. Why do we insist on letting people expose themselves to toxins and then think we should just offer up some heroic and expensive treatment. I mean we can head off most cancer before it starts with just some common sense and low cost programs."

"Such as?"

"We know most people are exposed to cancer in the workplace, while cleaning the home with various products, or by ingesting various carcinogens. We need to work on all of these fronts simultaneously. There is so much we can do that is not being done. We need to make sure we get the chlorine out of water before people actually drink the stuff or shower in it. We need to get the hazardous chemicals out of our cosmetics, our food, our medicine, etc. Most people do not realize that almost half of our current medications may be cancer-causing if taken long enough. All vaccines should have to be tested for this as well. We need to stop exposing people to excess radiation, air pollution, pesticides, and on and on. We already know what needs to be done. It is just not popular since it will initially cost money, cause massive change with how we conduct certain business, and it will cost some businesses to lose substantial profits. Yet, what we are spending on cancer care in this country far exceeds the costs I speak of, so all things being even, we would save a huge sum over the coming decades. It is much harder to treat disease after it has manifested itself than to prevent it in the first place. Of course, look at all the steps we have discussed already, David. Take care of your diet, your body, and your mind and good health will follow in almost all cases."

"What else can we do to keep costs down, Doc?"

"First, eliminate the third-party payment system. When you have people collecting from others, all kinds of mischief goes on. Plus, you create overhead, hassles and paperwork. Simply having people pay directly for services rendered would keep costs down dramatically."

"Come on, Doctor, that isn't going to happen anytime soon. I mean look at Medicare; it is a huge third-party system. And no one I know wants to give up their Medicare benefits."

"I suppose you are right, David. So we could do some other simple fixes to reduce costs."

"Such as?"

"David, just look at history to see why those costs went up so high in the first place. Too many people are making too much money from modern medicine and its care. So reverse some of the trends. Keep doctors from being sued for such high amounts for simple mistakes that will happen over time. If a doctor is grossly incompetent then pull their license. Doctors should have the right to have patients sign arbitration forms just as most securities brokers do. It doesn't keep a client or patient from pursing action it just keep it out of the regular legal system that tends to be much more adversarial and expensive. Doctors need to know that there will be system in place that will be reasonable and not bankrupt them every time someone has a complaint."

"And more?

"Of course. Let's look at the past before the American Medical Association became so strong and took over most of medicine. In many countries, pharmacists can issue various prescriptions on the spot based on a person giving an intelligent and detailed request for such drugs. This would, of course, exclude narcotics, but why can't someone get an antibiotic from a pharmacist after describing their symptoms to them? Of course, the pharmacist will have to educate the person that not all disorders require antibiotics, but that is very easy to explain. It will be no worse than what is occurring now. Many people are given antibiotics by their doctors when it is not even a bacteria infection but a virus, which will not respond to antibiotics anyways. In years past, pharmacists were able to provide this standard of care in this area and in many other areas. It saved people from having to go to a doctor in the first place, and would really free up a lot of our emergency room traffic. And saying that, I have seen in many Latin American countries where this works very nicely and people are able to have access to medicine quickly. Also, since we are talking about letting highly educated pharmacists issue various prescriptions on the spot for various disorders or refills of current medicines, I would allow most registered nurses with at least five years experience the same privilege. In addition, I would urge an increase in the amount of doctors in family medicine, geriatrics, and pediatrics. A 30% increase would be a nice start. If the schools won't allow more students in their schools so we can have more family doctors, then I would encourage the government to get involved immediately, mandating more medical schools. Competition will bring down cost quickly."

"Doctor, I have to tell you that I have not heard that from anyone else before. Any other suggestions?"

"Yes, open up medicine to others in the alternative medical field and give people more choice of health care. In addition, I would urge the government to impose a small deductible to every medical insurance plan out there. Only when people have to pay the first hundred dollars of a bill will they really question everything that is being proposed. Testing clinics would be set up all over the country offering lower-cost medical tests if this was initiated. EKGs, stress tests, various other heart tests, MRI imaging tests, and various other tests would quickly drop in price. Overall expenses would plummet within three years of doing these simple actions alone. And finally, let people buy their drugs and prescriptions from any country they wish. As long as that company or drug as been stamped with an approval process by someone equivalent to our FDA and is periodically tested for safety."

David responded, "Would that be enough to drive prices down?"

"I think so, David, but if not, and if private and public hospitals do not cooperate, then probably the most controversial thing I would implement if I had any say is to make our Veterans Hospital network open to all Americans."

"Really? How would that work?"

"If you do not have adequate coverage we could make veterans hospitals a safety net for everyone. We would have to expand and vastly improve that system but we could do it intelligently. Let's say for every current veterans hospital we could have them establish a series of ten urgent care clinics attached to them as satellite offices. People would go there first and possibly be treated cheaply before ever needing an actual hospital. I am not saying this so that these veterans hospitals would compete with regular hospitals, I am just saying we need a large safety net of care networks out here so no one goes without treatment."

"Would they be free?" asked David.

Replying, the doctor said, "Flexible payment plans could be made right then and there, people could commit to a small amount being paid over time based on their actual current income. So a person needing extensive treatment would not be turned away or bankrupt by an illness. Let's assume someone just had open heart bypass or other serious illness. This would wipe out most people, financially speaking, without insurance. To prevent this from wiping them out financially, we need a payment method based on ability to pay, not on what a hospital wants to charge. Someone not making a lot would only have to forfeit 5%-10% of their take-home pay over a maximum time frame of five years instead of owing a huge sum for the rest of their life. The same would apply to someone making a good living who decided to go with out insurance. The most they would risk is having 5%-10% taken from their pay for the next five years instead of being wiped out. They pay a fair amount based on what they earn. It would be fair."

"Doc, that does sound fair to me. It is very easy for people to go bankrupt over the huge amounts that can be run up in regular hospitals, with or with out proper insurance in place."

The doctor added, "We must get big business's high costs and profits out of our healthcare system. Otherwise, we will see these expenses bankrupt our country. They charge outrageous fees for simple things like an aspirin pill or a box of facial tissues. It is not sustainable. It is insane. After all, if we can mandate that people have to pay income tax on their hard-earned wages, why can we mandate that those hard-working taxpayers have access to top medical care at a reasonable price? If we are forced to pay taxes then force our government to give us a safety net of health care."

"Is that moving us to a socialist environment?" asked David.

Smiling, the doctor replied, "No, not really, David, there is nothing socialist about it. Do you consider the public library to be a socialist institution? How about public schools? It's no more socialistic than having police and fire protection provided by your community or airport security provided by the government. I have many other thoughts, David, but our time today has come to an end."

"Doctor, I can't wait until we meet again."

KEY POINTS

- Modern medicine does not have all the answers.

- Historically, various forms of healing offer less harmful treatments.

- Modern medicine, or heroic medicine, has been tamed somewhat by the gentle healers of the past, but more needs to be done to reign in its harmful effects.

- Current health care practices in the U.S. are expensive and unsustainable. Something needs to be done.

22
The Great Balancing Act

"OK, Doc, I think I have it. You've seen in your lifetime a huge reduction in people dying from syphilis, pneumonia, smallpox, TB and diphtheria. You have seen continuous improvements. What else would you recommend for extending our lives?"

"David, I have several more theories of aging that will really help, but before we get into them, we need to cover 'The Great Balancing Act.'"

"What's that, Doc?"

"Our hormones. We are doing so many things wrong today that are disrupting our hormones that most of us are experiencing hormone problems that are impacting our health and longevity."

"That sounds interesting."

"It is, David. We will cover it at our next meeting and what you can do about it. I have an outline of what to do, what supplements to take, and maybe more importantly, what not to do."

"Can you give me a hint, Doctor?"

"Let me just say that after hearing about this, you may never have your lawn sprayed more than once a year or drink from plastic bottles. Also, David, more importantly, I wish to discuss one of the greatest potential area of research for extending life which is gene therapy. I feel gene therapy holds the greatest value for extending longevity for future generations. We will continue to develop ways to turn-on or turn-off various genes. In animal studies this has doubled various animals' life expectancies. This I feel will really be the holy grail of combating aging. But it can all wait, David. We have covered enough for today."

"You have my full attention, Doctor. I feel I have a good handle on your twelve theories of aging. I just hope I can communicate their importance to my readers."

"So do I, David, so do I."

KEY POINTS

- Positive manipulation of our DNA holds tremendous possibilities.

- Hormones are crucial to our health and are ignored by too many people.

Epilogue

WHEN DAVID RETURNED to visit with Dr. Tessler he was surprised to see the doctor's house sitting empty. There were several tapes of different colors criss-crossing the door and several notices posted. They all read similar and stated that this office was closed to such and such violation. It appeared that several government agencies coordinated their attack on his office to ensure he closed his doors to the public and remain closed. David had the thought that this must have happened before to the doctor, especially considering his methods.

The state of Virginia wanted to speak with Dr. Tessler, as it seemed too many of his patients were claiming religious exemptions from vaccines. They did not like it. The Virginia Department of Health had spent years getting people to comply with their vaccines strategy. They would lead people to believe that attending school was impossible without these vaccines and so parents by the thousands had their children inoculated at very young ages imposing all kinds of toxic substances into their systems.

Never were these vaccines questioned. If the U.S. government felt they were safe, who were the state medical authorities to argue? Virginia even had a special panel formed with physicians to inform and pressure parents into getting many vaccines. The reason? They felt that too many parents were being misinformed about the safety of vaccines and misguided into thinking that vaccines could cause autism and adverse effects. This committee felt vaccines were the most important duty physicians could have to their patients. So our children's health and welfare are left to a group of people who don't even question the possibility of harm being done in the name of public health and service.

Many of these doctors, especially the pediatricians, will shun patients who question their viewpoint or their vaccine schedule, often sending parents that question their authority to the nearest hospital emergency ward when their children are sick, where they would pay four times the going rate for an office visit, just to get their children treated for a common infection like strep throat, which inoculation wouldn't address anyways. Why? Because these parents question them about vaccines and opted out of having so many vaccines done, and done so often and early. Parents are led to believe in a most strong way that they must comply.

In regards to nutrition advice, the same old garbage is being peddled by the FDA, Department of Agriculture, and the American Medical Association. Most of which are very critical of all things not anointed with the M.D. initials after it. The AMA still states to 'see your doctor' for nutrition advice. After all, they did study nutrition in school, maybe? These medical doctors, and the nutritional consultants they refer people to, are the same ones that have failed to halt the huge amount of ill health occurring in this country. Their advice simply does not work. Many registered dieticians often offer different advice than what they were taught in school, as what they were taught doesn't work too well.

The American Medical Association does not approve of anything deemed alternative. They do not recommend homeopathy, herbology, alternative cancer therapies, etc. Their view can be summarized easily as, "Far better to die from cancer than be cured by a dubious source."

The state medical board also was seeking out Dr. Tessler. It seems his medical license showed his age to be 104 years. That would have made him one of the oldest practicing physicians in the country, superseding the previously oldest doctor known to have been practicing: Dr. Leila Denmark of Athens, Georgia, who practiced medicine until age 103. David recalled that she lived to age 114, dying in 2012. So she had started her journey back in the late 1800s. One of her mottos was, "No milk after the baby is weaned!" They wondered if Dr. Tessler was really alive or was, perhaps, his son using his medical license. After all, according to all reports, Dr. Tessler looked to be in his early 60s. When David heard that he smiled to himself as he thought, "There is no doubt that Dr. Tessler was indeed a doctor." In fact, one of the best ones he had ever encountered.

It is the hope of this author that every person will strive for the best health possible. Sometimes just knowing it is a possibility is enough incentive. In the words of the famous Benjamin Franklin, "Those who will not be counseled, cannot be helped."

KEY POINTS

- Delegate your health care to caring and reasonable people, but never abdicate it!

- You must take charge of your own personal health care. Become your own personal Chief Executive Officer. Hire various medical people as needed and let go of those medical people who are not serving you.

Helpful Notes

If IMPLEMENTING THE supplements mentioned in the book, I suggest you do not use most of them every day. It would prove expensive and, in my view, unnecessary. Americans have a belief that if a little of something is good for you, then more must be better. That's not recommended.

Various supplements that contain multiple ingredients can be purchased, and that is a good move. Other supplements such as multiple vitamins can be used several days a week but not every day. Also a good consideration.

What can seem overwhelming in regards to various supplements can become relatively easy if taken on different days.

I personally divide my supplements up into three groups. On the first day, I take from the first group, then the next day, from the second group, and finally on the third day, I take from the third group. I then repeat the pattern. Otherwise, you will find your self trying to swallow forty pills a day.

GROUP ONE

- Vitamin C (1000 mg) & Magnesium (100% RDA), both taken twice a day

- Carnosine 500 mg twice a day

- DMAE 200 mg taken twice a day

- Krill oil or fish oil capsules, take four gel capsules twice on that day

- Q-10 supplement, 100 mg soft gel

- Vitamin D3 with K2, in normal amounts giving you the RDA of each; increase if your blood levels of vitamin D test low. Always take with food, preferably a meal containing fat

- Natural Vitamin E (Alpha & Gamma), with mixed tocopherols

GROUP TWO

- Vitamin C & Magnesium (see above)

- A combo synergistic antioxidant product for your mitochondria like:

  - Life Extension's product called *Mitochondrial Energy Optimizer*, which contains: Vitamin B6, Carnosine, Acetyl-L-carnitine, benfotiamine, R-Lipoic acid, BioPQQ, and luteolin

  - Or use Solaray's product instead, called *Acetyl L-Carnitine, Alpha Lipoic Acid*, also containing N-Acetyl-Cysteine, resveratrol, vitamin D3, vitamin E (mixed tocopherol), tart cherry, bromelain, nattokinase, and quercetin

    I like both products. Take the recommended amount listed on the supplement, but only use on the day that you have decided. So you would be using this product only once every three days, not every day.

GROUP THREE

- Vitamin C

- A good multiple vitamin. Make sure it contains real folate, zinc, and a good form of selenium derived from yeast or other source, not just in the selenium selenate form.

  Once again, I prefer *Life Extension's Mix Capsules* containing a host of ingredients along with their *Super Booster* soft gels, which contain a mixture of ingredients. This brand contains 100% or more of many vitamins and minerals.

Other helpful supplements such as quercetin, niacin, Pycnogenol, apple polyphenols, milk thistle, TMG, turmeric and spirulina can be worked in by adding them to one of your groups but never to all three groups at the same time. Note, the only supplements I take each and every day is vitamin C and magnesium, and melatonin at night. Not a mega-dose but a normal dose. All of the other supplements I only take as I rotate from group one, group two, or group three. So at most, you will be taking from these groups only twice a week and sometimes for one group, three times. By the way, if you decide not to take supplements one day a week, then for sure you will only be taking each group just twice in a given week.

Action needed

Take control of your body as you are its Chief Executive Officer or CEO. Work with your physician to determine your current biomarkers. Make sure to inquire on costs before moving ahead, as there is a lot of leeway in this area. However, discuss this important issue before doing medical tests, not after. Getting your blood work done through Life Extension (www.lef.org) out of Florida is a cost effective way to proceed. You can get your blood work done through them and present it to your doctor. Many times, they are impressed that you have taken this important step in finding out what is truly going on within your body. Your physician can be one of the most important players in maintaining your health. However, remember you are the number one person who is responsible for your health. Don't delegate that responsibility to anyone else. Use medical professionals as they should be utilized, as important people that can help you reach your health goals.

For updates on our informative content and nutritional protocols, please visit our website at http://www.12theories.com

Recommended Sites & Sources

12 Theories of Aging
http://www.12theories.com

International Antiaging Systems (IAS)
http://www.antiaging-systems.com

Life Extension
http://www.lef.org

Weston A. Price Foundation
http://www.westonaprice.org

Think Twice Global Vaccine Institute
http://www.thinktwice.com

Key Points

CHAPTER 2
THE COMMITMENT

• First, do no harm. Keep this in mind when dealing with medical personnel. Often, they get so wrapped up with processes and procedures that they exceed boundaries of safety, reasonableness and common sense.

• Watch out for assumed consent. Many times medical staff use this technique to proceed with procedures or tests without explaining all the real risks. This also pertains to financial costs involved. Most patients are never told up front what the true costs will be.

• Take a knowlegable and trusted friend or family member with you when you are being asked to do an invasive test, surgical procedure, or before undergoing radiation treatments or chemotherapy. In all of these cases, seek a second and third medical opinion.

• Ask about all risks and all costs of any procedure or treatment beforehand and keep detailed records. Only by keeping the medical system accountable in both of these areas can we affect meaningful change.

CHAPTER 3
IMMUNIZATIONS

• Vaccines are miracle tools, but like most tools, they must be used correctly.

• The medical community is under pressure from the drug companies to vaccinate children while they are young. The reason? Vaccine manufacturers are protected more due to federal law against the effects of a vaccines given to a minor. Children also can't speak up for themselves.

• Consider practicing watchful waiting. Observe your child after receiving a vaccine. Give it some time (two to three months). If no negative reactions are seen, it may be deemed safer to proceed. This is only recommended if there are no deadly outbreaks currently occurring.

CHAPTER 4
QUICKSILVER

• Mercury is still used in the medical field. It is unsafe in any amount.

• Avoid unnecessary medical tests.

• Keep always in mind that you are in charge of your own health. Delegate tasks but never abdicate total authority to medical staff. Yes, you may have to place yourself in their hands for life-saving procedures. However, make sure you are making an informed decision and not reacting to needless pressure. It's not easy to speak out and politely demand that everything be explained to you in simple English, but the reward can be less medical procedures and less risk from those procedures.

CHAPTER 5
POLIO SCARE

• Many older adults were exposed to polio vaccines containing active monkey viruses as both the dead polio type vaccine and live type vaccine were grown within monkeys' kidneys. These viruses, including SV40, have been found in many cancerous tumors and could also be the cause for several severe medical disorders. These contaminated vaccines occurred during the years 1955 through 1963. Even today, polio vaccine manufacturers still use monkey kidneys to culture polio vaccines, but they do inactivate potential viruses by using powerful agents to kill them. Hopefully, that is enough. Thousands of monkeys have been killed in the manufacturing of the polio virus and millions of humans have been exposed to viruses that previously only were found in monkeys. You have to question the science and the justification of all of this.

• Generally, you are best to avoid new vaccines until you have had the time to analyze the risk and return of such vaccines. Also, wait until researches have had time to see what the real long-term effects of any vaccine are going to be. Don't always assume your doctor knows best, as your doctor may have been misled by misinformation, conflicting studies, drug companies and sales people.

CHAPTER 6
GREAT MYSTERIES SOLVED

• Diseases have plagued humankind throughout history. Great discoveries and research have allowed humankind to overcome many killer ailments. However, apathy and a loss of respect for some of these diseases may cause a virulent resurgence.

• Our medical community may be focusing on the wrong vaccines to be given and ignoring the real threats.

CHAPTER 7
PREVENTION THEORY

• First, do no harm.

• Eat real foods, which consist of good fats, good carbs, and good sources of protein.

• Eat close to the earth, which means avoiding most processed food.

• Never forget where we as a species came from. That alone should lead you to enjoying real food and not the processed stuff they want you to believe is food.

• Food is supposed to be free of preservatives, pesticides, fungicides and other harmful ingredients.

• Health nuts may not be nuts but everyone else truly is for eating the horrible way they do. It simply is not natural nor is it healthy.

• Keep in mind, what is your vibrant health really worth to you?

• Drink pure water, free of chlorine, fluoride, arsenic and other contaminants.

• Don't assume anything when it comes to medical care or treatment. The cure may kill you even if the initial medical condition does not.

• Never forget cause and effect.

• Think differently than your friends, family and community.

• Make your own lifestyle decisions.

• Allow time each day to commune with nature, such as walking outside.

• We all have lead in our systems. Why? Leaded gas was used for years around the world (it allowed gasoline engines to run smoother), along with lead-based paints used in homes. Many of us have been overexposed to these harmful lead products and have accumulated lead in our systems. Keep your current exposure to lead to a minimum by not using lead products and not removing harmful lead paint found in older homes. Also, consider ways of getting lead out of your system, such as chelation. People that have used chelation therapy have far less cancer.

• Trace minerals are important. Kelp tablets are an excellent source of iodine. Iodine and selenium, in small amounts, can be protective. Large amounts, however, can be toxic.

• Take a quality vitamin and mineral supplement several times a week.

• Observe your digestion and digestive track and take steps to improve digestion, assimilation and elimination.

• Do not overconsume the preformed source of vitamin A that is contained in most supplements, as too much may cause more harm than good. Too much vitamin A, often listed as retinyl acetate or retinyl palmitate, may interfere with proper vitamin D utilization. This reason alone should cause you to limit your intake of multiple vitamins on a daily basis. Natural vitamin A, also called retinol, can be found in fatty fish, fish liver oil, eggs, and liver. Heat, air, and light readily destroy vitamin A. Plant sources contain beta carotene, which the body can convert to vitamin A. Stating this, you should get vitamin A from both sources: fish, eggs, liver, and plants.

• Get your own blood work done before seeing doctors. Life Extension (www.lef.org) offers the ability to do so.

CHAPTER 8
CALORIC RESTRICTION THEORY

• Follow the previous steps outlined for prevention as they apply to caloric restriction as well.

• Always undereat compared to the norm. Most people consume way too many calories each day.

• Only consume nutrient-dense food that contains wholesome ingredients and are known to be good for you.

• Avoid all processed food since it is health destroying. This includes most products that have added sugar, added fat, fried foods, processed meat, most flour products, and products with additional sodium added, etc. Avoid overly processed food found in a jar, prepackaged food, and canned food with some exceptions (sardines). Note many prepackaged soups only look healthy but in fact are laced with artificial taste enhancers and sodium. These taste enhancers damage the brain.

• Shop around the outer rim of the grocery store buying only fresh vegetables, frozen organic vegetables, fresh fruit, and low-fat meat products (if consuming meat). Frozen fish is good, but make sure it was caught in Alaska, Iceland, or other northern cold waters. Consume fish such as cod, salmon, sardines, etc.

• Avoid tuna, swordfish, battered fish (which usually contain flavor enhancers and trans fat oils), most farm raised seafood such as farm-raised salmon, tilapia, or shrimp. Consume lake fish rarely, as it usually is high in contaminants.

• Avoid using too much heavy cream, butter and fat containing sauces like cheese sauce, Alfredo sauce, etc.

• Avoid all processed oils, which mean that they have been hydroge-nated or heat-treated to last longer. These are also known as trans fatty acids or partially hydrogenated oils. Food companies like to sneak them into their products since it extends the shelf life of those products. Many bakeries continue to use these same cheap oils for the same reasons.

• Focus on using only good cold press oils for cooking or for adding to salads and recipes. Keep olive oil on hand for salads. Don't deep fry, as that will convert any healthy oil into unhealthy oil due to its high temperature. If stir frying, then consider non-hydrogenated nut oils like peanut oil or macadamia oil for that. Unprocessed coconut oil is good as a skin cream, on toast, and for baking as well. Also, real butter can be used for baking, as can non-hydrogenated palm shortening.

• Even when consuming healthy oils, do not consume more than 2 to 3 tablespoons total per day. Afterall, fat is fat and always higher in calories than carbohydrates and proteins.

• Shop for organic goods to reduce your toxic exposure to so many heavily sprayed food items. Food companies have convinced people that the abnormal act of spraying pesticides, fungicides and other toxins is normal.

• Load up on wholesome food such as salads, homemade coleslaws, fresh fruit platters, avocados, nut spreads, lightly steamed vegetables, interesting side dishes such as hummus, tabouli, lentils, bean dishes, brown rice, wild rice, and root vegetables of all types.

• Avoid packaged products entirely that are promoted as low fat, no cholesterol, etc. Notice that many of them are cheap carbohydrate products mixed with cheap oils, lots of flour, lots of sodium, and dangerous flavoring agents known as MSG, yeast extract, spices, autolyzed plant protein, hydrolyzed plant protein, textured protein extract, etc., which damage the brain.

• Do use small plates and bowls to serve food. Many people do not know that plates used today are far larger than dishes that were used even forty years ago.

• Avoid using processed food or heavily laden restaurant food in a social setting or as a personal reward. Instead, focus on having a good cup of herbal tea, green tea, oolong tea, or black tea. Coffee is good in moderation but avoid overconsuming as it then drives up cortisol levels mitigating its good effects such as clearing the liver, initiating bowel movements, and helping blood sugar.

• Consider using a supplement called trans-resveratrol. Many studies point to it as a supplement that may mimic caloric restriction by activating some of the same genes such as the SIRT1 gene and the SIRT3 gene. It also seems to positively affect sugar levels, reducing the risk of diabetes, and it may even help reduce beta amyloid plaque, which may lead to Alzheimer's disease, along with protecting against other neuro-degeneration diseases in the brain. Note that more of this supplement is not better; you simply want some exposure to this each

347

day or every other day.

• Commune with nature by taking daily outside walks. Caloric restriction works best when doing a moderate amount of physical activity and consuming real food in its natural state.

• Saturated fats are derived from three sources: animal products, coconuts, and vegetables oils that have been hydrogenated. These hydrogenated vegetable oils are called partially hydrogenated oils, or trans fatty oils. The body can handle a fair amount of saturated fat from animal products and coconuts, but it cannot handle hydrogenated or heat-treated oils that are created by the hydrogenation of normal vegetable oils. While normally most vegetable oils are considered unsaturated or monounsaturated, once you hydrogenated them they can become a very harmful type of saturated oil. The human body has a hard time processing these oils. Likewise, coconut oil is normally a healthy saturated oil, but is turned into an unhealthy saturated oil when hydrogenated. Avoid all hydrogenated oils for this reason.

• Eat a wide variety of food. Most people only consume about 20 different foods, month in and month out.

• Eating eggs and meat, especially fish, several times a week is OK. Your body will need the protein and vitamin B-12. Most people only need 15% to 20% of their diet to consist of protein. However, on a caloric restriction diet, you will need to increase your protein levels since you are consuming less calories overall. Your body stills need enough protein to repair itself. To make sure you have enough protein on a caloric restricted diet, consider moving your protein percentage up from 15% to 20%, to around 25%.

CHAPTER 9
ALTERNATIVE TREATMENTS

• Prevention is much better than needing a cure.

• Always have a back up plan. Too many cancer patients wait and rely on conventional doctors to cure them. What happens if their treatments fail or are deemed ineffective for your type of cancer? Have several alternative plans of action ready to go. Do your own research as well, as the life you may save could be your own.

CHAPTER 10
FREE RADICAL THEORY

• Follow the previous steps outlined for Prevention and Caloric Restriction as they apply to Free Radicals as well.

• Consume a diet rich in colorful vegetables and fruits. Use various grains and beans, along with nuts and berries. All of these contain natural antioxidants. Include daily vegetables from the mustard family which include cabbages, watercress, cauliflower, Brussels sprouts, broccoli, kale, and collard greens, to name a few.

• Do drink a small amount of real fruit juice that is made without added sugars, as it is a potent source of antioxidants. Fresh vegetable juice can be consumed more often as it tends to have less sugar. The need for such juices cannot be overstated. They flood your body with what it really needs: chlorophyll, antioxidants, flavonoids and minerals.

• Supplement wisely. Use supplements that have numerous antioxidants instead of those usually containing only one. That way you can get some synergy along with less filler material. This also saves you money. Buy on quality, not just on price.

• Vitamin C with quercetin and other bioflavonoids is good along with a full spectrum vitamin E supplement. The vitamin has to be natural not synthetic or else it may do more harm than good. For example, a good vitamin E would contain gamma-Tocopherol along with other mixed Tocopherol. The combination of vitamin C, which is a water soluble vitamin, is good along with a fat soluble vitamin E.

349

• Research has shown that many vitamin supplements are now available and affordable such as Q-10, lipoic acid, and vitamins D and K. Include trace minerals such as selenium.

• Don't overconsume overcooked food products, especially fried foods. They create glycation within the body.

• Don't consume foods with a high glycemic index. These include sugar, soda, fruit juices and drinks, and most snack products and junk food.

• Consume antioxidants along with a well rounded natural balanced diet. Consider a balanced B supplement every few days and make sure it contains real folate.

• Consider adding spices like turmeric to your diet. Turmeric is absorbed best when combined with ginger.

• If you are taking fish oil or krill oil, always take a taste test when you first get them. You need to bite into a capsule to make sure it is not rancid. Otherwise you will be doing more harm than good.

• Consider using a zinc supplement periodically.

  • Good forms of zinc:
    • zinc monomethionine
    • zinc picolinate
    • zinc orotate
    • zinc aspartate
    • zinc citrate

  • Forms of zinc to avoid:
    • zinc gluconate
    • zinc oxide
    • zinc sulfate

• Don't overconsume zinc, as it displaces copper.

CHAPTER 11
OTHER THEORIES OF AGING

• Causes of aging have been ignored throughout history. However, many are waking up to the fact that something can really be done to delay its effects and impact.

• Only by shifting our attention from that of acceptance on aging to what can be done about it, will we see real progress being made.

• Take care of yourself and follow any steps you can to preserve what time you have left so you can also benefit from new or future breakthroughs.

CHAPTER 12
MEMBRANE THEORY

• Follow the previous steps outlined for Prevention, Caloric Restriction, and Free Radicals, as they apply to Membrane Theory as well.

• Consume a clean diet of healthy food.

• Consume good fats such as monosaturated fats like olive oil or avocado fat, a small amount of saturated fat from fish, lean meats, or coconuts, as long as they are not processed, and a small amount of polyunsaturated fats from fish and nuts.

• Consume non-contaminated fish like sardines or salmon.

• Use supplements that aid in protecting your cell membranes like natural vitamin E, alpha-lipoic acid or if available the better form called R-lipoic acid, acetyl-L-carnitine, carnosine & DMAE.

• Eat smaller meals and less often. Place food servings on plates and store the rest of the food away to avoid second servings.

• Stop eating when 80% full. To do this, eat slower.

• Fast periodically, as it helps your body cleans up its waste.

• Avoid too much sugar.

• Never ever consume processed oil. Oil processed through a hydrogenation process is referred to as partially hydrogenated trans fat. These are toxic, leading to cancer, heart disease and diabetes.

• Stop using plastic bottles or containers, especially those containing BPA.

• Drink clean water often.

CHAPTER 13
MITOCHONDRIA THEORY

• Follow the previous steps outlined for Prevention, Caloric Restriction, Free Radicals, and Membrane Theory as they apply to Mitochondria Theory as well.

• Foremost for mitochondria protection and energy are R-lipoic acid and acetyl-L-carnitine. If R-lipoic acid is not available, use alpha-lipoic acid. R-lipoic acid is usually twice as strong as alpha-lipoic acid due to the chemical configuration. Lipoic acid is important, as it provides antioxidant protection both to water soluble parts of the body and fat soluble. Lipoic acid may aid in proper sugar metabolism. Using lipoic acid and acetyl-L-carnitine together gives it more synergy in providing mitochondria protection.

• Hint: Look for supplements that contain both of these ingredients together. For example, Life Extension Company offers a product that contains several ingredients such as R-lipoic acid, acetyl-L-carnitine, benfotiamine (a unique form of vitamin B1), and carnosine. All in all, a tremendous way to take all of these supplements together in a synergistic fashion and with a cost savings. Solaway Vitamin Company also has a similar product which contains alpha-lipoic acid, acetyl-L-carnitine, resveratrol, and N-acetyl cysteine.

- N-acetyl cysteine and vitamin C may be a good second defense.

- Protect your liver since your liver produces so much of the bodies' glutathione. So what protects your liver? Healthy food along with various supplements like vitamin C, melatonin, turmeric extract, milk thistle, coenzyme Q10.

- Q10 also protects your mitochondria. Life Extension offers a synergystic supplement that includes PQQ.

- Avoid toxic food such as white flour, sugar, high fructose corn syrup, simple sugars added to processed foods, and preservatives. Avoid all processed meat products, and foods covered in pesticides. Weight gain can lead to a fatty liver, and that equates to a liver that cannot protect itself much longer or the body.

- Don't overeat.

- Do aerobic exercise at least four times a week for at least 30 minutes each session.

- Avoid taking Tylenol on a long term basis. When using Tylenol avoid alcohol.

- Avoid mercury.

CHAPTER 14
GLYCOGEN CROSS LINKING THEORY

• Follow all the steps mentioned previously to reduce damage on the cellular level.

• Avoid all added sugar food and drink products.

• Avoid refined food products and hydrogenated oils and hydrogenated fat.

• Never consume fried foods of any type.

• Avoid consuming overcooked food of all types, especially fried eggs, barbecued meats, charred food, and processed baked products.

• Watch your oxidative load and don't overdue oxidative damage by consuming a processed food diet or by over exposing yourself to too much sun, excess radiation from medical body scans and airport check-in body scanner machines, too many medical X-rays, radon gas, or by using oxidative agents like excess alcohol or any tobacco product in any amount.

• Avoid all pesticides, solvents or other toxic chemicals.

• Consider supplements like carnosine, DMAE, cinnamon, chromium polynicotinate (nicotinate, chromium bound to niacin), and benfotiamine (B1), all in moderation.

• A dosage of carnosine, 500 mg per day, should work well with 200 mg of DMAE per day. Many people double those amounts a few days a week.

• Avoid excessive doses of common cinnamon (*Cinnamomum cassia*). A small amount each day is helpful for blood sugar, but an excessive amount may inflame the liver.

- Avoid cheap chromium picolinate. It has been shown to be destructive to DNA when tested in test tubes. Get chromium from food sources or use chromium polynicotinate or the brand ChromeMate.

- Take a brisk 20 minute walk after meals to reduce glucose levels.

CHAPTER 15
TELOMERE THEORY

- Follow all the steps to anti-aging such as prevention, caloric restriction, antioxidants for free radical damage, protecting your cells' membranes, preserving your mitochondria, and preventing excess cellular, tissue, and organ cross linking damage via the glycogen cross-linking theory.

- Tame inflammation.

- Keep stress in your life to a minimum. Use tools like exercise, long walks, yoga, meditation, communing with nature. Establish a network of friends, be realistic about issues, and in dealing with people don't be a perfectionist. Practice forgiving others and yourself for mistakes that will always be made.

- Monitor your homocysteine levels and reduce them if necessary. Consider using the supplement TMG (trimethylglycine) to help.

- Telomeres affect cells' ability to replicate so it may go a long way in preserving and extending your life. Various supplements may help such as TA-65 offered by a company named Geron. As of yet, no real studies have been published on the effects or safety of TA-65.

- Take vitamin C each day. At least 1000 mg twice a day.

- Consider a quality magnesium supplement and take daily.

- Strive to consume natural, non-synthetic versions of vitamins B, C and E.

- Exercise on a regular basis.

- Everyday consume some fresh vegetable juice that contains green plants.

CHAPTER 16
INFLAMMATION THEORY

- It's crucial to follow all the previous steps outlined to tame inflammation.

- Avoid processed food.

- Avoid too much sugar.

- Avoid all trans fats, partially hydrogenated fats, or rancid fats. All of these processed fats are toxic. Heat-treated fats are unnatural to the body and will quickly make any body inflammatory.

- The start for reducing inflammation within your body starts with diet. Reduce all simple carbs, such as sugar, processed food, packaged foods, fried foods, fast foods, junk food, white flour, soda pops of all types including diet, canned or bottled fruit juice, which are usually just sugary fruit imitations, excess alcohol, etc. Ditch these simple carbs, as they cause inflammation.

- Balance the good fats you consume by making sure you are consuming, in moderation, the best omega-6 fats, such as nuts, flax seed, cereals, avocado, borage oil, sunflower and pumpkin seeds. It's crucial to include an adequate amount of omega-3 fats as well such as flax seed, chia seed, quinoa grain, and walnuts and cold water fish. Many oil and fats, such as olive oil, are neutral; these are called monosaturated. Consider fresh avocados and cold processed coconut oil as additions to your diet.

- Monitor your inner terrain. Bad diets, stress, and lack of exercise can make your body inflammatory. A bad lifestyle will allow various bacteria and fungus to take over too much of your biological territory or your inner terrain as it is also called. This can result in a host of problems such as H. pylori bacteria giving you ulcers, yeast infections, fungus disorders, leaky gut syndrome, autoimmune disorders, and a host of other afflictions. You need to consume a minimally processed diet of real foods in their natural state and consume a diet that is mostly alkaline.

• Never smoke and limit your exposure to polluted air, water or food.

• Take steps to distress such as long walks, quiet times, meditation, gardening, hobbies and sports. Prolonged exercise, if not taken to excess, will reduce inflammation within the body.

• Avoid toxic people. These are people who are negative, gossip constantly, complain too much, or belittle others. People that constantly doubt or demand that you prove something can be energy draining. These people lower your immune system while also driving up your cortisol levels, a major stress indicator.

• Exercise on a consistent basis, walking at least 30 minutes minimum each day.

• Use supplements like turmeric, ginger, vitamin C, green tea, and a good source of omega-3 oils from cold water fish or krill capsules.

• Consume raw food with any cooked food to garner some natural enzyme potential. Supplement with digestive enzymes with meals and between meals to tame inflammation.

• Use a magnesium supplement most days to tame excess chronic inflammation. Best forms are magnesium citrate, magnesium orotate, magnesium glycinate, and magnesium chloride.

CHAPTER 17
THYMUS THEORY

• Follow all the previous steps as outlined as they will all benefit your immune system.

• Consume a natural diet heavy in uncooked food consisting mostly of vegetables, fruit and berries.

• Consume lean sources of protein never over cooked.

• Consume fat in its natural state, never hydrogenated. Avocado, olive and coconut oils that have not been hydrogenated or heat-treated are good for the body in moderation.

• Sprout grains and nuts before consuming by soaking in water overnight. This biologically activates the enzymes and makes the food more bio-available and nutritious. It also keeps your body from using its own enzymes purely for the digestive process.

• Exercise often, jogging, fast walking, doing jumping jacks, or using a mini trampoline. These stimulate the lymph system.

• Reduce stress in your life. High cortisol levels greatly diminish your immune system.

• Periodically take micronutrients like zinc. Safely use up to 50 mg per day. If taking everyday, however, add 2 mg copper since too much zinc will deplete copper.

• Consider thymus extract if your immune system remains weak for a prolonged period. Make sure you select extracts made from cows from Argentina or New Zealand, two countries free of any mad cow disease-causing prions.

• Do supplement with probiotics in capsule form or, if consuming dairy, have yogurt and kefir several times a week. Much of our immune system lies in our digestive tract.

• Supplement with vitamin C and other antioxidants.

• Sleep in a dark room and, as you age, consider a melatonin supplement.

• The herb astragalus helps wake up the immune system, especially the thymus gland. Use in moderation and cycle on-and-off. Never take a herbal preparation on a neverending basis.

• Various mushroom supplements may aid in boosting your immune system. One such supplement includes three types: maitake, reshie, and shiitake.

• Use the supplement IP-6 periodically.

• Use ginseng for increased immune strength. It also is known to protect against cancer and is used for males as a sexual aid. Cycle on and off with this herb; this simply means to use ginseng for a month or two and then take a month off. If you are 55 or older then you can usually continually take ginseng on an even more consistent basis, as you will usually derive more benefit than possible side effects. However, to be safe it is always wise to cycle on and off of any herb, as this will lessen the possibility of having too much build up in your system and also will allow your body to keep getting a response from the herb. People with high blood pressure must monitor themselves well while taking ginseng, as it can raise blood pressure in many people. Panax ginseng also called Korean ginseng may work best, but many people use American ginseng as well.

CHAPTER 18
ACIDIFICATION THEORY

• Follow all the other previous steps mentioned.

- Our bodies have a multiple buffering system. One uses our body's minerals to neutralize this acid. This can lead to mineral depletion with the negative effects of our system being too acidic and also our bodies then have fewer minerals within our systems for other needs.

- Food consumption needs to be mostly alkaline versus acidic. Most people should consume about 80% alkaline and 20% acidic foods. Liquids are included in this, too.

- All the previous steps to anti-aging covered lead to a naturally alkaline body.

- In the words of a famous biologist and scientist Henry G. Bieler, "Germs seek their natural habitat—diseased tissue—rather than being the cause of diseased tissue." This may be at odds with modern germ theory but explains a lot of sickness and disease.

- Arm your body with the tools it needs. Consume mineral-rich food such as vegetables and fruits. Organic food usually contains more of these minerals.

CHAPTER 19
ENZYME THEORY

- Follow all the previous steps mentioned.

- Investigate what foods can be eaten raw.

- Learn to sprout grains, nuts and seeds before consuming. According to Dr. Howell, squirrels bury nuts not to hide them but to germinate them, thereby releasing the maximum food value.

- Consider quality digestive enzymes. They can be taken with meals and in between meals.

- If you eat like everyone else, you can expect the same results. Eat close to the earth by saying no to processed food.

• Pasteurization is a heat treatment therefore modern milk and cheese products are sold without their true enzyme potential.

• Eat less, as that uses less of your enzymes and also allows your enzymes to repair your body.

• If eating cooked food, incorporate raw food with them.

• Chew your food thoroughly.

CHAPTER 20
MINERAL OVERLOAD THEORY

• Follow all the previous steps mentioned.

• Avoid fluoride, as it can cause severe pineal gland disfunction.

• Consume some vitamin D-3 and K-2 together, several days a week.

• Don't over use calcium supplements. If using, make sure they contain equal amounts of magnesium.

• Obtain most of your vitamin A through food, not supplements.

• Do not consume rice grown in the southern U.S.A. daily, due to a possibly high arsenic contamination.

• Do not overconsume shellfish and shrimp from the Gulf of Mexico, as it may contain cadmium and other toxins. Limit these items to twice a week.

• Get your iron levels checked first. *If above normal*, use the following steps:

- Consume less red meat.

- Donate blood at least four to six times a year.

- Don't take vitamin C with your meals but instead take it in between meals.

- Drink tea with main meals as it may reduce iron availability.

- Drink alcohol in moderation, if at all.

- Consider taking a baby aspirin daily.

- Exercise since sweat contains iron.

- Don't use cookware that exposes your food to direct contact with iron, aluminum, copper or non-stick coatings. Do not use glazed containers, especially with acid foods.

- Don't use iron supplements or use multiple vitamins that contain iron, or consume iron-rich food like fortified cereal product.

CHAPTER 21
ANY OTHER SURPRISES?

- Modern medicine does not have all the answers.

- Historically, various forms of healing offer less harmful treatments.

- Modern medicine, or heroic medicine, has been tamed somewhat by the gentle healers of the past, but more needs to be done to reign in its harmful effects.

- Current health care practices in the U.S. are expensive and unsustainable. Something needs to be done.

CHAPTER 22
THE GREAT BALANCING ACT

- Positive manipulation of our DNA holds tremendous possibilities.

- Hormones are crucial to our health and are ignored by too many people.

EPILOGUE

- Delegate your health care to caring and reasonable people, but never abdicate it!

- You must take charge of your own personal health care. Become your own personal Chief Executive Officer. Hire various medical people as needed and let go of those medical people who are not serving you.

Glossary

A1C/Glycated hemoglobin: A form of haemoglobin that is measured primarily to identify the average plasma glucose concentration over prolonged periods of time.

acetyl-L-carnitine: An acetylated form of L-carnitine. It is a dietary supplement and naturally occurs in plants and animals. ALCAR has the ability to cross the blood–brain barrier and get to the brain blood circulation, where it acts as a powerful antioxidant, which helps in prevention of the brain cells' deterioration.

acrylamide: A known lethal neurotoxin and animal carcinogen. Its discovery in some cooked starchy foods in 2002 prompted concerns about the carcinogenicity of those foods. Acrylamide was accidentally discovered in foods in April 2002 by scientists in Sweden when they found the chemical in starchy foods that had been heated. It was not found in food that had been boiled or in foods that were not heated.

aldehyde: An organic compound formed by the oxidation of alcohols. When heated to frying temperature for extended periods, some oils produce aldehydes, which may be associated with some neurodegenerative diseases.

ADP/adenosine diphosphate: A nucleotide, the result of adenosine triphosphate (ATP) losing a phosphate group in metabolism. ADP can be converted, or powered back, to ATP through the process of releasing the chemical energy available in food; in humans this is constantly performed via aerobic respiration in the mitochondria.

AGE/advanced glyc[osyl]ation end-product: The result of a chain of chemical reactions after an initial glycation reaction. AGEs may be formed external to the body (exogenously) by heating (e.g., cooking); or inside the body (endogenously) through normal metabolism and aging. Under certain pathologic conditions (e.g., oxidative stress due to hyperglycemia in patients with diabetes), AGE formation can be increased beyond normal levels. The formation and accumulation of advanced glycation end-products (AGEs) has been implicated in the progression of age-related diseases. AGEs have been implicated in Alzheimer's disease, cardiovascular disease, and stroke. The mechanism by which AGEs induce damage is through a process called cross-linking that causes intracellular damage and apoptosis. They form photosensitizers in the crystalline lens, which has implications for cataract development. Reduced muscle function is also associated with AGEs.

allopathy: A traditional medical method or treatment.

alpha-lipoic acid: A fat- and water-soluble antioxidant created by the body and found in every cell. Evidence suggests that alpha-lipoic acid may help regenerate other antioxidants and make them active again. It is found in red meat, organ meats (liver), and yeast, particularly brewer's yeast. Also available in supplement form.

antioxidant: One of a group of vitamins that act against the effects of free radicals.

astaxanthin: A xanthophyll pigment that occurs widely in plants and animals, especially crustaceans. Research shows that, due to astaxanthin's potent antioxidant activity, it may be beneficial in cardiovascular, immune, inflammatory and neurodegenerative diseases.

Atkins Diet: A low-carbohydrate diet created by Robert Atkins from a research paper he read in the Journal of the American Medical Association published by Gordon Azar and Walter Lyons Bloom. The Atkins diet involves limited consumption of carbohydrates to switch the body's metabolism from metabolizing glucose as energy over to converting stored body fat to energy.

ATP/adenosine triphosphate: A nucleotide that occurs in muscle tissue, and is used as a source of energy in cellular reactions, and in the synthesis of nucleic acids. It is often called the "molecular unit of currency" of intracellular energy transfer.

Benfotiamine: A derivative of thiamine (vitamin B1) used to treat sciatica and other painful nerve conditions. Benfotiamine may be useful for the treatment of diabetic retinopathy, neuropathy and nephropathy.

biomarker: An indicator of a biological state. It is a characteristic that is objectively measured and evaluated as an indicator of normal biological processes, pathogenic processes, or pharmacologic responses to a therapeutic intervention. It is used in many scientific fields.

bloodletting/releasing humours: The archaic practice of treating illness by removing some blood, believed to be tainted, from the stricken person. Bloodletting was based on an ancient system of medicine in which blood and other bodily fluid were regarded as humors that had to remain in proper balance to maintain health. It was the most common medical practice performed by physicians from antiquity until the late 19th century, a span of almost 2,000 years.

BPA/Bisphenol A: An organic compound used in the manufacture of certain plastics. BPA exhibits hormone-like properties that raise concern about its suitability in consumer products and food containers. It is thought to be an endocrine disruptor which can mimic estrogen and may lead to negative health effects.

caloric restriction: A dietary regimen that restricts calorie intake, where the baseline for the restriction varies, usually being the previous, unrestricted, intake of the subjects. CR without malnutrition is one of the few dietary interventions shown to increase both median and maximum lifespan in a variety of species, among them yeast, fish, rodents and dogs.

carbohydrate: A sugar, starch or cellulose that is a food source of energy for an animal or plant; a saccharide.

carnosine: A dipeptide of the amino acids beta-alanine and histidine. It is highly concentrated in muscle and brain tissues. Carnosine can oppose glycation and it can chelate divalent metal ions. Chronic glycolysis is suspected to accelerate aging. Carnosine was found to inhibit diabetic nephropathy by protecting the podocytes and mesangial cells. Because of its antioxidant, antiglycator and metal chelator properties, carnosine supplements have been proposed as a general anti-aging therapy. Carnosine containing products are also used in topical preparations to reduce wrinkles on the skin.

catalase: An enzyme found in the liver that catalyses the decomposition of hydrogen peroxide, a harmful byproduct of normal metabolic processes, to water and oxygen.

chemotherapy: Chemical treatment to kill or halt the replication and/or spread of cancerous cells in a patient. Chemotherapy may be given with a curative intent or it may aim to prolong life or to palliate symptoms. It is often used in conjunction with other cancer treatments, such as radiation therapy or surgery. Traditional chemotherapeutic agents act by killing cells that divide rapidly, one of the main properties of most cancer cells. This means that chemotherapy also harms cells that divide rapidly under normal circumstances – cells in the bone marrow, digestive tract, and hair follicles.

cholesterol: A sterol lipid synthesized by the liver and transported in the bloodstream to the membranes of all animal cells; it plays a central role in many biochemical processes and, as a lipoprotein that coats the walls of blood vessels, is associated with cardiovascular disease. Although cholesterol is important and necessary for human health, high levels of cholesterol in the blood have been linked to damage to arteries and cardiovascular disease.

coenzyme Q10: A 1,4-benzoquinone, where Q refers to the quinone chemical group, and 10 refers to the number of isoprenyl chemical subunits in its tail. Helps to maintain a healthy cardiovascular system.

C-reactive protein: A protein found in the blood, whose levels rise in response to infection or inflammation.

DHEA/dehydroepiandrosterone: An important endogenous steroid hormone. The most abundant circulating steroid in humans. It is produced in the adrenal glands, the gonads, and the brain.

DIM/diindolylmethane: A compound derived from the digestion of indole-3-carbinol, found in cruciferous vegetables such as broccoli, Brussels sprouts, cabbage and kale. The reputation of Brassica vegetables as healthy foods rests in part on the activities of diindolylmethane. Promotes a beneficial estrogen metabolism in both women and men.

DNA/deoxyribonucleic acid: A substance in living beings which determines their form and can be used to uniquely identify a person.

endocrine system: The system of glands, each of which secretes different types of hormones directly into the bloodstream (some of which are transported along nerve tracts) to regulate the body. The endocrine system is in contrast to the exocrine system, which secretes its chemicals using ducts.

digestive enzyme: Enzymes that break down polymeric macromolecules into their smaller building blocks, in order to facilitate their absorption by the body. Digestive enzymes are diverse and are found in the saliva secreted by the salivary glands, in the stomach secreted by cells lining the stomach, in the pancreatic juice secreted by pancreatic exocrine cells, and in the intestinal (small and large) secretions, or as part of the lining of the gastrointestinal tract.

fiber: Any substance, generally of plant origin, which is undigested on passage through the human alimentary tract – consists mostly of complex carbohydrates.

folate/folic acid: A polycyclic heterocyclic carboxylic acid, one of the vitamin B complex, essential for cell growth and reproduction. The human body needs folate to synthesize DNA, repair DNA, and methylate DNA as well as to act as a cofactor in certain biological reactions. It is especially important in aiding rapid cell division and growth, such as in infancy and pregnancy. Children and adults both require folic acid to produce healthy red blood cells and prevent anemia.

free radicals: Any molecule, ion or atom that has one or more unpaired electrons; they are generally highly reactive and often only occur as transient species. Excessive amounts of these free radicals can lead to cell injury and death, which may contribute to many diseases such as cancer, stroke, myocardial infarction, diabetes and major disorders.

glutathione: A tripeptide formed from glutamic acid, cysteine and glycine, that is active in many biological redox reactions.

glycation: A reaction that takes place when simple sugar molecules become attached to proteins or lipid fats without the moderation of an enzyme. This results in the formation of rogue molecules known as advanced glycation end-products (AGEs).

GSH-PX/Glutathione peroxidase: The general name of an enzyme family with peroxidase activity whose main biological role is to protect the organism from oxidative damage.

Hayflick limit: The number of times a normal human cell population will divide until cell division stops. Empirical evidence shows that the telomeres associated with each cell's DNA will get slightly shorter with each new cell division until they shorten to a critical length.

HDL/high-density lipoprotein: A class of lipoprotein that transports cholesterol to the liver from other tissue; high levels may decrease the risk of coronary heart disease.

heart disease: The narrowing or blockage of the coronary arteries, usually caused by atherosclerosis. Atherosclerosis (sometimes called "hardening" or "clogging" of the arteries) is the buildup of cholesterol and fatty deposits (called plaques) on the inner walls of the arteries. These plaques can restrict blood flow to the heart muscle by physically clogging the artery or by causing abnormal artery tone and function.

high-fructose corn syrup: Comprises any of a group of corn syrups that has undergone enzymatic processing to convert some of its glucose into fructose to produce a desired sweetness. In the United States, consumer foods and products typically use high-fructose corn syrup as a sweetener. It has become very common in processed foods and beverages, including breads, cereals, breakfast bars, lunch meats, yogurts, soups, and condiments.

Hippocratic Oath: An oath sworn by newly-qualified physicians that they will observe the medical ethics that derived from Hippocrates.

homeopathy: A system of treating diseases with small amounts of substances which, in larger amounts, would produce the observed symptoms.

homocysteine: An amino acid that is monitored in the blood to estimate risk of cardiovascular disease.

hormesis: Stimulation by the use of a low concentration of a toxin.

hydrogenation: Occurs when infused hydrogen gas is moved through oil, often under high pressure and with a catalyst. High heat will not hydrogenate oil, but will cause oxidation, causing it become unhealthy or rancid, making it very unhealthy.

hyperkalemia: An abnormally high concentration of potassium in the blood.

immunization: The process by which an individual is exposed to a material that is designed to prime his or her immune system against that material.

indole-3-carbinol: Produced by the breakdown of the glucosinolate glucobrassicin, which can be found at relatively high levels in cruciferous vegetables such as broccoli, cabbage, cauliflower, Brussels sprouts, collard greens and kale. I3C is also available in a dietary supplement. Indole-3-carbinol is the subject of on-going Biomedical research into its possible anticarcinogenic, antioxidant, and anti-atherogenic effects.

inflammation: A condition of any part of the body, consisting in congestion of the blood vessels, with obstruction of the blood current, and growth of morbid tissue. It is manifested outwardly by redness and swelling, attended with heat and pain. Chronic inflammation can also lead to a host of diseases, such as hay fever, periodontitis, atherosclerosis, rheumatoid arthritis, and even cancer. It is for that reason that inflammation is normally closely regulated by the body.

L-cysteine: A sulphur-containing nonessential amino acid found in most animal proteins; it readily oxidizes to cystine. One of the main functions of l-cysteine is the promotion of stomach lining health and also the correction of situations where the absorption of essential nutrients from food sources takes place. L-cysteine can be found in a number of foods ranging from meats to dairy and vegetable sources.

LDL/low-density lipoprotein: A class of lipoprotein that transports cholesterol around the bloodstream; high levels may increase the risk of coronary heart disease.

lipofuscin: The name given to finely granular yellow-brown pigment granules composed of lipid-containing residues of lysosomal digestion. It is considered one of the aging or "wear-and-tear" pigments, found in the liver, kidney, heart muscle, adrenals, nerve cells, and ganglion cells.

longevity: The quality of being long-lasting, especially of life.

lutein: A naturally occurring antioxidant found in a wide range of fruits and vegetables. Classified as a carotenoid, this nutrient has a reputation for helping the eyes to function properly, both in terms of general health and their ability to process blue light. This antioxidant can be found in a number of different foods, notably dark green leafy vegetables such as kale and collards.

Maillard reaction: The condensation reaction of an amino acid and a reducing sugar, followed by polymerization to form brown pigments – melanoidins; one of the causes of browning during cooking.

Mediterranean Diet: A modern nutritional recommendation inspired by the traditional dietary patterns of Portugal, Spain, southern Italy, southern France, Greece and specifically the Greek island of Crete, and parts of the Middle East. The principal aspects of this diet include high olive oil consumption, high consumption of legumes, high consumption of unrefined cereals, high consumption of fruits, high consumption of vegetables, moderate consumption of dairy products (mostly as cheese and yogurt), moderate to high consumption of fish, low consumption of meat and meat products, and moderate wine consumption.

melatonin: A naturally occurring hormone in humans and animals. In humans, melatonin is produced by the pineal gland, a small endocrine gland located in the center of the brain but outside the blood–brain barrier. The melatonin signal forms part of the system that regulates the sleep-wake cycle by chemically causing drowsiness and lowering the body temperature. Production of melatonin by the pineal gland is inhibited by light to the retina and permitted by darkness. Its onset each evening is called the dim-light melatonin onset (DLMO).

mineral: Any inorganic element that is essential to nutrition. Minerals in order of abundance in the human body include the seven major minerals calcium, phosphorus, potassium, sulfur, sodium, chlorine and magnesium. Important "trace" or minor minerals, necessary for mammalian life, include iron, cobalt, copper, zinc, molybdenum, iodine and selenium.

monounsaturated fat: Fatty acids that have one double bond in the fatty acid chain and all of the remainder of the carbon atoms in the chain are single-bonded. Sources include olive oil, macadamia nut oil, grapeseed oil, peanut oil, sesame oil, corn oil, popcorn, whole grain wheat, cereal, oatmeal, safflower oil, almond oil, sunflower oil, tea-oil Camellia, and avocado oil.

N-acetyl cysteine: A pharmaceutical drug and nutritional supplement used primarily as a mucolytic agent and in the management of paracetamol (acetaminophen/Tylenol) overdose. Other uses include sulfate repletion in conditions, such as autism, where cysteine and related sulfur amino acids may be depleted.

naturopathy: A system of therapy that avoids drugs and surgery and emphasizes the use of natural remedies (air, water, heat, sunshine) and physical means (massage, electrical treatment) to treat illness.

nixtamalization: A process for the preparation of maize (corn) in which the grain is soaked and cooked in an alkaline solution, usually limewater, and hulled.

omega-3 fatty acid: Any polyunsaturated fatty acid having a double bond between the third and fourth carbon atoms from the end of the molecule farthest from the carboxylic acid. They are essential fatty acids, and seem to be beneficial in reducing the risk of heart disease. Common sources of omega–3 fatty acids include fish oils, algal oil, squid oil, and some plant oils such as echium oil and flaxseed oil.

omega-6 fatty acid: A family of unsaturated fatty acids that have in common a final carbon–carbon double bond in the omega-6 position, that is, the sixth bond, counting from the methyl end. Some medical research suggests that excessive levels of certain omega-6 fatty acids, relative to certain omega-3 fatty acids, may increase the probability of a number of diseases. Modern Western diets typically have ratios of omega-6 to omega-3 in excess of 10 to 1, some as high as 30 to 1. Humans are thought to have evolved with a diet of a 1 to 1 ratio of omega-6 to omega-3 and the optimal ratio is thought to be 4 to 1 or lower, and it is even better if there is more omega-3 than omega-6.

omega-9 fatty acid: A family of unsaturated fatty acids which have in common a final carbon–carbon double bond in the omega-9 position; that is, the ninth bond from the methyl end of the fatty acid. Unlike omega-3 and omega-6 fatty acids, omega-9 fatty acids are not classed as essential fatty acids (EFA). This is both because they can be created by the human body from unsaturated fat, and are therefore not essential in the diet, and because the lack of an omega-6 double bond keeps them from participating in the reactions that form the eicosanoids.

organelle: A specialized subunit within a cell that has a specific function, and it is usually separately enclosed within its own lipid bilayer.

oxalate: Any salt or ester of oxalic acid. The toxicity of oxalic acid is due to kidney failure, which arises because it causes precipitation of solid calcium oxalate, the main component of kidney stones. Oxalic acid can also cause joint pain due to the formation of similar precipitates in the joints.

Paleolithic Diet (paleo/caveman diet): A modern nutritional plan based on the presumed ancient diet of wild plants and animals that various hominid species habitually consumed during the Paleolithic era that ended with the development of agriculture and grain-based diets. First popularized in the mid-1970s by gastroenterologist Walter L. Voegtlin.

placebo: A dummy medicine containing no active ingredients.

polyunsaturated fat: A fat or oil, almost exclusively from vegetable sources, containing a high proportion of polyunsaturated fatty acids; will typically be liquid at room temperature. Sources include walnuts, sunflower seeds, sesame seeds, chia seeds, peanuts, peanut butter, olive oil, seaweed, sardines, soybeans, tuna and wild salmon.

PQQ: Pyrroloquinoline quinone: known as a redox cofactor. It is similar to CoQ10 (CoEnzyme Q10) in the sense that it aids with oxidation and reduction reactions and associates itself with proteins, but rather than being located in the mitochondria's electron transport chain, PQQ is located in the cells cytoplasm and forms what is known as a "water-soluble electron transport chain" (a non-legitimate term, used to demonstrate the point of PQQ conducting many REDOX reactions). It is amazingly potent at doing this, being able to conduct 1000-10,000 more REDOX cycles than the standard Vitamin C.

quinine: A bitter-tasting, colorless drug derived from the bark of certain cinchona trees and used medicinally to treat malaria. For hundreds of years quinine was the only drug known to effectively combat malarial infection. It has since been largely replaced by synthetic compounds that not only relieve the symptoms of malaria but also rid the body of the malarial parasite, which quinine does not do.

radiation therapy: The medical use of ionizing radiation, generally as part of cancer treatment to control or kill malignant cells. Radiation therapy may be curative in a number of types of cancer if they are localized to one area of the body.

resveratrol: Occurs in some fruits, nuts and in red wine, that has antioxidant and other beneficial properties.

R-lipoic acid: The carboxylic acid 5-[(3R)-dithiolan-3-yl]pentanoic acid, one enantiomer of which is an essential cofactor for many enzyme complexes. Widely available as an over-the-counter nutritional supplement in the United States in the form of capsules, tablets and aqueous liquids, and has been branded as antioxidants.

ROS/reactive oxygen species: Chemically reactive molecules containing oxygen such as superoxide, hydrogen peroxide, and hydroxyl radical and are associated with cell damage. ROSs form as a natural by-product of the normal metabolism of oxygen and have important roles in cell signaling.

saturated fat: A fat or oil, from either animal or vegetable sources, containing a high proportion of saturated fatty acids; will typically be solid at room temperature. A diet high in saturated rather than unsaturated fats is thought to contribute to higher levels of cholesterol in the blood.

SOD/Superoxide dismutase: Enzymes that catalyze the dismutation of superoxide into oxygen and hydrogen peroxide. Thus, they are an important antioxidant defense in nearly all cells exposed to oxygen.

Sonoma Diet: Developed by Connie Guttersen, it is a derivation of the Mediterranean diet. The diet plan consists managing portion sizes and eating approved foods centered around 10 items known as the "power foods." According to the creator of the diet, these foods were chosen for their nutritional value and intense flavors. The power foods are whole grains, almonds, bell peppers, tomatoes, broccoli, grapes, spinach, blueberries, strawberries and olive oil.

South Beach Diet: Designed by cardiologist Arthur Agatston and dietician Marie Almon as an alternative to low-fat approaches such as the Ornish Diet and the Pritikin Diet advocated by the American Heart Association in the 1980s. It focuses on the glycemic impact (short-term change in blood glucose) of foods.

telomere: A region of repetitive nucleotide sequences at each end of a chromosome, which protects the end of the chromosome from deterioration or from fusion with neighboring chromosomes. Telomere regions deter the degradation of genes near the ends of chromosomes by allowing chromosome ends to shorten, which necessarily occurs during chromosome replication. Over time, due to each cell division, the telomere ends shorten.

trans fat: An unsaturated fat with carbon-carbon double bonds in the trans configuration, especially one prepared by partial hydrogenation, associated with an elevated risk of coronary heart disease. These partially hydrogenated fats have displaced natural solid fats and liquid oils in many areas, the most notable ones being in the fast food, snack food, fried food, and baked goods industries.

triglyceride: An ester derived from glycerol and three fatty acids. There are many triglycerides: depending on the oil source, some are highly unsaturated, some less so. Triglycerides are the main constituents of vegetable oil (typically more unsaturated) and animal fats (typically more saturated). In humans, triglycerides are a mechanism for storing unused calories, and their high concentration in blood correlates with the consumption of starchy and other high carbohydrate foods. In the human body, high levels of triglycerides in the bloodstream have been linked to atherosclerosis and, by extension, the risk of heart disease and stroke.

unsaturated fat: A fat or oil, from either animal or vegetable sources, containing a high proportion of unsaturated fatty acids; will typically be liquid at room temperature. A diet high in unsaturated rather than saturated fats is thought to contribute to lower levels of cholesterol in the blood.

vaccine: A substance given to stimulate the body's production of antibodies and provide immunity against a disease, prepared from the agent that causes the disease, or a synthetic substitute.

vitamin: Any of a specific group of organic compounds essential in small quantities for healthy human growth, metabolism, development, and body function; found in minute amounts in plant and animal foods or sometimes produced synthetically; deficiencies of specific vitamins produce specific disorders.

zeaxanthin: One of the most common carotenoid alcohols found in nature. It is important in the xanthophyll cycle. Synthesized in plants and some micro-organisms, it is the pigment that gives paprika (made from bell peppers), corn, saffron, wolfberries, and many other plants and microbes their characteristic color. Zeaxanthin supplements are used to treat different disorders, mainly with affecting the eyes. There are no reported side effects from taking zeaxanthin supplements. However, there is a decreased absorption rate when taken with Orlistat, mineral oil, and Chitosan.

Zone Diet: Popularized in books by biochemist Barry Sears. It advocates consuming calories on a 40:30:30 ratio of carbohydrates, proteins and fats, respectively.

Bibliography

CHAPTER 3

Conis, Elena. (2014). *Vaccine Nation: America's changing relationship with immunization.* Chicago, IL: University of Chicago Press.

Habakus, L. K., & Holland, M. (Eds.). (2013). *Vaccine epidemic: How corporate greed, biased science, and coercive government threaten our human rights, our health, and our children.* Skyhorse Publishing, Inc.

Mendelsohn, R. S. (1987). *How to Raise a Healthy Child: In Spite of Your Doctor.* Ballantine Books.

Sears, R. W. (2011). *The vaccine book: making the right decision for your child.* Little, Brown.

Mendelsohn, R. S. (1980). *Confessions of a medical heretic.* Lebanon, IN: Warner Books.

Native Americans and The Smallpox Epidemic. (n.d.). Retrieved April 13, 2016, from http://www.earlyamerica.com/early-america-review/volume-11/native-americans-smallpox/

3_3 European Disease in the New World. (n.d.). Retrieved April 13, 2016, from http://www.uic.edu/classes/osci/osci590/3_3%20European%20Disease%20in%20the%20New%20World.htm

American History Myths Debunked. (n.d.). [Text]. Retrieved April 13, 2016, from http://indiancountrytodaymedianetwork.com/tags/american-history-myths-debunked

Native American Netroots. (n.d.). Retrieved from http://nativeamericannetroots.net/

CHAPTER 4

Exquemelin, Alexander. (2008). *The illustrated pirate diaries: A remarkable eyewitness account of captain morgan and the buccaneers.* (T. Breverton, Ed.) New York City, NY: HarperCollins. (Original work published 1678)

Billings, Frank. (1903). *Presidential Address.* 54th Annual Session of the American Medical Association.

Edwards, Rob. (1999, June 12). Shadow of a doubt. *New Scientist,* (2190), 23. Retrieved from http://www.newscientist.com/article/mg16221903.800-shadow-of-a-doubt.html

Rodgers, C. (2006). Questions about prenatal ultrasound and the alarming increase in autism. *Midwifery Today, 80,* 16.

Kirby, D. (2007). *Evidence of harm: Mercury in vaccines and the autism epidemic: A medical controversy.* Macmillan.

Moritz, A. (2011). *Vaccine-Nation: Poisoning the Population, One Shot at a Time.* Ener-Chi Wellness Center.

International Programme on Chemical Safety. Environmental Health Criteria 22. Ultrasound. (1982). United Nations Environment Programme, International Labour Organisation and International Radiation Protection Association. http://www.inchem.org/documents/ehc/ehc/ehc22.htm

Kieler, H., Cnattingius, S., Haglund, B., Palmgren, J., & Axelsson, O. (2001). Sinistrality—a side-effect of prenatal sonography: A comparative study of young men. *Epidemiology, 12*(6), 618-623.

Ang, E. S., Gluncic, V., Duque, A., Schafer, M. E., & Rakic, P. (2006). Prenatal exposure to ultrasound waves impacts neuronal migration in mice. *Proceedings of the National Academy of Sciences, 103*(34), 12903-12910.

Rados, C. (2005). FDA cautions against ultrasound" keepsake" images. *FDA Consumer Magazine. www. fda. gov/fdac/features/2004/104_images. html. Accessed, 11.*

Samuel, E. (2001, December 4). Fetuses can hear ultrasound examinations. *New Scientist.* https://www.newscientist.com/article/dn1639-fetuses-can-hear-ultrasound-examinations/

Miller, M. W., Nyborg, W. L., Dewey, W. C., Edwards, M. J., Abramowicz, J. S., & Brayman, A. A. (2002). Hyperthermic teratogenicity, thermal dose and diagnostic ultrasound during pregnancy: implications of new standards on tissue heating. *International journal of hyperthermia, 18*(5), 361-384.

Graham, J. M., Edwards, M. J., & Edwards, M. J. (1998). Teratogen update: gestational effects of maternal hyperthermia due to febrile illnesses and resultant patterns of defects in humans. *Teratology, 58*(5), 209-221.

Barnett, S. B. (1998). Can diagnostic ultrasound heat tissue and cause biological effects? *Safety of Diagnostic Ultrasound.* UK: Parthenon Publising.

Edwards, M. J. (1998). Apoptosis, the heat shock response, hyperthermia, birth defects, disease and cancer. Where are the common links?. *Cell stress & chaperones, 3*(4), 213.

Edwards, M. J., Saunders, R. D., & Shiota, K. (2003). Effects of heat on embryos and foetuses. *International journal of hyperthermia, 19*(3), 295-324.

Milunsky, A., Ulcickas, M., Rothman, K. J., Willett, W., Jick, S. S., & Jick, H. (1992). Maternal heat exposure and neural tube defects. *Jama, 268*(7), 882-885.

Honda, H., Shimizu, Y., & Rutter, M. (2005). No effect of MMR withdrawal on the incidence of autism: a total population study. *Journal of Child Psychology and Psychiatry, 46*(6), 572-579.

Bricker, L., & Neilson, J. P. (2000). Routine Doppler ultrasound in pregnancy. *The Cochrane Library.*

New research offers clues to prevent brain damage in premature babies. (2006). *Medical News Today.* http://www.medicalnewstoday.com/medicalnews.php?newsid=28786.

Ewigman, B. G., Crane, J. P., Frigoletto, F. D., LeFevre, M. L., Bain, R. P., & McNellis, D. (1993). Effect of prenatal ultrasound screening on perinatal outcome. *New England journal of medicine, 329*(12), 821-827.

CHAPTER 5

SV40 Cancer Foundation. http://www.sv40foundation.org/

Sears, Robert. (2011). *The vaccine book: Making the right decision for your child.* (Rev Upd ed.). New York, NY: Little, Brown and Company.

Ingram, Cass. (2008). *The cause for cancer revealed: The vaccine connection.* Vernon Hills, IL: Knowledge House Publishers.

Bernice Eddy (& Sarah Stewart), speech and research on SV40 virus and lung and brain tumors

McKee, M. (2004, March 30). Monkey virus link to human cancers. Retrieved from https://www.newscientist.com/article/dn4830-monkey-virus-link-to-human-cancers/

CHAPTER 6

Kraut, Alan. (n.d.). Dr. *Joseph Goldberger & the war on pellagra*. Retrieved from http://history.nih.gov/exhibits/goldberger/index.html

Koehn, Jr., C. J., & Elvehjem, C. A. (1937). Further studies on the concentration of the antipellagra factor. *The Journal of Biological Chemistry*, (118), 693-699. Retrieved from http://www.jbc.org/content/118/3/693

Holmgren, I. (1934, December 10). *Physiology or medicine 1934 - presentation speech*. Retrieved from http://www.nobelprize.org/nobel_prizes/medicine/laureates/1934/press.html

Christiaan Eijkman, Beriberi and Vitamin B1. (n.d.). Retrieved May 4, 2016, from http://www.nobelprize.org/educational/medicine/vitamin_b1/eijkman.html

Boring, W. I. (2014, May 31). Eating Too Much Rice Almost Sank the Japanese Navy — War Is Boring. Retrieved May 4, 2016, from https://warisboring.com/eating-too-much-rice-almost-sank-the-japanese-navy-f985772c81a6

Sugiyama, Y., & Seita, A. (2013). Kanehiro Takaki and the control of beriberi in the Japanese Navy. Journal of the Royal Society of Medicine, 106(8), 332–334. http://doi.org/10.1177/0141076813497889

Hawk, A. (2006). The great disease enemy, Kak'ke (beriberi) and the Imperial Japanese Army. Military Medicine, 171(4), 333–339.

Jandl, James. (n.d.). *William B. Castle: Biographical memoir.* Retrieved from http://www.nap.edu/readingroom/books/biomems/wcastle.html

Shampo, M.A., Kyle, R.A., Steensma, D.P. (2006). William Murphy: Nobel prize for the treatment of pernicious anemia. *Mayo Clinic proceedings, Mayo Clinic*, 81, (6), 726. Retrieved from http://www.mayoclinicproceedings.org/article/S0025-6196%2811%2961724-2/fulltext

Woodward, R. B. (1973). The total synthesis of vitamin b12. *Pure and Applied Chemistry*, 33(1), 145-178. doi:10.1351/pac197333010145

Schatz, A., Bugle, E., Waksman, S.A. (1944). Streptomycin, a substance exhibiting antibiotic activity against gram-positive and gramnegative bacteria. *Experimental Biology and Medicine*, 55(1), 66-69. doi:10.3181/00379727-55-14461

Johnson, Steven. (2006). *The ghost map: The story of London's most terrifying epidemic and how it changed science, cities and the modern world.* New York, NY: Riverhead Books.

CHAPTER 7

McNamara, J., Molot, M., Stremple, J., & Cutting, R. (1971). Coronary artery disease in combat casualties in vietnam. *JAMA*, 216(7), 1185-1187. doi: 10.1001/jama.1971.03180330061012

Framingham heart study. (n.d.). In *Wikipedia*. Retrieved November 8, 2013, from http://en.wikipedia.org/wiki/Framingham_Heart_Study

Framingham heart study. http://www.framinghamheartstudy.org

Campbell, T. C., & Campbell, T. M. (2005). *The China study: Startling implications for diet, weight loss and long-term health.* Dallas, TX: BenBella Books.

CHAPTER 8

Keys, A.B., & Keys, M. (1975). *How to eat well and stay well the Mediterranean way.* New York City, NY: Doubleday.

Walford, Roy L. (1987). *The 120 year diet: How to double your vital years.* New York City, NY: Simon & Schuster.

McCay, C. M., Crowell, Mary F. (1934) Prolonging the Life Span. *The Scientific Monthly,* 39(5), 405-414. doi: 10.2307/15813

Exquemelin, Alexander (2000). *The buccaneers of america* (A. Brown, Trans.). Mineola, NY: Dover. (Original work published 1678)

McCay, Clive M. (1940). *Cornell bread.* Retrieved from http://www.cornell.edu/search/index.cfm?tab=facts&id=188

Wallach, Joel D., Lan, Ma. (2004). *Dead doctors don't lie.* Wellness Publications

Walford, Roy L. (2005). *The anti-aging plan: The nutrient-rich, low-calorie way of eating for a longer life.* (10th ed.). Cambridge, MA: Da Capo Press.

Robbins, John. (1987). *Diet for a new america.* HJ Kramer.

Balance test: How to improve your balance. (2009, August). Retrieved from http://www.sharecare.com/health/fitness-exercise/article/improve-your-balance

CHAPTER 9

Wolford, D. (2013, May 22). Milk Showdown: Cow vs. Sheep vs. Goat - Which is best? Retrieved from http://www.weedemandreap.com/milk-showdown-cow-sheep-goat/

CHAPTER 10

Harman, Denham. (1956). Aging: A theory based on free radical and radiation chemistry. *Journal of Gerontology*, 11(3), 298-300. doi: 10.1093/geronj/11.3.298

Gerschman, R., Gilbert, D. L., Nye, S. W., Dwyer, P., Fenn, W. O. (1954). Oxygen poisoning and x-irradiation: a mechanism in common. *Science* 119(3097), 623-626. doi: 10.1126/science.119.3097.623

Burk, Dean. (1976, July 21). *Congressional record*. Retrieved from http://www.cancer.org/aboutus/drlensblog/post/2008/04/11/60-minutes-and-the-cancer-cure.aspx

Carper, Jean. (1994). *Food: Your miracle medicine*. New York City, NY: HarperCollins.

Fuhrman, Joel. (n.d.). *Do not take multivitamins that contain folic acid*. Retrieved from http://www.drfuhrman.com/library/folic_acid_dangers_and_prenatal_vitamins.aspx

Kim, Y.-I. (2006). Does a high folate intake increase the risk of breast cancer? Nutrition Reviews, 64(10 Pt 1), 468–475.

Baggott, J. E., Oster, R. A., & Tamura, T. (2012). Meta-analysis of cancer risk in folic acid supplementation trials. Cancer Epidemiology, 36(1), 78–81. http://doi.org/10.1016/j.canep.2011.05.003

Ebbing, M., Bønaa, K. H., Nygård, O., Arnesen, E., Ueland, P. M., Nordrehaug, J. E., ... Vollset, S. E. (2009). Cancer incidence and mortality after treatment with folic acid and vitamin B12. JAMA, 302(19), 2119–2126. http://doi.org/10.1001/jama.2009.1622

Ulrich, C. M. (2007). Folate and cancer prevention: a closer look at a complex picture. The American Journal of Clinical Nutrition, 86(2), 271–273.

Hirsch, S., Sanchez, H., Albala, C., de la Maza, M. P., Barrera, G., Leiva, L., & Bunout, D. (2009). Colon cancer in Chile before and after the start of the flour fortification program with folic acid. European Journal of Gastroenterology & Hepatology, 21(4), 436–439. http://doi.org/10.1097/MEG.0b013e328306ccdb

Kwan, M. L., Jensen, C. D., Block, G., Hudes, M. L., Chu, L. W., & Buffler, P. A. (2009). Maternal diet and risk of childhood acute lymphoblastic leukemia. Public Health Reports (Washington, D.C.: 1974), 124(4), 503–514.

Kim, Y.-I. (2007). Folic acid fortification and supplementation--good for some but not so good for others. Nutrition Reviews, 65(11), 504–511.

Tso, Mark O.M., Lam, Tim-tak. (1996). *US Patent No. 5527533*. Washington, DC: U.S. Patent and Trademark Office.

Faure, P., Rossini, E., Lafond, J. L., Richard, M. J., Favier, A., & Halimi, S. (1997). Vitamin E improves the free radical defense system potential and insulin sensitivity of rats fed high fructose diets. *The Journal of nutrition, 127*(1), 103-107.

Alberts, B., Johnson, A., Lewis, J., Raff, M., Roberts, K., & Walter, P. (2002). The Preventable Causes of Cancer.

Cooper, G. M. (2000). The Development and Causes of Cancer.

CHAPTER 11

de Grey, Aubrey. (n.d.). *A reimagined research strategy for aging*. Retrieved from http://www.sens.org/research/introduction-to-sens-research

Dilman, Vladimir. (1954). *Data regarding the origin of climacteric and the role of age-associated "perestroika" in the elevation of blood pressure, blood cholesterol levels, and body weight*. Master's Thesis. Leningrad.

CHAPTER 12

Zs.-Nagy, Imre. (1994). *The membrane hypothesis of aging.* Boca Raton, FL: CRC Press.

Zs.-Nagy, Imre. (1989). On the role of intracellular physicochemistry in quantitative gene expression during aging and the effect of centrophenoxine. a review. *Archives of gerontology and geriatrics, 9*(3), 215-229.

The membrane theory of aging. (n.d.). *Anti-Aging Today.* Retrieved from http://www.anti-aging-today.org/research/aging/theory/membrane.htm

Gold, Campbell M. (2009). *DMAE (dimethylaminoethanol).* Retrieved from http://www.campbellmgold.com/archive_health/dmae.pdf

CHAPTER 13

Miquel, J., Economos, A. C., Fleming, J., & Johnson Jr., J. E. (1980). Mitochondrial role in cell aging. *Experimental Gerontology, 15*(6), 575–591. doi:10.1016/0531-5565(80)90010-8

Hagen, T. M., Liu, J., Lykkesfeldt, J., Wehr, C. M., Ingersoll, R. T., Vinarsky, V., … Ames, B. N. (2002). Feeding acetyl-l-carnitine and lipoic acid to old rats significantly improves metabolic function while decreasing oxidative stress. *Proceedings of the National Academy of Sciences, 99*(4), 1870–1875. doi:10.1073/pnas.261708898

CHAPTER 14

Maillard. Louis Camille. (1912). Action of amino acids on sugars. Formation of melanoidins in a methodical way. *Comptes rendus de l'Académie des sciences 154*(66), 1554–1556.

Bjorksten Johan (1968). The crosslinkage theory of aging. *Journal of the American Geriatrics Society,16*(4), 408–427.

Guillén, M. D., & Uriarte, P. S. (2012). Aldehydes contained in edible oils of a very different nature after prolonged heating at frying temperature: Presence of toxic oxygenated α,β unsaturated aldehydes. *Food Chemistry, 131*(3), 915–926. doi:10.1016/j.foodchem.2011.09.079

Tareke, E., Rydberg, P., Karlsson, P., Eriksson, S., & Törnqvist, M. (2002). Analysis of Acrylamide, a Carcinogen Formed in Heated Foodstuffs. *Journal of Agricultural and Food Chemistry, 50*(17), 4998–5006. doi:10.1021/jf020302f

Benfotiamine. (n.d.). Retrieved March 3, 2014, from http://www.benfotiamine. org/FAQ.htm

Boaz, Levi and Moshe J. Werman. (1998) Long-Term Fructose Consumption Accelerates Glycation and Several Age-Related Variables in Male Rats. *Journal of Nutrition. 128*(9), 1442-1449.

Dills, W. L. (1993). Protein fructosylation: fructose and the Maillard reaction. The American Journal of Clinical Nutrition, 58(5 Suppl), 779S–787S.

Havel PJ, Elliott S, Keim NL, Rader D, Krauss R, Teff K. (2003) Short-term and long-term consumption of high fructose, but not high glucose, diets increases postprandial triglycerides and apo-lipoprotein-B in women. *J Invest Med.* 51(suppl):S163 (abstr)

McPherson, J. D., Shilton, B. H., & Walton, D. J. (1988). Role of fructose in glycation and cross-linking of proteins. *Biochemistry, 27*(6), 1901-1907.

CHAPTER 15

Hayflick, L., & Moorhead, P. S. (1961). The serial cultivation of human diploid cell strains. *Experimental Cell Research, 25*(3), 585–621. doi:10.1016/0014-4827(61)90192-6

Cold Spring Harbor Laboratory (2009, May 5). Specific Small RNA Pathways Protect Germ Line From Transposons. *ScienceDaily*. Retrieved November 13, 2013, from http://www.sciencedaily.com/releases/2009/05/090505153631.htm

Olovnikov, Alexy. (1973). A theory of marginotomy. The incomplete copying of template margin in enzymic synthesis of polynucleotides and biological significance of the phenomenon. *Journal of Theoretical Biology, 41*(1), 181-190.

Greider, Carol W., & Blackburn, Elizabeth H. (1985). Identification of a specific telomere terminal transferase activity in tetrahymena extracts. *Cell 43*(2), 405-413. doi:10.1016/0092-8674(85)90170-9

Blackburn, Elizabeth. (n.d.). *Blackburn lab research - public lectures*. Retrieved from http://biochemistry.ucsf.edu/labs/blackburn/

Moini, H., Packer, L., & Saris, N.-E. L. (2002). Antioxidant and prooxidant activities of α-lipoic acid and dihydrolipoic acid. *Toxicology and Applied Pharmacology, 182*(1), 84–90. doi:10.1006/taap.2002.9437

Packer, Lester, & Colman, Carol. (1999). *The antioxidant miracle: Your complete plan for total health and healing*. New York, NY: Wiley.

Homocysteine reduction. (n.d.). *Life Extension*. Retrieved February 7, 2014, from http://www.lef.org/protocols/heart_circulatory/homocysteine_reduction_01.htm

Cysteine. (2013). *University of Maryland Medical Center's Complementary and Alternative Medicine Guide*. Retrieved February 7, 2014, from http://umm.edu/health/medical/altmed/supplement/cysteine

Ames, Bruce N. (1999). Micronutrient deficiencies: A major cause of DNA damage. *Annals of the New York Academy of Sciences, 889*, 87-106.

Garlick, Peter J. (2006). Toxicity of methionine in humans. *The Journal of Nutrition, 136*(6), 1722S–1725S.

Ipatenco, S. (n.d.). How to Reverse Calcium Buildup in the Heart. Retrieved May 24, 2016, from http://www.livestrong.com/article/553994-how-to-reverse-calcium-buildup-in-the-heart/

CHAPTER 16

Simopoulos, A. P. (2002). The importance of the ratio of omega-6/omega-3 essential fatty acids. Biomedicine & Pharmacotherapy = Biomédecine & Pharmacothérapie, 56(8), 365–379.

Food Ingredients and Inflammation | Slideshows | ArthritisToday.org. (n.d.). Retrieved May 24, 2016, from http://www.arthritis.org/living-with-arthritis/arthritis-diet/foods-to-avoid-limit/food-ingredients-and-inflammation.php

Boston, 677 Huntington Avenue, & +1495 1000, M. 02115. (n.d.). Shining the Spotlight on Trans Fats – The Nutrition Source – Harvard T.H. Chan School of Public Health. Retrieved from http://www.hsph.harvard.edu/nutritionsource/transfats/

Fighting Inflammation. (n.d.). Retrieved May 24, 2016, from http://www.cspinet.org/nah/articles/fighting_inflammation.html

Inflammatory Remarks About Arachidonic Acid | NutritionFacts.org. (n.d.). Retrieved from http://nutritionfacts.org/video/inflammatory-remarks-about-arachidonic-acid/

Nutrition, C. for F. S. and A. (n.d.). Labeling & Nutrition - Guidance for Industry: Trans Fatty Acids in Nutrition Labeling, Nutrient Content Claims, Health Claims; Small Entity Compliance Guide [WebContent]. Retrieved May 25, 2016, from http://www.fda.gov/Food/GuidanceRegulation/GuidanceDocumentsRegulatoryInformation/LabelingNutrition/ucm053479.htm

Ascherio, A., Hennekens, C. H., Buring, J. E., Master, C., Stampfer, M. J., & Willett, W. C. (1994). Trans-fatty acids intake and risk of myocardial infarction. Circulation, 89(1), 94–101.

Willett, W. C., Stampfer, M. J., Manson, J. E., Colditz, G. A., Speizer, F. E., Rosner, B. A., ... Hennekens, C. H. (1993). Intake of trans fatty acids and risk of coronary heart disease among women. Lancet (London, England), 341(8845), 581–585.

Katan, M. B., Zock, P. L., & Mensink, R. P. (1995). Trans fatty acids and their effects on lipoproteins in humans. Annual Review of Nutrition, 15, 473–493. http://doi.org/10.1146/annurev.nu.15.070195.002353

Thomas, L. H., Jones, P. R., Winter, J. A., & Smith, H. (1981). Hydrogenated oils and fats: the presence of chemically-modified fatty acids in human adipose tissue. The American Journal of Clinical Nutrition, 34(5), 877–886.

Mozaffarian, D., Pischon, T., Hankinson, S. E., Rifai, N., Joshipura, K., Willett, W. C., & Rimm, E. B. (2004). Dietary intake of trans fatty acids and systemic inflammation in women. The American Journal of Clinical Nutrition, 79(4), 606–612.

Mozaffarian, D., Katan, M. B., Ascherio, A., Stampfer, M. J., & Willett, W. C. (2006). Trans fatty acids and cardiovascular disease. The New England Journal of Medicine, 354(15), 1601–1613. http://doi.org/10.1056/NEJMra054035

CHAPTER 17

Cumming, Elaine, & Henry, William E. (1961). *Growing old: The process of disengagement.* New York, NY: Basic.

Miller, Jacques F. A. P. (1961). Immunological function of the thymus. *The Lancet, 278*(7205), 748–749.

Peat, R. (1996). *Coconut oil.* Retrieved from http://raypeat.com/articles/
articles/coconut-oil.shtml

Tian, Y.-M., Zhang, G.-Y., & Dai, Y.-R. (2003). Melatonin rejuvenates
degenerated thymus and redresses peripheral immune functions in
aged mice. *Immunology Letters, 88*(2), 101–104. doi:10.1016/S0165-
2478(03)00068-3

Mocchegiani, E., et al. (1994). The immuno-reconstituting effect of melatonin
or pineal grafting and its relation to zinc pool in aging mice. *Journal of
Neuroimmunology, 53*(2), 189-201. doi:10.1016/0165-5728(94)90029-9

Sánchez-Hidalgo, M., Lee, M., de la Lastra, C. A., Guerrero, J. M., & Packham,
G. (2012). Melatonin inhibits cell proliferation and induces caspase
activation and apoptosis in human malignant lymphoid cell lines.
Journal of Pineal Research, 53(4), 366–373. doi:10.1111/j.1600-
079X.2012.01006.x

Feychting, M., Osterlund, B., Ahlbom, A. (1998). Reduced cancer incidence
among the blind. *Epidemiology, 9*(5), 490-494. doi:10.1097/00001648-
199809000-00004

Pukkala, E., Verkasalo, P.K., Ojamo, M., Rudanko, S.L. (1999). Visual
impairment and cancer: a population-based cohort study in Finland.
Cancer Causes & Control, 10(1), 13-20. doi:10.1023/A:1008897317401

Shiitake mushroom. (n.d.). *American Cancer Society.* Retrieved March 3, 2014,
from http://www.cancer.org/treatment/treatmentsandsideeffects/
complementaryandalternativemedicine/dietandnutrition/shiitake-
mushroom

Kay, Leslie K. (2010, November). From A to shiitake: Japanese mushrooms
may offer certain benefits. *Today's Dietitian, 12*(11), 20. Retrieved from
http://www.todaysdietitian.com/newarchives/110310p20.shtml

Maitake mushrooms. (n.d.). *American Cancer Society.* Retrieved March 3, 2014, from http://www.cancer.org/treatment/treatmentsandsideeffects/ complementaryandalternativemedicine/dietandnutrition/maitake-mushrooms

Reishi mushroom. (n.d.). *Memorial Sloan Kettering Cancer Center.* Retrieved March 3, 2014, from http://www.mskcc.org/cancer-care/herb/reishi-mushroom

CHAPTER 19

Howell, Edward, (1985). *Enzyme nutrition: The food enzyme concept.* New York, NY: Avery.

Meyer, J., Golden, J. S., Steiner, N. and Necheles, H. (1937). The ptyalin content of human saliva in old age. *American Journal of Physiology – Legacy Content, 119*(3), 600-602

Stefansson, Vilhjalmur. (1935, November). Adventures in diet. *Harper's Magazine,* Retrieved from http://www.biblelife.org/stefansson1.htm

Fletcher, Horace. (1913). *Fletcherism: What it is; or, how I became young at sixty.* New York, NY: Frederick A. Stokes Company.

Beard, John. (1911). *The enzyme treatment of cancer and its scientific basis.* London: Chatto & Windus.

Kelley, William Donald. (1997). *One answer to cancer: Reviewed after 30 years, 1967-1997: The metabolic approach to the successful resolution of malignancy.* Mineral Wells, TX: Cancer Coalition.

Gonzalez, Nicholas J. (2010). *One man alone: An investigation of nutrition, cancer, and William Donald Kelley.* New York, NY: New Spring Press.

Gonzalez, Nicholas J., Isaacs, Linda L. (2009). *The trophoblast and the origins of cancer: One solution to the medical enigma of our time*. New York, NY: New Spring Press.

CHAPTER 20

Weinberg, E. D. (2004). *Exposing the hidden dangers of iron: what every medical professional should know about the impact of iron on the disease process*. Nashville, TN: Cumberland House Publishing.

O'Neill, G., & Sullivan, J. (1996). Iron-heart disease link. *Sunday-Herald Sun*. Retrieved from http://www.americanhs.org/ah00072.htm

Sardi, Bill. (2007, January 03). *A unifying theory of aging*. Retrieved from http://www.longevinext.com/articles/a-unifying-theory-of-aging-part1

Fallon, S., & Enig, M. G. (2000, January 01). *Vitamin primer*. Retrieved from http://www.westonaprice.org/vitamins-and-minerals/vitamin-primer

Micronutrient deficiencies. (n.d.). Retrieved February 7, 2014, from http://www.who.int/nutrition/topics/vad/en

Vitamin A deficiency. (n.d.). In *Wikipedia*. Retrieved February 7, 2014, from http://en.wikipedia.org/wiki/Vitamin_A_deficiency

CHAPTER 21

Arndt–Schulz rule. (n.d.). In *Wikipedia*. Retrieved November 19, 2013, from http://en.wikipedia.org/wiki/Arndt–Schulz_rule

Southam, C.M., Ehrlich, J. (1943). Effects of extract of western red cedar heartwood on certain wood-decaying fungi in culture. *Phytopathology, 33*(6), 517-524.

Giuliano, Vince. (n.d.). *Aging Sciences – Anti-Aging Firewalls*. Retrieved from http://www.anti-agingfirewalls.com/

Jones, I. G. (1857). *The American eclectic practice of medicine*. Cincinnati, OH: Moore, Wilstach, Keys & Co. Retrieved from https://archive.org/details/americaneclectic01jone

Thomas, Rolla L. (1906). *The eclectic practice of medicine*. Cincinnati, OH: Scudder Brothers Company. Retrieved from https://archive.org/details/eclecticpractic00thomgoog

Index

SYMBOLS

A

B

C

D

E

F

G

L

M

N

O

P

Q

R

S

T

U

V

W

X

Y

Z

A Personal Story from the Author

As a young ten year old, I found myself at the lake with a group of much older boys. The boys decided to swim out to a large floating raft far away from the shore. With all the excitement I joined in and after a long swim found myself sitting on top of that floating raft enjoying the warmth of the sun. However, the other boys soon decided to swim back to the shore. Not fully recovered from the long swim, I stupidly joined them in the return. They swam much faster than me and I found myself alone deep in the lake, short of breath, tired, and in a panic. I started flailing my arms and yelling for help while attempting to tread water. Panic washed over me and my vision filled with large black spots. I was going up and down in the water catching long glances of nothing but the lake water as I was looking up at the surface and then catching brief glimpse of the shoreline as I managed to push my head above the surface for brief moments. In short, I was drowning. My muffled yells were barely heard as I was too far out and the few adults that seemed to be looking my way thought I was just fooling around. Water started entering my nose, my throat, and I felt my life would soon be over. Shortly, I realized that I was too far away from any other person and that no one could rescue me. No one could save me, but me! Composing myself somehow, and beating down the panic, I slowly managed to get back to more shallow water. Walking out to the shore, I realized how close I came to being just another drowning statistic.

How does this story relate to your health? In more ways than you may think. You see, we all at one time or another will face a crisis maybe even death. While it would be nice for others to take care of us, to protect us or even to save us, many times we cannot expect that nor should we wait for that to occur. In short, we must save ourselves from drowning.

I feel we all would benefit if we accept the premise that we are our own best caretaker and take steps to protect, preserve, and save ourselves. Too many people nowadays want some medical professional to rescue us when, in reality, most of us need to save ourselves. My whole motivation of this book is to get people to wake up to the fact that only we as individuals have our best interest at heart and only we can be truly responsible for our own health and wellbeing. So, use medical personnel, clinics, and hospitals to take care of your health needs but always keep in mind that you are the boss. Do not let others take over your personal responsibility for your wellbeing as they may have a totally different agenda. Often others will use language, props, customs, misdirection, intimidation, confusion, or pressure to sway us to their ways, but we all must decide what is truly best for us. Your future health indeed lies within your own hands and therefore we all need to educate ourselves on what's in our own best interest. It may take a lot of work but the reward will be a life based on personal responsibility and a knowledge that you did the most you could do for yourself for the brief time you are on this earth.

C.E.O.

Good luck in that endeavor and I wish you the longest life possible with the least amount of ills. By following the concepts in this book I hope you also find that your life is much improved since you should find yourself full of more energy and good health. Take some time and effort to become your own Chief Executive Officer, C.E.O., of your health and make your life everything it should be. After all, what could possibly be more important than the health and welfare of yourself and your family? Focus on wellness, not illness.

About the Author

HAVING SEVERAL DECADES of experience as a financial advisor investigating potential companies suitable for investment, Terence L. Reed, CFP®, discovered how our medical system really works. Corporate interests have established a world where we are treated but seldom cured. This is the age of pharmaceutical drugs, which all started with the patent medical craze back in the 18th and 19th centuries.

The author noted two major observations. The first observation was that clients coming to him for investment and estate advice often would discuss the loss of a loved one. When reading the death certificate, the author often noted what was listed on the death certificate stated one thing, such as heart attack, but the deceased's family would comment that it was in fact, something else that really killed the person. Often, he heard that the wrong medication was given, a medical procedure was botched, or that a hospital infection actually killed their loved ones.

The second observation was when the author experienced the death of both of his parents via the traditional medical system. Prescribed drugs destroyed his father's heart, and a strong prescription hormone induced cancer within his mother and led to her demise. In both cases, he was astounded by the wrong-headed treatment, high costs, and total disregard for the truth. Side by side with his sick parents, the author experienced and saw the agony of misguided medical treatments for over eight years.

In addition to his extensive financial background and experience, Terence went on to obtain a bachelor's of science degree in holistic nutrition and has received certification as a clinical nutritionist, herbalist and personal fitness trainer.

www.ingramcontent.com/pod-product-compliance
Lightning Source LLC
Chambersburg PA
CBHW080406290526
45791CB00008BA/2170